Radiographic Imaging

D. NOREEN CHESNEY
F.C.R. T.E. S.R.R.

Group Superintendent Radiographer
Coventry and Warwickshire Hospital

AND

MURIEL O. CHESNEY
F.C.R. T.E. S.R.R.

Principal, Central Birmingham School of Radiography
General Hospital, Birmingham

FOURTH EDITION

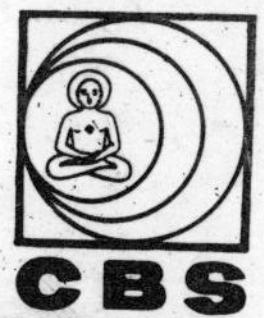

CBS PUBLISHERS & DISTRIBUTORS PVT. LTD.
New Delhi • Bangalore • Pune • Cochin • Chennai (India)

ISBN : 81-239-0997-7

First Indian Edition : 1994
Reprint : 1998, 1999, 2003, 2004

Copyright © 1965, Blackwell Scientific Publication, UK

Reprinted in India by CBS Publishers & Distributors in arrangement with
Blackwell Scientific Publication, UK

Published by Satish Kumar Jain and produced by V.K. Jain for
CBS Publishers & Distributors Pvt. Ltd.,
CBS Plaza, 4819/XI Prahlad Street, 24 Ansari Road, Daryaganj,
New Delhi - 110002, India.   • Website: www.cbspd.com
e-mail: delhi@cbspd.com, cbspubs@airtelmail.in
Ph.: 23289259, 23266861, 23266867   • Fax: 011-23243014

Branches:
• *Bengaluru:* Seema House, 2975, 17th Cross, K.R. Road,
  Bansankari 2nd Stage, Bengaluru - 560070   Ph.: +91-80-26771678/79
  Fax: +91-80-26771680   • E-mail: cbsbng@gmail.com,
  bangalore@cbspd.com
• *Pune:* Bhuruk Prestige, Sr. No. 52/12/2+1+3/2,
  Narhe, Haveli (Near Katraj-Dehu Road By-pass), Pune - 411051
  Ph.: +91-20-64704058/59, 32342277   • E-mail: pune@cbspd.com
• *Kochi:* 36/14, Kalluvilakam, Lissie Hospital Road,
  Kochi - 682018, Kerala • Ph.: +91-484-4059061-65
  Fax: +91-484-4059065   • E-mail: cochin@cbspd.com
• *Chennai:* 20, West Park Road, Shenoy Nagar, Chennai - 600030
  Ph.: +91-44-26260666, 26208620   • Fax: +91-44-42032115
  E-mail: chennai@cbspd.com

Printed at :
Nazia Printers, Delhi

Contents

List of Illustrations

List of Illustrations

Preface to Fourth Edition

A funny thing happened to *Radiographic Photography* on its way to the publisher. The book's journey was slow, from a distant past in the heads of its authors to a terminus at the premises of Blackwell Scientific Publications, beside the river in Osney Mead, Oxford. Somewhere, along some 60 miles of road and the uncountable reaches of our cerebral pathways, *Radiographic Photography* became a different book.

When its 3rd printing ran out, the third edition of *Radiographic Photography* was almost 10 years old. This—in its authors' sight, as no doubt in others'—made it overdue for retirement, since if a textbook is advanced in years it cannot be advanced; it enters that unacceptable era when it possesses neither the truth of authenticity nor the tranquil appeal of antiquity.

During the decade since we wrote the third edition, radiographers and their patients have not changed: radiographers have remained—and will remain—caring makers of images. What have changed are the materials and equipments available for the practice of our profession; and indeed our very thinking about radiographic images and the recurrent assessments which we make of them within our schools of radiography and radiodiagnostic departments. In *Radiographic Imaging* we have attempted to salute these changes. Much of the book is fresh and we believe that it deserves a fresh title.

New chapters in this book include one on the storage of unexposed and exposed materials and another on daylight film-handling systems. Extensive revisions have been made to the chapters on intensifying screens and film now in use in radiodiagnostic departments. Chapter 17 has been re-written entirely, in order to include xeroradiography and modern materials for radiographic duplicating and subtraction.

What used to be the darkroom is now considered as part of a larger concept, the dispensing/processing/viewing area. Processing theory and practice, methods of silver recovery and evaluations of the radiographic image all have new faces and have been extensively up-dated. We have also described systematic tests for product control in a radiodiagnostic department.

Recognising changes in the syllabuses of the College of Radiographers, we have shortened the parts of the book concerned with optics and the camera; and we have made a new approach to fluorography which includes techniques for image storage and which we hope will have revitalised the subject.

This book may be different from its predecessor but it is the same in two fundamental respects. The first of these is our 'non-mathematical' attitude. Radiographic imaging unquestionably is an applied science; but its practitioners in medical diagnosis generally are not scientists, nor conversant with chemical, electronic and mathematical languages. We have tried to make this book consistently comprehensible to those who are likely to consult it and hope that the readers of *Radiographic Photography* will not now hesitate to open our new pages, because of possibly 'difficult bits'. We assure you that there are none.

Secondly, *Radiographic Imaging* shares fully with its predecessor the indebtedness of its authors to a number of people, without whose co-operation the book's journey to its publisher could not have begun with any confidence in its success. It is a pleasure now to give outlet to our overflowing appreciation to the following: Mr R. F. Farr, of the Central Birmingham Health District, who read and commented upon part of Chapter 12; Mr Fraser Sanders, of Du Pont (UK) Ltd, who gave us generously of his knowledge and time in support of Chapter 13; and Mr Alan Waller, of Ilford Ltd, who likewise made journeys in order to educate us and gave skilled attention to Chapter 5.

Our thanks are extended to others, too, who have been interested agents on our behalf and instrumental in making available to us either current information or their companies' permission to use certain material. We are happily grateful to the following of our friends for their active concern: Du Pont's Chris Nathan and Peter Ranger; Ilford's John Hale; Kodak's John Bennett, Keith Dandy and Don Martin; 3M's Brian Brandon; Medical X-ray Supplies' Bill Mead; and Siemens' Ernie Orme.

We are pleased to acknowledge the courtesy of the following organisations in allowing us to reproduce certain illustrations of which they hold the copyright: Du Pont (UK) Ltd; GEC Medical Equipment Ltd; Ilford Ltd; Kodak Ltd; 3M United Kingdom Ltd; Radiation Measurements Inc.; Siemens Ltd; Wardray Products (Clerkenwell) Ltd.

Finally, we offer appreciation to the Department of Medical Illustration of Birmingham Dental Hospital for successfully undertaking another 'rush job' on 4 of our diagrams; and not least we say 'Thank you' to Mr Per Saugman of Blackwell Scientific Publications who has displayed patience whilst waiting for this book to be written.

1981

D.N.C.
M.O.C.

Preface to
First Edition

This book is not about photography; it is about a number of subjects which are grouped together under the title Radiographic Photography in the syllabus of training for the Membership Diploma of the Society of Radiographers. The word camera appears in this book comparatively seldom and those who would seek in its pages for light on their studio lighting must remain perpetually unillumined.

In the first and last analyses, we should recognize that good radiography, though it may depend upon a knowledge of theoretical concepts, in fact is a practical skill. The subjects in their syllabus of training, summarized in the term radiographic photography, are important to radiographers because they are realistic subjects: knowledge and appreciation of them significantly affect the quality of the end-product—the radiograph. It seems strange that no textbook has yet been written for radiographers about radiographic photography and that their teachers must build courses of instruction on manufacturers pamphlets and photographic manuals in a wider category. The authors hope that this book may fill what appears to be a gap among the aids to those who must learn and the tools of those who must teach.

In attempting to meet the needs of student radiographers, as we believe that they are not scientists and may have only irregular knowledge of chemistry, we have kept to a minimum the appearance of mathematical expressions and have avoided chemical formulae. Of great convenience to those in the know, such shorthand can be only profoundly baffling to those who are not. We hope that we have made to radiographic photography the practical approach which its character deserves.

The syllabus of training for the M.S.R. Diploma has directed the selection of material for this book. While it has been written for the education of student radiographers, we know that in some places greater detail is given than may be required for the M.S.R. course. It seems a proper principle to include in a textbook something more than the minimum demanded by a particular course of study; perhaps especially so in a field of knowledge which is fertile of development. This aspect of the book may attract at least some post-graduate readers who wish to prepare for the Higher Examination of the Society of Radiographers.

From inclusions to an omission. This book has given no space to the reproduction of photographic faults in radiographs. Possibly this may appear a serious defect to its critics. However, it must be evident to radiographers of experience that if the catalogue of such errors is to be usefully extensive, apart from any attempt to make it complete, a large number of illustrations is necessarily required: even then it is certain that someone at some time would be confronted in the viewing room with a bizarre radiographic appearance for which no reference here would enable the radiographer to account. Reproduction on paper of certain classic faults is much less satisfactory than their visualization on original films. We would suggest that for student radiographers a more useful exercise than looking at such copies is always the handling and examination of the real material. Why should they not be permitted some limited experiment from which to form their own library of malpractices in handling radiographs?

No man is an island and, perhaps more than many others, authors of textbooks are dependent on links with certain mainlands of learning and material. We are aware that the substance of this book has been strengthened because a number of people each have given to us generous measures of their knowledge, ability and not least of their time. We are glad of an opportunity to offer to them an expression of our thanks, though the small gesture is incommensurate with the gift received.

We are grateful to Dr D. M. Alexander, consultant radiologist at the Coventry and Warwickshire Hospital, for reading Chapter 14 and discussing it with us; and to Miss A. L. Hebden, medical photographer at the same hospital, who took photographs, with most welcome expedition, of a step-wedge and of parts of the Odelca and Hansen equipment. Dr J. F. K. Hutton, consultant radiologist at the General Hospital, Birmingham, receives our thanks for kindly reading Chapters 12 and 13 and giving his comments. Mr W. Hurt, medical photographer at the Birmingham Children's Hospital, came to our aid at very short notice and provided illustrations to show the appearance of a granular pattern at different degrees of photographic enlargement.

From Mr K. W. Goddard we have had the stimulus of early interest in the project and we appreciate his help in reading the MS of Chapters 11, 6 and 7 and in mobilizing for us some of the resources of Kodak Ltd who have loaned many illustrations and supplied other material. With Kodak we must associate Mr Sydney Marshall who has been most helpful as informant, reader and commentator.

We would like to thank Mr John Bennett and Mr R. Greenway, each of whom supplied a personal communication of immeasurable value on automatic processing and respectively read Chapters 6, 7 and 8, and 9. We are grateful also to Mr R. J. Hercock for his kindness in giving close attention to nearly a third of the manuscript and to us so much of his time.

It has been necessary in some parts of this book to provide working descriptions of certain equipment. In the absence of practical contact with the apparatus concerned such accounts may be troublesome to follow, but they are no less than impossible to write. With this problem we have appreciated energetic help from Mr C. W. Mead who has made available opportunities to examine certain fluorographic equipment, supplied technical data and given useful commentary on the resultant chapters of the MS. We are grateful too to Mr P. Spencer for having so willingly put us on similar good terms with a Ken-X processor and for freely loaning relevant material. Finally we owe to the knowledge and helpfulness of Dr George Parker, who read Chapters 15 and 16, the reassurance that our own pristine ignorance of some photographic optics has been successfully eliminated.

This book would have been poorly illustrated had it depended solely on the artistic ability of either of its authors. Nearly all the diagrams and photographs have been given to us through the courtesy of certain manufacturers, learned journals and publishers, and to these collectively we are most grateful for such practical assistance, in some cases on a very generous scale. We give sincere appreciation to the following: Cuthbert Andrews; The Fountain Press; Ilford Ltd, particularly Mr J. James of X-ray Sales and Mr D. H. O. John of the Techno-Commercial Dept (X-ray Division); the *Journal of Photographic Science*; Kodak Ltd, particularly Mr K. W. Goddard of the Medical Sales Division; N.V. Optische Industrie, De Oude Delft, Holland; Pako Corporation, Minneapolis, U.S.A.; D. Pennellier and Co Ltd; Philips Electrical Ltd; Philips Technical Library; *Radiography*, the Journal of the Society of Radiographers; Theratronics Ltd; Watson and Sons (Electro-Medical) Ltd, particularly Mr G. R. Woodall, Publicity Manager; X-ray Sales Division, Eastman Kodak Co, Rochester, New York.

D.N.C.
M.O.C.

Chapter 1
The Photographic Process

VISIBLE LIGHT IMAGES

Photography is a record made by means of light. Three separate processes can be distinguished.

(i) The formation of an image. In general photography this is an optical image produced when *divergent* rays coming from a subject are made to *converge* by means of a lens. In radiography it is a shadow image produced when interposed objects attenuate an X-ray beam.

(ii) Recording the image. In the first instance the image exists as a hidden one within the material used for the record; this must be a substance which reacts to light.

(iii) The production of the image in permanent form. This involves the action of a chemical agent to make the hidden image visible. This stage is known as *development*, and it is followed by further chemical processes which fix the image and make it into a permanent record.

Photographic history is the story of discovery of physical and chemical processes by which an image is formed, recorded, and made permanent. It has extended over a long period of time. The science of optics, for example, is a very old one, and the 'pinhole camera' which has pleased many of us in our schooldays is a device by no means new; Aristotle referred to pinhole images as long ago as 350 B.C. Yet it was not until the nineteenth century that real progress was made in obtaining permanent record for photographic images.

In the search for a means by which to make such records, the action of light on certain materials was noticed. That light can produce change is common knowledge to us all. Curtains and carpets fade under the action of sunlight; some human bodies turn agreeably brown. It is not within the intended scope of this book to recount the evolution of photographic processes, attractive though such by-ways may be. We are concerned at present with the light-sensitive materials encountered by radiographers in their work. These are materials which on exposure to light are found, after chemical development, to have darkened where the light has reached them.

A photographic material recording an image receives more light from the brighter parts of the subject. If the material reacts to light by becoming *darker*, it follows that in the developed result those parts of the subject which were bright to the eye are dark in the recorded image. Those parts of the subject which are dark to the eye are light in the recorded image. This image with reversed tones constitutes a *photographic negative* (Fig. 1.1).

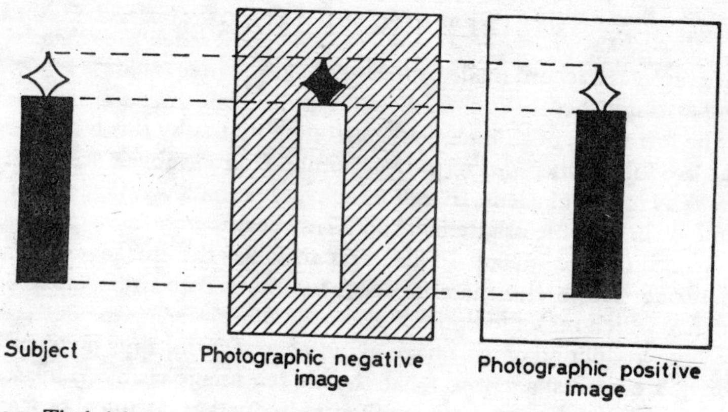

Fig. 1.1. The bright parts of the subject (e.g. the candle-flame) in the first photographic image (a negative one) are dark. From the negative, a positive can be made. The dark parts of the negative transmit less light, and in the positive these parts correspond in tone to the bright parts of the original subject.

From this negative another positive image can be made quite simply. If the negative image is on a transparent film or glass base, it will allow light to pass. Obviously the dark parts of the image will allow less light to pass than do the light parts of the image. The procedure then is to pass light through the negative image on to another piece of photographic material which, like the first, responds to light by becoming black after development. The two photographic materials may be in contact with each other, or the image may be projected from the one to the other. The light parts of the negative transmit more light to blacken the second piece of material than do the dark parts of the negative. The second image is therefore dark in areas corresponding to the dark parts of the subject, and light in areas corresponding to the light areas of the subject. The recorded image is therefore in the same tones (or it may be expressed that the record is in the same sense) as the original. This type of photographic image is called a *positive*.

IMAGES PRODUCED BY X RADIATION

Radiography is the making of images by means of X rays. The light-sensitive materials used in photography respond to X radiation as they do to light. Given exposure to X rays and then developed, they are seen to have darkened where the radiation reached them.

When an X-ray beam passes through a body, some of the radiation is absorbed and some is transmitted. The subject will transmit the beam to a varying amount depending on the penetrating power of the radiation, and upon the atomic number and density and upon the thickness of the material traversed. When the subject consists of tissues which are of different atomic numbers, there is difference of absorption. The emergent radiation shows this difference, and a pattern of varying amounts of radiation reaches the film (Fig. 1.2).

This is closely analogous to the varying amounts of light reflected from a subject in ordinary photography. Some parts of the radiographic subject transmit more radiation and correspond to the bright parts of a photographic subject. Some parts of a radiographic subject transmit less radiation or no radiation, and they therefore correspond to the dark parts of a photographic subject. The radiographic image appearing on X-ray films, with the partially radiopaque bony structures appearing white and the radioparent gas-filled organs appearing black, is considered to be a negative image (Figs. 1.2 & 1.3).

This negative image can be used to make a positive image with reversed tones in precisely the same way as a photographic negative can be used. Radiographic reproductions in the positive image have been used to illustrate textbooks. The student should note that the image seen on a fluorescent screen during fluoroscopy is a *positive* one (Fig. 1.4). This is because the response of the screen to radiation is the opposite response of a photographic material; the screen becomes *bright* when radiation falls on it, the photographic material becomes *dark*. Thus the radiolucent parts of the subject are light upon the screen, dark on the film, and the radiopaque parts are dark upon the screen, light upon the film.

LIGHT-SENSITIVE PHOTOGRAPHIC MATERIALS

Radiography is a specialized application of the photographic process and, as has been seen, certain fundamentals are common both to the wider

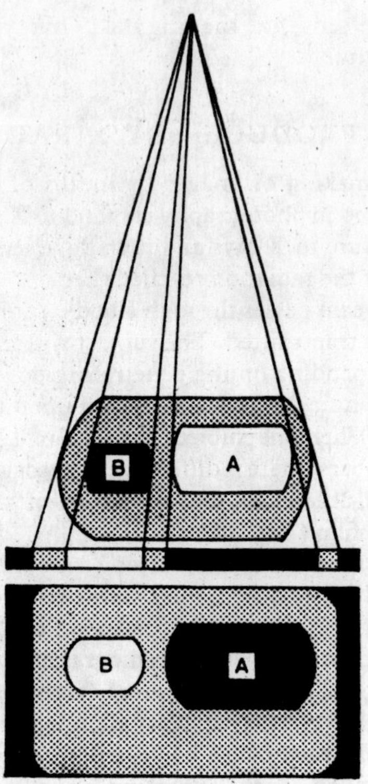

Fig. 1.2. B represents a bone which is relatively opaque to X rays and therefore allows least radiation to reach the film. The film is light underneath it. A represents a hollow gas-filled organ which allows most radiation to reach the film. The film is dark underneath it. The bone and the organ are surrounded by soft-tissue allowing some radiation to reach the film, which is therefore an intermediate tone. At the edges of the film there is nothing in the way of the radiation. The radiographic image is a pattern of varying amounts of radiation transmitted through the subject to the film.

science and to this special branch. One of these fundamentals is the general character of the light-sensitive materials used.

The group of elements known as the halogens—bromine, chlorine, and iodine—combine with silver to form salts, which are silver bromide, silver chloride, and silver iodide. These salts undergo a change when exposed to light or X rays which enables them to form a photographic image.

Photographic materials may be divided into those which are intended to produce negatives (this group includes X-ray films), and those which are intended to produce positive images. Virtually all negative materials

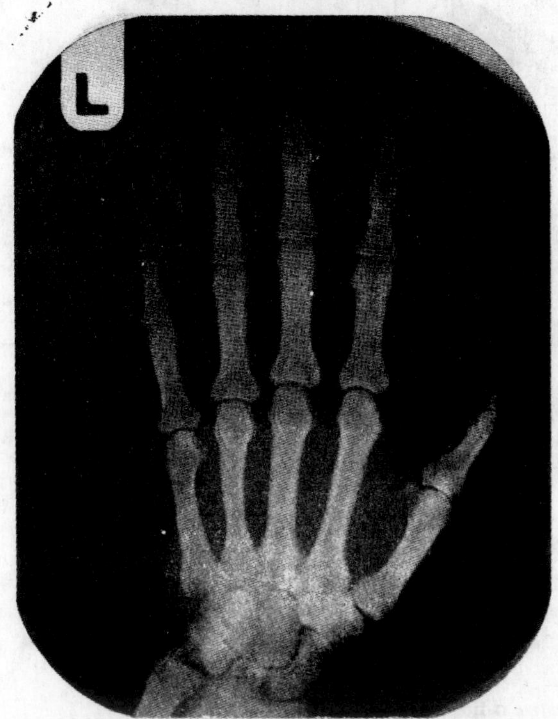

Fig. 1.3. A negative radiographic image.

use silver bromide as the light-sensitive salt. Silver iodide is never used alone, but in combination with silver bromide; the iodide is added to the bromide as a very small proportion of the order of 2–3 per cent. Certain positive materials use silver chloride (which has low sensitivity) or silver bromide, or a combination of the two, according to the type of response which is required.

PHOTOGRAPHIC EMULSIONS

In order to use any silver halide in a photographic material, it is necessary to prepare it in a form which can be coated upon a support; this support is called a *base*. It may be a transparent base which is film, or it may be paper. The form the silver halide takes for this purpose is a suspension of tiny crystals of the salt in a suitable binding agent. This suspension, as it should properly be called, is termed in photography a *photographic emulsion.*

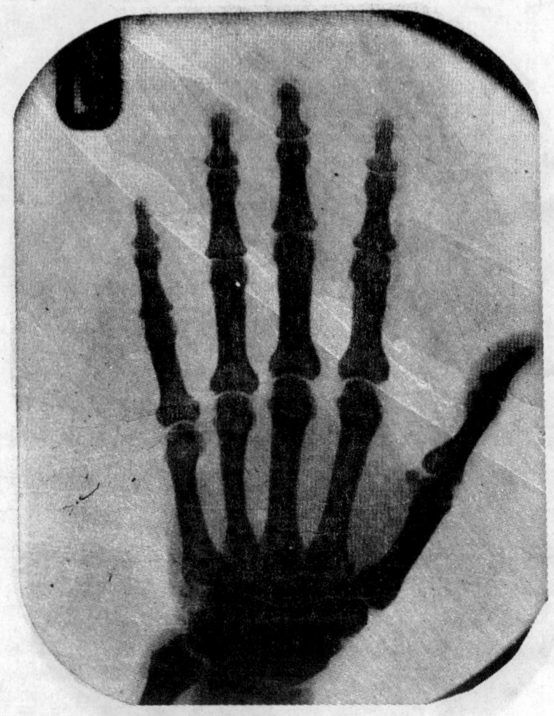

Fig. 1.4. A positive radiographic image.

CHARACTERISTICS OF SENSITIVE EMULSIONS

Any photographic material has certain characteristics which are important to the photographer who is to use it. One of these is the *speed* of the material; this determines whether the material needs more or less exposure to light in comparison with another material in order to produce a similar picture.

Another important characteristic is *contrast*. This refers to the way in which the material reacts to a range of exposures by showing on development a number of different densities: these range from a maximum density which is the darkest tone in the image to a minimum density which is the lightest tone. If the material is of high contrast, the difference between the maximum and minimum densities is great; that is, the range is from 'black' to 'white' with only a few intermediate steps. If the material is of low contrast, the difference between the maximum and minimum densities is not great and there are many steps between the two; that is, the image is composed of various shades of grey. This low-contrast image looks very different from the 'soot and whitewash' effect of the high-contrast image.

A material which is of low contrast has wide exposure latitude. This means that a wide range of exposures can be given and the resultant image (be it pictorial or radiographic) will continue to look correctly exposed; it will be neither too dark nor too light. Material of high contrast has the opposite characteristic of little exposure latitude and if the image is to look correctly exposed (neither too dark nor too light) then the range of exposures which is acceptable is narrow.

TABLE 1

In any given emulsion, the grains are of various sizes. The characteristics of the grains and the resultant photographic characteristics of the materials are tabulated below.

Grain sizes	Features of the material
On average, large	Material is fast (high speed)
On average, small	Material is slow (fine grain)
Range of sizes is narrow	Contrast is moderately high, with narrow exposure latitude
Range of sizes is wider	Contrast is low with wide exposure latitude
Only one size of grain is present	Contrast is very high with very narrow exposure latitude

These characteristics—speed and contrast—are determined when the photographic emulsion is made. Speed depends on the size of the silver halide crystals (which are called 'grains'), the preparation of the emulsion, the nature of the radiation used for the exposure, and the development given. Contrast depends on the distribution of size and sensitivity of the grains, and on development.

In any given emulsion the grains are of various sizes. If most of the grains in an emulsion are small, the sensitive material is then said to be of fine grain, and it is usually of high contrast and low speed. Photographic materials which are of high speed are of large grain size, and are of relatively lower contrast.

MAKING A PHOTOGRAPHIC EMULSION

It has been explained that the emulsion consists of silver halide crystals or grains suspended in a suitable agent. This agent is extremely important. The one chosen is gelatin, and it has certain valuable characteristics as a suspending and binding agent for the silver halide grains.

(i) It is a suitable medium in which to form the silver halide crystals. These are produced in a chemical reaction between solutions of silver nitrate and alkaline halides, as a result of which the insoluble silver halide crystals are formed; they remain suspended in the gelatin, finely dispersed.

(ii) It maintains the silver halide crystals evenly distributed within the suspension.

(iii) When warmed, the gelatin forms a solution which will flow over the base on to which it is to be coated.

(iv) When cooled it forms a firm jelly which sets on the base. It can then be dried, when it has some resistance to moderate mechanical stress, such as abrasion. It is a flexible transparent layer on the base.

(v) It allows solutions to penetrate the emulsion when, at a subsequent stage in its life, the material is chemically processed after photographic or radiographic exposure.

(vi) Some of the constituents of gelatin act on the silver halides as sensitizers and influence the speed of the emulsion. Others act as restrainers and reduce fog.

(vii) On exposure to light, change takes place in the silver halide grains. It is believed that gelatin helps to prevent any reversal of this change, which would of course reduce the effect of the exposure.

Manufacturers producing photographic materials choose the gelatin very carefully and test it stringently. The making of an emulsion is a complex process, carried out with close control of the materials, and of each stage of the procedures involved. The characteristics of the emulsion are precisely regulated. Today there is a great range of photographic materials available of various speeds and different contrast. That this should be so, and that all these diverse materials should be consistent in performance and physical character are indications of the advances which have been achieved, and of the fine control in the processes of manufacture.

The chemical process by which the photographic material is produced is precipitation. Silver nitrate and an alkali halide are combined, together with gelatin. The reactions result in insoluble silver halide grains being dispersed through the gelatin.

In following stages of manufacture, the sensitivity of the grains is controlled (with other features of the final product) and sensitivity specks are encouraged to form within the grains. These sensitivity specks are important in producing the hidden image (called the latent image) which is formed in the photographic material by the actions of light or X rays upon it; the latent image is more fully explained in Chapter 6.

Eventually the photographic emulsion is coated on a base which is usually film or paper. In radiographic applications the base is almost always film and hence is transparent and flexible.

Since light-sensitive materials are affected by such factors as moisture, temperature, presence of impurities, exposure to certain gases, airborne fluff and dust, static electricity, and by mechanical stress, it is clear that the difficulties of manufacture are great. A very high standard of control and general cleanliness must be vigilantly maintained.

THE PHOTOGRAPHIC LATENT IMAGE

It has been seen that the basis of photography is a sensitive emulsion containing silver halide which undergoes change when exposed to light (or to X radiation). This change is the decomposition of the silver halide into its two constituents. These are metallic silver and whichever halogen (chlorine, bromine, or iodine) has been in combination with the metal. This metallic silver is in a finely divided state, and it is black in colour. Its presence accounts for the darkened appearance of the photographic material on development after exposure to light.

The light-initiated change, which is a minute one, is amplified many million times by the chemical developer. This acts rapidly on the silver halide grains which have received exposure, and produces a visible image. The exposed grains and the change existing in them before development constitute the *photographic latent image*; this and the action of the developer are considered fully in Chapter 6 of this book.

POSITIVE PROCESSES

THE NEGATIVE-POSITIVE PROCESS

It will be understood from the opening section of this chapter that the first stage in making a photograph yields an image in which the tones of the original are reversed, and this is described as a photographic negative. Only in certain special applications are negative images accepted as an end in themselves. We know that they are so accepted in radiography, and the practice also applies in some types of document copying.

However, every student will realize from previous common experience that pictorial records in which the tones are reversed are not acceptable at all. Even the brunettes among us who yearn to be blondes would hardly care for portraits which totally reversed the tones of skin and hair, and a landscape with ashen trees and jet sky does not impress us as realistic. In general therefore negatives exist as the first stage towards obtaining a positive image in which the tones correspond to those of the original subject. As was indicated previously, in order to obtain a positive two stages may be necessary—(i) obtaining the negative image, and (ii) using this negative to make a positive image. This process of making a negative first and using it to make a positive is known as the *negative–positive process*.

Colour photography involves specialized work beyond the intended scope of this book. In black-and-white photography the positives used are of two main types.

(i) Positive images on transparent bases, known as *transparencies* or *diapositives*. They may be projected. This group includes lantern slides, film strips, and cine films.

(ii) Positive images on paper base are called *reflection positives*, but to most of us the term *paper prints* is more familiar. They are viewed by reflected light.

Although the necessity for two stages may seem to add to the difficulty of the negative–positive process, at the same time it has certain practical advantages for the general amateur and professional user. For example, many prints can be made easily from a single negative, which can be used repeatedly at different times. Furthermore, the second stage of the process gives opportunity for closer control of the result; this is important to the pictorial photographer who aims for a beautiful and striking picture.

It seems reasonable that the student should have some understanding of the negative–positive process as it applies to radiographs.

A radiograph is a negative image. If the radiograph is used, as a photographic negative is used, to print another image on to a paper base, the result is a *positive print*. If it is used to print on to a transparent base, the result is a *positive transparency*. The positive print on paper and the positive transparency, it is clear, are both second-stage results from the radiographic negative.

The positive print may be used to illustrate a book, but today authors prefer their radiographic illustrations to be negatives, that is in the same sense as the originals; or it may be that what is wanted is a *copy* of the original radiograph, that is a negative image on a transparent base. In using the negative–positive process to obtain either of these, it is necessary to proceed to a *third* stage. The *positive transparency* must now be used as the negative was used, and a print must be made from it on to a paper or film material. If the print is made on a paper material, the result is a *negative image print* with the tones of the original radiograph; if the print is made on a film material, the result is a *negative image transparency* just as the original radiograph was, and it is in fact a copy or facsimile of the first.

OTHER POSITIVE PROCESSES

Procedures have been devised which give positive images in a single operation, eliminating the two stages of the negative–positive process. Radiographers encounter some of them in certain applications within the X-ray department.

DIRECT POSITIVE MATERIALS

Direct positive materials yield a positive instead of a negative image. Use is made of a specially prepared emulsion. If this film is chemically developed in the ordinary way, it emerges from the developer a uniform black from a deposit of metallic silver. If it is given a photographic exposure before development, the blackening *decreases* with increased exposure—exactly the reverse of the normal photographic process. The resultant image is therefore a positive one.

Film material of this type, although too slow for ordinary photographic purposes, can be used to make copies in the same sense directly from original radiographs, eliminating the tedious and time-consuming stage of the intermediate positive transparency. Manufacturers are supplying such material to X-ray departments for this purpose, and radiographers who are asked to copy radiographs use it. Some details of a copying technique are given in Chapter 17. To sum up, this method consists of special material given ordinary development.

REVERSAL DEVELOPMENT

An ordinary photographic emulsion can be used to obtain a positive result instead of a negative one if it is given special processing. This technique is called *reversal processing*. It is used in some forms of cinematography and also in colour photography to obtain a positive image directly from negative material exposed in the camera, the result in both cases being a positive transparency. To sum up, this method consists of ordinary material given special development.

IMAGE TRANSFER SYSTEM

The image transfer system is called the diffusion transfer reversal process, which is a long but reasonable name; it is reasonable because the system involves a diffusion process, it achieves the transference of an image from one piece of sensitive material to another, and it gives reversal of the image.

The two pieces of material involved are one which is sensitive to light (photo-sensitive) and one which is sensitive not to light but to chemicals. A negative image is produced in the photo-sensitive material in the ordinary way by the exposure to light. At the time of development, the sheet of photo-sensitive material is put in close contact with the chemically sensitive one, which is known as the transfer or receiving paper.

At this stage therefore three things are brought together:
(i) the photo-sensitive material with a latent image in it;
(ii) the developer;
(iii) the receiving material which is chemically sensitive.

The latent image in the photo-sensitive material is acted upon by the developer and the exposed silver halide is reduced to black silver, giving a negative image in the usual way. At the same time the special developing agents also act upon the unexposed silver halide and free silver atoms in it. These silver atoms in the unexposed parts are free to diffuse into the receiving layer (while those in the exposed parts are not free), and they

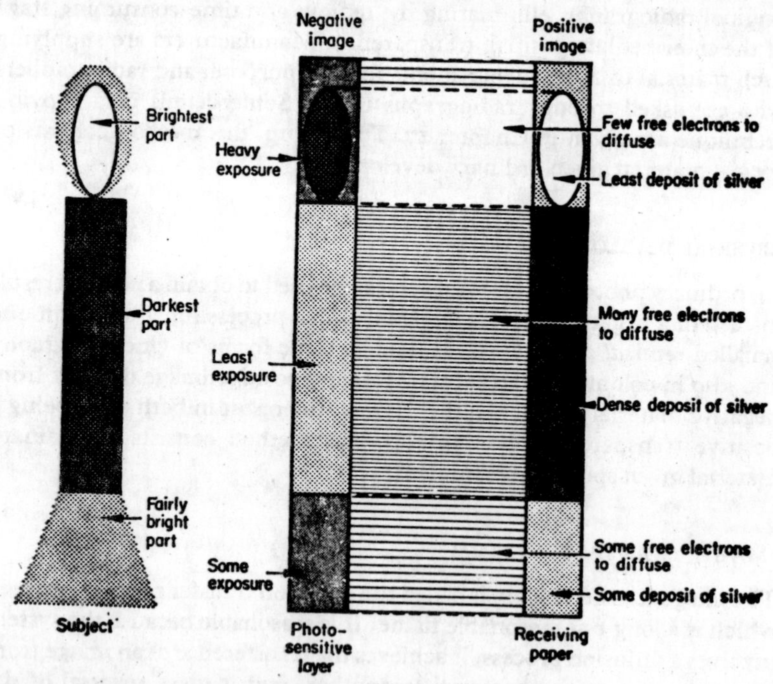

Fig. 1.5. Diffusion transfer reversal process.

form a black deposit on the receiving material, attaching themselves to minute silver particles which are already there. Fig. 1.5 is a diagram indicating how the process takes place in the different parts of the image.

The result is a positive image developing in the receiving layer at the same time as the negative image is developing in the photo-sensitive layer.

This transfer method has been used in various ways for document copying. It is the basis of the Polaroid-Land camera; this is a specially designed hand-camera providing a finished picture in the positive image some seconds after the exposure is made. In this camera, the sensitive paper and the receiving paper are both in rolls. The chemical agents for the processing are in plastic pods. After the exposure, both papers are brought out together through rollers which keep them in contact, break the pods, and spread the chemicals between the papers.

Chapter 2
Film Materials in X-ray Departments

The film materials used in X-ray departments are now to be considered in more detail. As a starting point, two main groups can be differentiated as follows:

(i) films which are to be exposed to X rays only or to a combination of X rays and light (these are X-ray films);

(ii) films which are to be exposed to light only and are to receive no exposure to X rays (these are mainly films for fluorography, which is photography of an image on a fluorescent screen, but the group also includes film materials to be used in copying radiographs and in techniques for subtraction).

For many years X-ray films have been available for two different techniques of exposure. The one method is to expose the film in a light-tight pack to X rays only. The other technique is to expose the film between a pair of intensifying screens which are activated by X rays and as a result produce light. The ability of X rays to penetrate materials is used to the full in forming the image; these X-ray films have a sensitive emulsion layer coated on both sides of a base and the X-ray beam produces an image in both emulsion layers simultaneously as can be seen in Fig. 2.1. Films which have a sensitive emulsion layer on both sides of a base are said to be duplitized.

If a film is to be exposed to light only, there is no point in putting a layer of emulsion on the side of the base which is further from the light source as no effective penetration takes place and no image could be produced in the second layer. So fluorographic films (like materials for copying radiographs and for subtraction) may be described by radiographers as *single-emulsion films* in order to distinguish them from the duplitized films with emulsion on both sides of the base. Perhaps *single-sided films* (not single-emulsion) would be a better description to avoid confusion with terms that photographers might use. A photographer takes single-sided film for granted since he is using it all the time and if he ever talks of a single-emulsion film he doubtless means a material

14

which is coated on one side of the base with only one sensitive emulsion. This is in contradistinction to his double-coated films which have two layers of emulsion coated one upon the other to make a fast negative material.

THE STRUCTURE OF DUPLITIZED X-RAY FILM

The structure is built up in layers upon the base which provides a support. The base will therefore be considered first.

THE BASE

Film base is made of substances derived from cellulose. Cellulose can be treated with acids to form cellulose salts, which are called cellulose esters, and for many years cellulose nitrate was used as film base. This is the cellulose ester produced by treating cellulose with nitric acid. It was in wide use as a film base, but had certain marked disadvantages, one of which was its readiness to burn. Not only did it burn very freely, giving off noxious gases as it did so, but it was liable to spontaneous combustion. It also disintegrated on prolonged storage.

Cellulose nitrate was long ago superseded by base made of cellulose acetate, cellulose triacetate, or similar related materials. These keep well and provide what is known as *safety base* that burns slowly if ignited and is not liable to spontaneous combustion. Today manufacturers sell X-ray films on a new synthetic base called 'polyester base'. It is made from polyethylene terephthalate resin. This base is flexible and so strong that it can be considered untearable. It is impermeable to water and processing solutions, and this makes it easier to transport through automatic processors as it remains firm when wet. An important advantage from the manufacturer's point of view is that this base can be made with hardly any risk of contamination from air-borne radioactive particles which eventually cause black spots of fog in an emulsion coating. The base presents a very clear appearance which is said to come from the degree of chemical purity which is maintained during its manufacture. Because a polyester base does not tear easily it can withstand considerable mechanical stress. But the very strong base can be a nuisance if films become jammed in an automatic film changer and can make their removal very difficult indeed.

The thickness of film base depends on the use for which the finished product is designed. The base constitutes the thickest layer of the complete film. X-ray film has a base which is 0·18 mm thick for a polyester base, the total thickness of the film being 0·2 to 0·4 mm.

The physical characteristics of the base are important and have increased in importance for X-ray films because of the precise requirements of automatic processing. The base must be entirely free from any defect or blemish and must be uniform in its thickness, since lack of uniformity here will lead to variations in the depth of the emulsion layer.

Since the base is required to transmit light, it must be uniform in its ability to do this. X-ray film base (whether cellulose acetate or polyester) is given a blue tone and is then described as *blue base film*. This blue tone inevitably diminishes to some extent the ability of the base to transmit light, but modern blue base film transmits about 85 per cent of the light falling on it. The blue tone is required to be uniform in colour, should show batch-to-batch consistency in colour, and should not change in colour with time. The blue tone gives intermediate densities in the image a more pleasing appearance and radiologists in the United Kindgom tend to object to its absence. In fact it has no effect on the properties of emulsion coated on to the base and it does nothing to improve the visibility of detail in the image. There seems little reason for its continuing use other than the maintenance of a tradition.

Film base must be sufficiently rigid to avoid kinking (which could occur very readily in the large film sizes if the base were not stiff enough), and yet it must not be too thick. In thickness and flexibility it must be just right to allow it to pass through and be conveyed by the closely-set moving rollers of automatic processors. The standards here are critical.

THE SUBSTRATUM LAYER

Before emulsion is coated upon it, film base must be prepared so that the emulsion will adhere to it well. The emulsion and its base do not behave in the same way when they become wet and are dried; the gelatin of the emulsion swells with moisture and contracts when dry to a degree that the base does not. There would therefore be a tendency in these conditions for the two to part from each other unless the base was specially prepared. This preparation consists of putting upon the base a very thin layer of a solution of cellulose ester and gelatin in water and acetone. The process eventually leaves on the surface of the base a deposit mainly of gelatin which constitutes the *substratum layer*. The technique of applying the substratum layer to the base is more elaborate for polyester than for acetate base. With a polyester base it may involve the use of coatings made of other synthetic resins. For an X-ray film this substratum layer is coated upon both sides of the base.

THE SENSITIVE EMULSION LAYER

The sensitive emulsion, coated upon the substratum on *both* sides of the base, constitutes the next layers of the film. As has been explained in Chapter 1, the sensitive emulsion consists of silver halide crystals suspended in gelatin. These undergo change under the action of light or X rays. The characteristics of the film material depend on the size of these silver halide grains, their size range, and their sensitivity range. The two emulsion layers on each of the X-ray film base are each 1/2000 in. thick and the film is said to be *double sided.*

ADVANTAGES OF TWO EMULSION LAYERS

Increase in Sensitivity. Since there is a sensitive emulsion on both sides of the film base, there are in fact two images formed one on each side of the base, each emulsion being exposed simultaneously with the other as is seen in Fig. 2.1. When X rays only are used in direct exposure, the beam penetrates the upper emulsion layer and the base to activate the lower emulsion layer as it has the upper one. When screens are used, each emulsion layer is in contact with the active aspect of an intensifying screen. The penetrating X-ray beam activates both emulsions and both screens, the screens being energized to give out light which is directed towards an emulsion layer. These two images are viewed by light transmitted through the film, and are thus seen as a single image formed by the two superimposed upon each other. The degree of blackness of

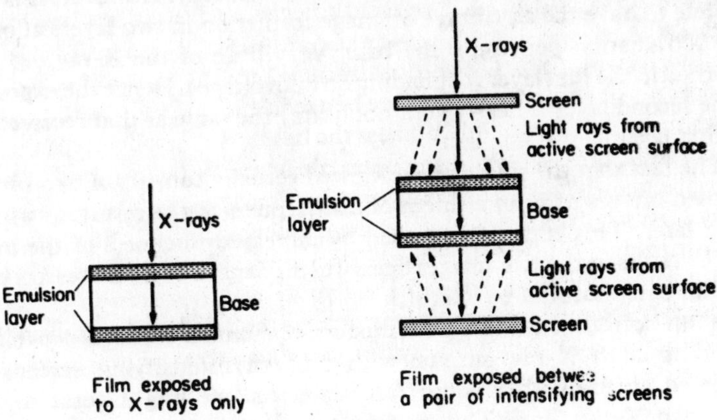

Fig. 2.1. Film exposed to X-rays only and between a pair of intensifying screens.

each silver image is therefore added to that of the other one. The two sides together consequently give an image which has twice the silver deposit obtained if a single-sided material were used. The efficiency of the process is about double what it would be with the use of a single-sided film. This enables much shorter exposure times to be used, with less risk of blurring from the movement of parts being radiographed, and with markedly less radiation dose to the patient.

Increase in contrast. Contrast in the image is difference between the degree of blackness of various regions. The blackness differences are greater for double-sided than for single-sided materials.

Another factor to be considered is the reduction in radiographic contrast that results from an increase in the X-ray tube voltage. As the radiation becomes more penetrating, the absorption differences in the various tissues of the subject become levelled. The result is an image of less contrast, and this effect could be very marked if a single-sided film were used. Double-sided film allows higher tube voltages to be employed without a deterioration in contrast beyond acceptable limits.

Production of an image in two layers. For X-ray film exposed in a cassette, the production of an image is achieved partly by X radiation but mainly by visible light produced by intensifying screens in the cassette. The fact that sensitive emulsion is coated on both sides of the base allows the film to be sandwiched between *two* screens, each screen producing an image on the emulsion surface nearer to it. This practice clearly doubles the efficiency of the process, and allows use of shorter times of exposure and reduction in radiation dose.

If a cassette and screens are not being used and the film is of the envelope-wrapped type to be exposed directly to X rays, then in this case the image is obviously produced by X radiation only. However, it is still possible to have the advantage of image formation in two layers at once. The X radiation penetrates the base. Very little of the X-ray beam is absorbed in the first layer (depending on kilovoltage). Hence the exposure of the second layer is nearly (but not quite) the same as that received by the first layer.

The fact that the single image viewed actually consists of two super-imposed images adds an element of unsharpness to the result, as will be noted later. This effect is increased by increased thickness of the base, which results in the two images being further apart. It is one reason why the film base must not be too thick.

It has been thought that with modern equipment which is capable of providing high X-ray output, with modern intensifying screens of increased speed, with modern fast materials, we might cease to use duplitized X-ray films. The argument is that the gain in speed is no longer needed and that it would be beneficial to eliminate from the finally viewed radiograph the unsharpness of two superimposed images. An economic benefit would be a saving in silver, which is an expensive and diminishing world resource.

CHARACTERISTICS OF THE EMULSION LAYER

The emulsion layer must be sufficiently flexible to allow the film to bend. Some bending will be required of it in use—for example in curved cassettes, in some types of film changer for angiography and in some automatic processing units.

When the film is processed there must be rapid and uniform dispersion of chemicals through the emulsion, so wetting agents are included in its manufacture. Chrome alum is added to harden the emulsion, for adequate hardness is important. This is particularly so in view of the widespread use of automatic processing. Soft emulsions absorb more water and will take longer to dry, so that quick drying in the processor becomes difficult. If the processing unit has rollers to transport the film, their grip on a soft emulsion may remove the gelatin with disastrous results, the unhardened emulsion being warmed by the high temperature at which the developer solution is used. At the other extreme too much hardening will impede dispersion of chemicals through the emulsion.

THE SUPERCOATING

The silver halide grains in a sensitive emulsion can be made developable by light pressure or abrasion. This results in such damaged areas appearing as dark spots or patches in the image. Since film has to be handled at many stages both in manufacture and in use, it is important that the sensitive emulsion should be protected as much as possible from this type of harm.

A thin layer of gelatin is therefore applied over it, and this protective gelatin is known as the *supercoat*, nonstress supercoat, or anti-abrasion layer. Since X-ray film has emulsion on both sides of the base, supercoating is applied to both emulsion layers.

The supercoat provides a shiny surface for the film which improves both its appearance and its durability. It must not be too shiny or the film cannot be marked with a pencil or white ink, methods of identification which may be used still in some departments. Furthermore radiologists are apt to find objectionable a highly glossed surface. Certain types of film changer for angiography require a slippery supercoat to the film to

Fig. 2.2. Diagram of an X-ray film in cross-section. The base is about 0·18 mm in thickness.

prevent its jamming as it is moved through the changer. To achieve this additives are in the supercoats for X-ray film.

The diagram in Fig. 2.2 shows all these layers built up, to form the duplitized complete X-ray film in cross section.

THE STRUCTURE OF SINGLE-SIDED FILMS

THE BASE, THE EMULSION LAYER, THE SUPERCOAT

What has been said of film base in relation to X-ray film applies also to single-sided materials, there being some difference in the thickness of the base according to the type of film being made. Films to be used flat generally have thicker base than roll film. The base is prepared to receive the emulsion by addition of a substratum layer, as already described, to ensure adhesion between the sensitive emulsion and the base. The distinguishing feature here between most X-ray film and general photographic materials is that in the case of film to be used for exposure to light, the emulsion is coated upon *one side only* of the base. This emulsion layer is covered with a protective layer of gelatin as previously described for X-ray film.

THE NON-CURL BACKING

It has been explained that photographic film has its emulsion layer coated upon one side only of the base. When this layer dries after processing there is a tendency for it to shrink, and this tendency results in the film curling, emulsion side inwards. In the case of duplitized film a tendency to curl does not exist, since the emulsion layers on both sides of the base shrink equally.

The curl on single-sided film can be prevented if the other side is given tendency either to curl in the opposite direction or to shrink. Base for flat and roll films is given a tendency to curl the other way by being coated with a layer of gelatin of the same thickness as the emulsion layer.

This anti-curl layer can be made to serve another purpose also, as will be seen in the next section. In order to ensure adhesion of this anti-curl layer, the base is given a substratum coating on this side just as if it were being prepared to receive emulsion.

In the case of 35 mm film for miniature cameras and cine film the problem of curl is solved in another way by giving the base a tendency to shrink. This can be done by treating it with solvents on the side opposite to the emulsion.

THE ANTI-HALO BACKING

Before it can be understood why anti-halo backing is required it is necessary to appreciate the results of light falling upon film. The emulsion layer is made of grains of silver halide, and when light strikes these grains there is some inter-reflection between them. This results in light being scattered sideways within the emulsion, an effect which is called *irradiation*. This scattered light does not form the image proper; it is a sideways spread of light beyond the boundaries of the image, and it is a source of unsharpness in the image. Thicker emulsion layers allow more irradiation than do thin ones of fine grain.

Some of the light falling on the film will pass through the emulsion layer and reach the base, being scattered into the base. According to the angle at which it strikes the base-air surface at the back of the film, it may either pass out of the base or be totally reflected back towards the emulsion (Fig. 2.3).

The light which is reflected back towards the emulsion produces another image separated from the proper image; this second image is known as *halation*. If the object being photographed is a small bright one such as a candle flame or naked light, halation takes the form of a ring or halo encircling the image and is then most readily observed. It can also be present with large areas of considerable brightness (Figs. 2.3 and 2.4).

Halation is most noticeable when the base is thick, as for example in a glass plate as opposed to film, since then the second image is at a greater distance from the primary image point and the 'halo' may not fuse with the true image but be entirely separated from it. Both halation and irradiation are most marked with bright images, such as naked light sources. This is because both effects show most in areas where the image is heavily exposed (that is, when plenty of light is reaching the film from the subject). Irradiation is least in emulsions which are thin. Where there is least irradiation there is also least risk of halation.

Halation can be prevented by adding a suitable dye to the gelatin of the non-curl backing on flat and roll films. Scattered light therefore

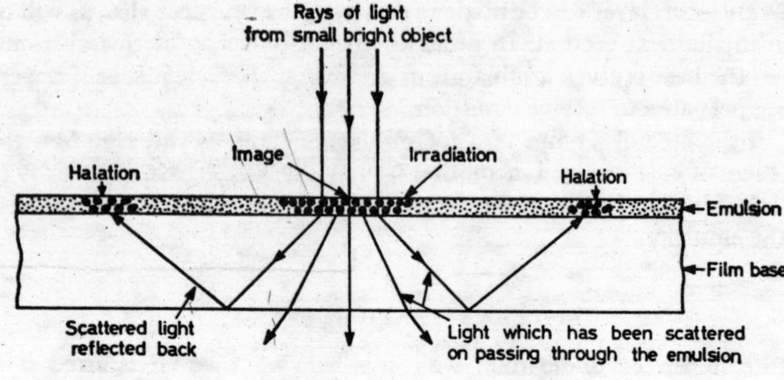

(a) Unbacked film

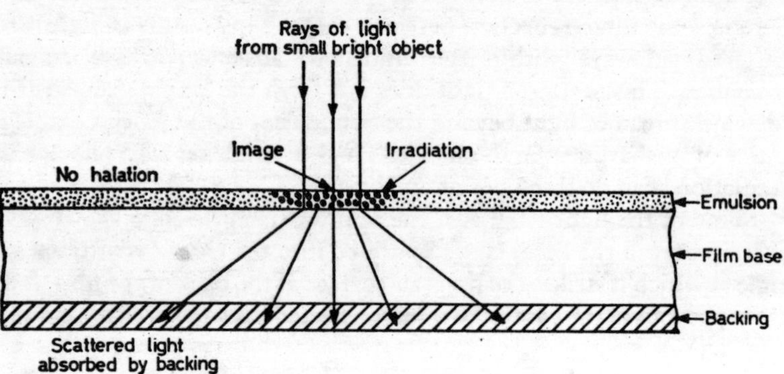

(b) Backed film

Fig. 2.3. Irradiation and halation. *By courtesy of Ilford Ltd.*

passes into the gelatin where it is absorbed by the dye. Thus the non-curl backing becomes anti-halo backing as well.

The dyes require to be carefully chosen for they must have no damaging effect on the emulsion and they must be removable during processing. If the film remained with a coloured back it would be difficult to use the negative for the production of prints. So dyes are used which will be bleached by processing solutions, and thus they disappear.

Cine films and 35 mm film for use in miniature cameras have no layer of gelatin as a non-curl back (Fig. 2.5) so in these cases a different answer must be found to the problem of halation. In these instances the dye is put into the film base itself, and the base is grey in colour. This dye cannot be removed in processing. Its density must therefore be selected so that it will prevent halation adequately without making it difficult to use the

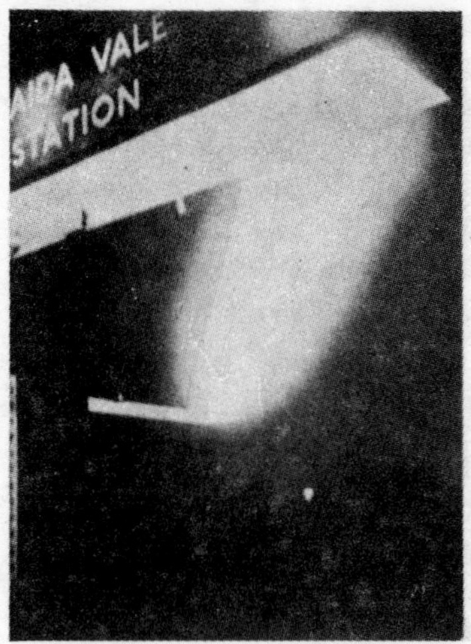

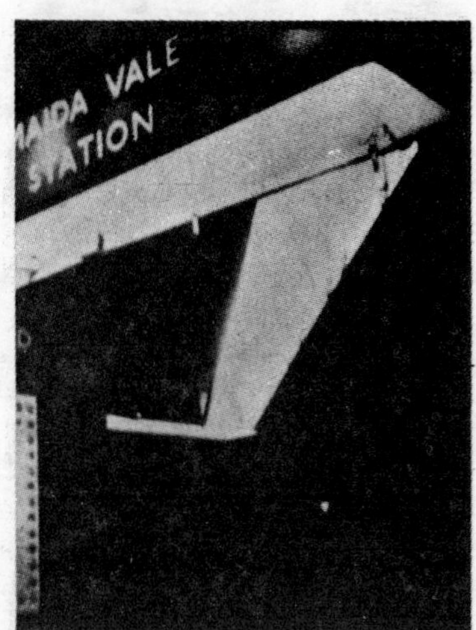

Fig. 2.4. (a) With halation (b) Without halation. *By courtesy of Ilford Ltd.*

negative in producing a print. This dye within the base does not *prevent* reflection of light from the base-air surface at the back, but it absorbs light as it goes through the base towards the back *and* as it comes back through the base towards the emulsion. The intensity of light is thus reduced and halation is prevented.

PHOTOGRAPHIC FILM IN RADIOGRAPHY

Single-sided films are used in X-ray departments for various applications as listed below.

(i) Single-sided X-ray film to be used with one intensifying screen, the emulsion surface of the film being in contact with the active surface of the screen. This single screen and film are sometimes held in a cassette which

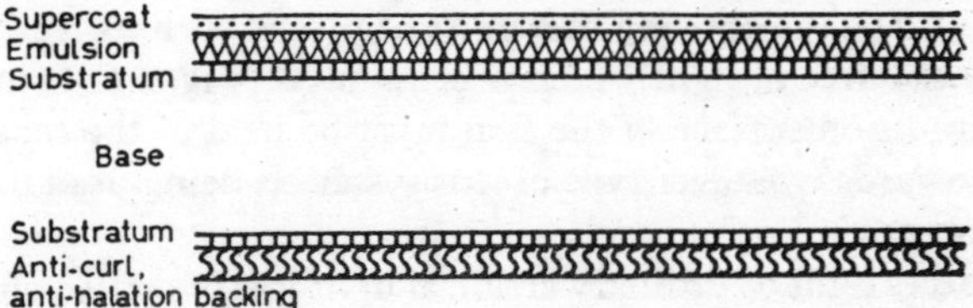

Fig. 2.5. Diagram of a photographic film in cross-section. The thickness of the base depends on whether it is flat film (8/1000 in.), roll film (3/1000 in.), or cine film (5/1000 in.).

is made of a soft plastic and can be positively evacuated of air by means of a pump so that the front and back surfaces of the cassette, the screen and the film are held in very close contact. Sometimes the single screen and film are put in a rigid cassette with a method of closure which helps to drive out air. This single-sided film and single intensifying screen are used for mammography. In this technique the object of using a single-sided film is to reduce to a minimum that amount of unsharpness in the image which is contributed by the recording system (in this case, the film/screen combination).

(ii) Single-sided film for fluorography.

(iii) Single-sided film to be used for making copies of radiographs.

(iv) Single-sided film to be used in a technique for subtraction.

(v) Single-sided film to be used in order to make a miniature reproduction of a full-sized radiograph. This miniaturization is a technique now practised in some X-ray departments to solve the problem of finding enough storage room for full-sized radiographs. These take up much space and furthermore are a considerable weight when large numbers of them are to be kept.

It is to be noted that the film mentioned in (i) is exposed to X rays and to light from the intensifying screen which the X rays elicit; it is X-ray film. The other films in (ii), (iii), (iv) and (v) are exposed to light sources only and receive no exposure from X rays. These films essentially are photographic films, photography being defined as making a record by means of light.

IDENTIFYING THE EMULSION ASPECT

Anyone using a single-sided film must be able to identify its emulsion-covered surface. In use this aspect must face towards the source of the energy which is to activate the film material. Thus for the X-ray film mentioned at the beginning of this section, the emulsion layer must be placed against the active surface of the intensifying screen since it is from this surface that the light will be emitted when the screen is energized by X rays (Fig. 2.6a); a copying film must be placed with its emulsion layer towards the source of light which is being used (Fig. 2.6b); in a camera unit the emulsion surface of the film must be held in the focal plane so that it is towards whatever type of lens system is being used to focus the image (Fig. 2.6c).

Under day light or ordinary artificial light it is of course quite easy to identify the emulsion-coated surface of a film. The emulsion layer is a pale colour, a somewhat dirty yellow-grey shade that as a colour makes no appeal at all. It is matt-finished, in contrast to the reverse side of the

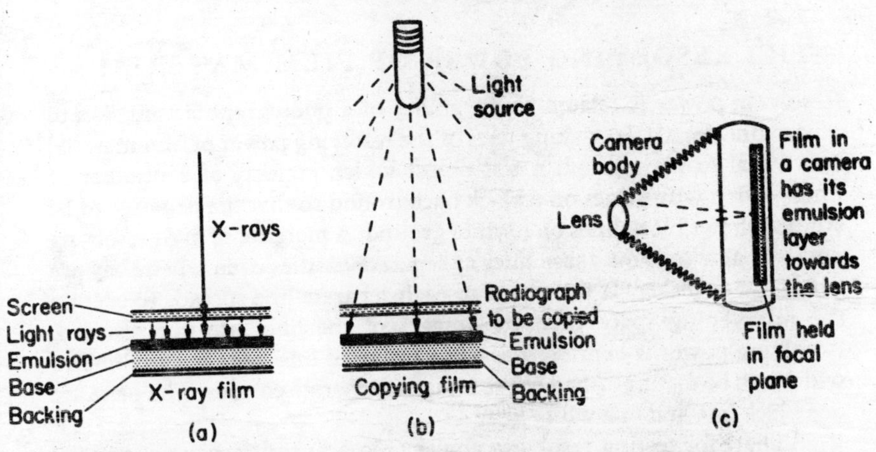

Fig. 2.6. Diagram to show single-sided materials in radiography, copying and fluorography.

film which is shiny and reflective and is in any case an entirely different colour; this might be magenta or dark plum-colour or green or blue.

However, if you blithely expose the film in full view under white light in order to identify its emulsion aspect, you will fog the film and will not be in a position to use the knowledge successfully when you have with certainty gained it. You must do the best you can under safelights or in complete darkness in some cases if the film is not to be spoiled for use.

The manufacturer usually helps you to orientate the film by touch. At one edge of the film there may be a notch or indentation in outline that can be felt when a finger is run lightly along the edges. The placing of this cut out portion can be keyed to the emulsion aspect of the film: for example, if you hold the film so that the indentation is in the top right-hand corner, the emulsion aspect of the film is facing towards you.

If there is no help from the manufacturer, you can discern under safelights the difference between the pale matt surface and the dark shiny reflective one. So you should inspect the film, holding it carefully with its edges against your fingers and tilting each surface in turn towards the safelight, making sure that you do not bring it too close to the light. You will soon see which is the darker shiny surface and which is the paler matt emulsion-covered surface.

Even in total darkness, if you must and are brave enough, you can find the emulsion aspect. For each surface in turn, gently moisten a tiny part of one corner with your tongue and slowly draw the moistened part across your lips. The emulsion surface is slightly sticky as the other is not.

THE RESOLVING POWER OF FILM MATERIALS

Resolving power is related to the ability of a photographic emulsion to record fine details. In making tests of the resolving power of film material it is usual to photograph a test object which consists of a number of lines—often white lines on a black background so that the negative to be studied shows black lines on a white ground. A material of high resolving power is able to show these lines as separate entities even when they are very close together. If the image of each separate line spreads to occupy the intervening space then the images of the lines are not resolved. Resolving power is expressed as the number of line pairs per millimetre which can be distinguished in the image as separate entities. The pairs are one black line and one white line.

A chart for testing resolving power (Fig 2.7) may consist of parallel lines separated by a space equal in width to the lines, the lines being arranged in groups of diminishing width. This is photographed with reduction in size and the image is then studied with magnification. The finest group of lines which is just resolved gives the resolving power of the emulsion.

The resolving power of an emulsion depends upon various factors such as grain size, contrast and the extent to which the emulsion absorbs and scatters light. The results of tests for resolving power of any given emulsion are influenced by such factors as the arrangement of the lines on the chart, the contrast between the tone of the lines and the tone of their

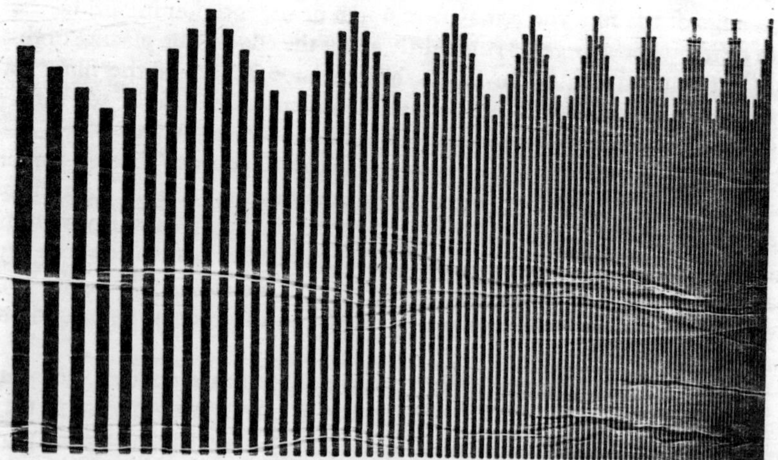

Fig. 2.7. A typical resolving power test chart. *By courtesy of Ilford Ltd.*

background, the wavelength of the light used to make the exposure, the exposure and development given to the film. The tests are made with specified standardization of these conditions using a camera lens of high resolving power. The resolving power of any photographic system as a whole is limited by the resolving power of the lens as well as that of the material; so these tests are made with a lens of resolving power much higher than that of the material being used.

Fast negative materials can resolve about 40–50 line pairs per millimetre, medium speed film about 70-100 line pairs per millimetre, and very slow emulsions designed for maximum resolution of detail may resolve over 1,000 line pairs per millimetre. In certain technical applications of photography the ability to resolve fine detail is most important.

The case of the resolving power of materials used for radiography is somewhat different. Here there are various factors which influence the resolving power of the system as a whole. Later in this book (Chapter 12), the features of the radiographic image will be considered more closely and it will be seen that there are many causes of image blur. These and not the resolving power of film materials are limiting factors in the resolution of the image. Cine radiography and fluorography entail the photography of an image on a fluorescent screen. The resolving power of the screen is very much less than that of the film materials used. The resolving power of the films used in radiography is therefore generally not a stringent consideration in the resolution of the images obtained although it may assume importance in cinefluorography.

GRAININESS OF FILM MATERIALS

If a photographic negative is viewed under sufficient magnification, the individual grains of silver which form the image can be seen by the eye. 'These grains are unevenly distributed through the emulsion. At lesser degrees of magnification the eye cannot resolve individual grains and the grains appear to be clumped together in colonies. This clumping gives rise to unevenness in density or a variation in photographic tone. The result is an impression of a granular pattern. This is known as *graininess* in the material (Figs. 2.8 and 2.9).

Graininess in photographic negatives is influenced by various factors, the most important one being the grain size of the film material used. If it is a fast emulsion with large average grain size, graininess will be more apparent than in the case of a slower emulsion with small average grain size. Another important consideration is the type of developing solution used. It is possible to obtain fine grain developers which act to reduce

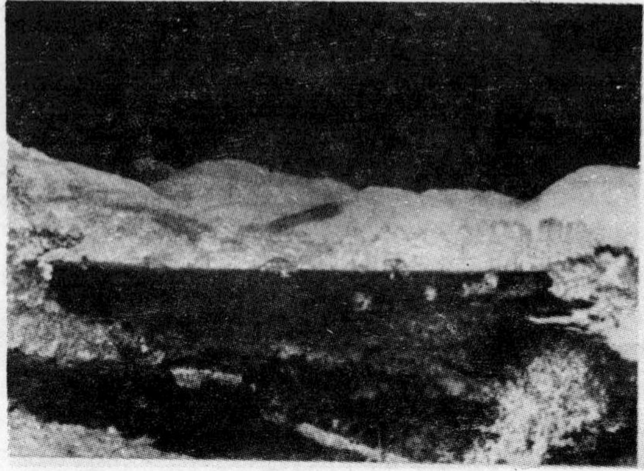

Fig. 2.8. Negative image without enlargement (original on fine grain panchromatic film).

graininess in the image. Exposure and degree of development also have some effect.

Graininess is insignificant in negatives which it is not intended to enlarge, for it is not apparent until some magnification has been given to the image. It may, however, be troublesome if the negative is to be projected as a slide or used to make an enlarged print, for the magnification thus given may be sufficient to reveal the grainy structure to an objectionable degree.

SPECTRAL SENSITIVITY OF FILM MATERIALS

Spectral sensitivity is the colour sensitivity of photographic films. It is important to realize that such materials are sensitive to colours in a different way from the human eye.

SPECTRAL SENSITIVITY OF FILM AND THE EYE

If white light is passed through a glass prism the various colours of which it is composed are separated. The human eye sees a spectrum of colours ranging from violet-blue through green, yellow and orange to red. The green-yellow part in the middle of this spectrum looks brighter than the violet-blue colours of the short-wavelength region and the red colour of the long-wavelength region at the ends of the spectrum. This is because the human eye is most sensitive to the green-yellow part of the spectrum. A sensitivity curve can be made for the eye in its response to the visible spectrum, and the curve will illustrate this fact (Fig. 2.10).

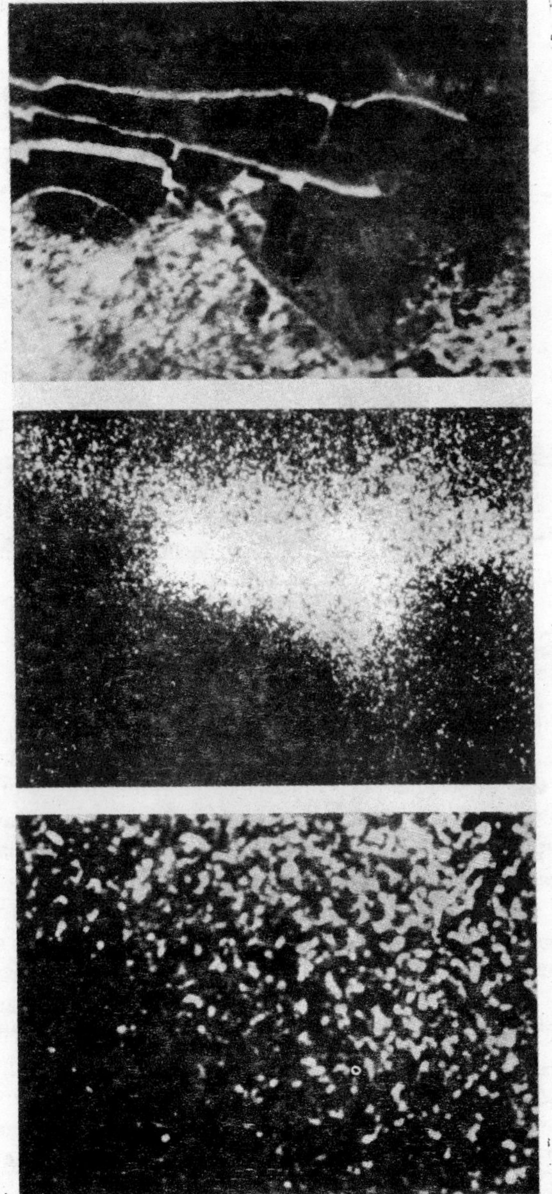

Fig. 2.9.
(a) A portion of the image with X 16 direct enlargement.
(b) X 198.
(c) X 850.
The granular pattern is perceptible at X 16 and is increasingly obvious at greater degrees
of enlargement.

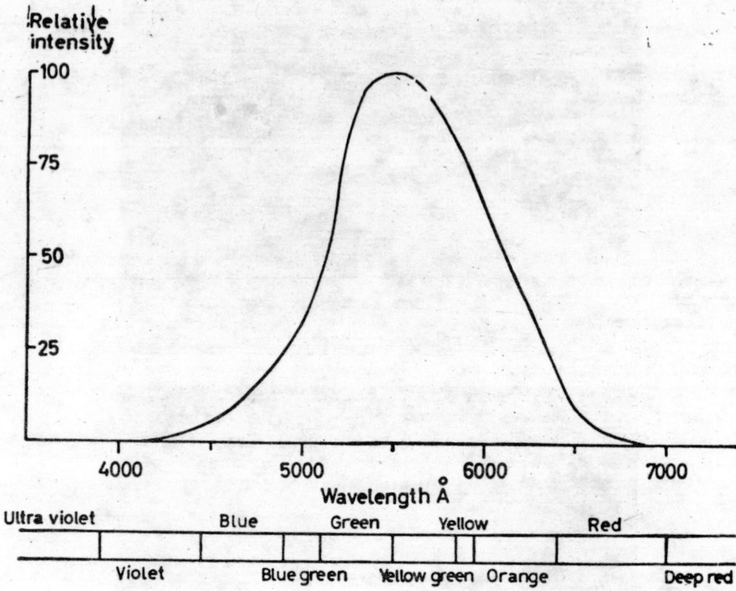

Fig. 2.10. Curve to show the sensitivity of the eye as a whole to different wave-lengths.

The response of photographic film to the colours of the visible spectrum is quite different. Untreated silver halide emulsions are very sensitive to the blue-violet parts of the spectrum but to none of the longer wavelengths, so that in this direction their sensitivity stops considerably short of that of the human eye. At the same time film materials are very sensitive to parts of the light spectrum in the short-wavelength range to which the eye is relatively insensitive. The photographic emulsion responds to ultra-violet light which the eye cannot see, and is sensitive to even shorter wavelengths (for example X rays) in the electro-magnetic spectrum of which the visible light spectrum is but a short part.

This explains the fact that X rays and gamma rays can be used for radiography. The photographic emulsion can in effect 'see' these radiations which the eye cannot.

If a sensitivity curve is drawn for the response of a photographic film to the same spectrum as given in the previous diagram, the difference between it and the eye can be shown (Figs 2.11A and 2.12)

It can be seen that the maximum sensitivity of the photographic emulsion is in the blue part of the spectrum. The response of the emulsion does not fall to nothing at the short ultra-violet end of the spectrum but will continue into regions of the electro-magnetic spectrum

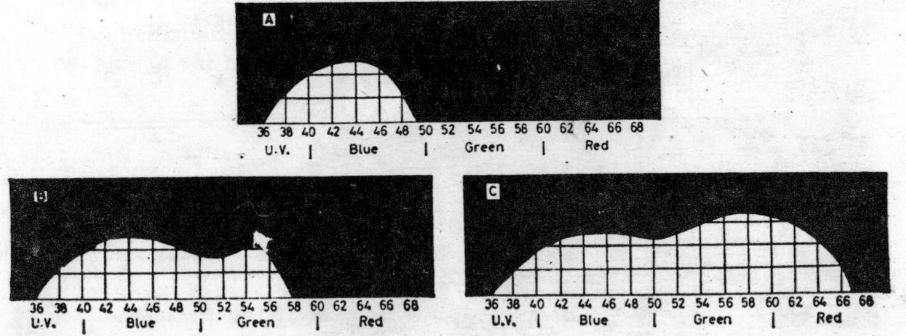

Fig. 2.11. (A) Curve to show the colour sensitivity of a non-colour-sensitive photographic emulsion.

(B) Curve to show the colour sensitivity of an orthochromatic photographic emulsion.

(C) Curve to show the colour sensitivity of a panchromatic photographic emulsion. *By courtesy of Kodak Ltd.*

which are much shorter in wavelength than visible light (and are not included in the range of wavelengths shown here).

THE IMPORTANCE OF SPECTRAL SENSITIVITY IN PHOTOGRAPHY

The sensitivity of photographic materials to blue light and (unless specially treated as below) their lack of sensitivity to other colours mean that they will not record an image as the eye sees it. A girl in a yellow dress standing against a 'royal blue' curtain impresses the eye as a light figure against a dark ground, for the eye is very sensitive to the green-yellow part of the spectrum and much less sensitive to the blue region. In a black-and-white photograph of this subject the eye will expect to see a light-toned dress against a dark-toned ground.

The photographic film, however, is markedly sensitive to blue and renders this as a light tone in the black-and-white photographic print. It is completely insensitive to yellow, so that in the photographic print this colour is rendered as a dark tone. The photograph therefore shows a girl in a dark dress standing against a light ground, and this cannot be accepted by the eye as a faithful reproduction of the original.

To make photographic film satisfactory from this point of view its colour sensitivity is extended into regions of the visible spectrum of wavelengths longer than the violet-blue range. This is done by adding suitable dyes to the emulsion, and the terms *dye sensitizing, optical sensitizing* or *colour sensitizing* are given to the process. This sensitizing extends the response of the emulsion to the longer wavelengths of the spectrum, while leaving unimpaired its original sensitivity to the short-

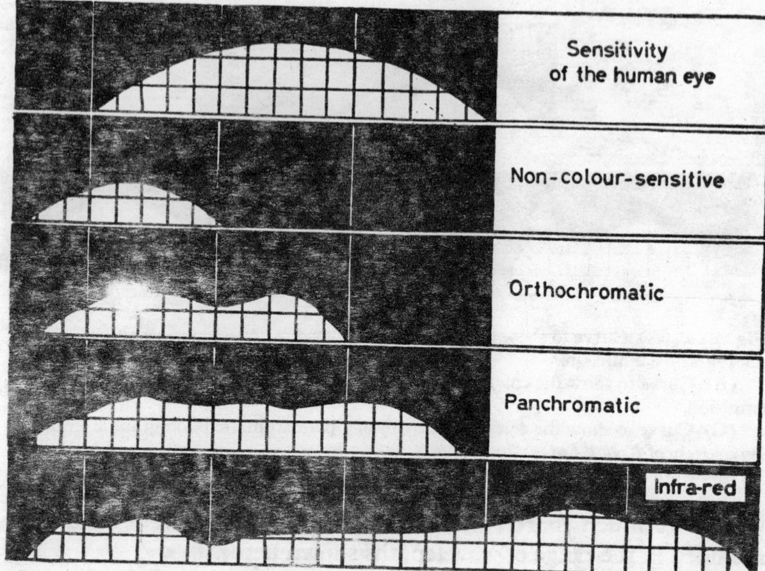

Fig. 2.12. Curves to show the spectral sensitivity of the human eye, and of various types of photographic material. It is shown that all the photographic materials respond to short wavelengths in the ultra-violet region to which the eye is insensitive. Radiations of the electromagnetic spectrum of shorter wavelengths than the ultra-violet range (such as X rays and gamma rays) are not included in the curves; photographic materials are of course sensitive to them and the eye is not.

wavelength regions—to blue, violet, and ultra-violet light and to the shorter wavelengths of X rays and gamma radiation beyond them. The high sensitivity to blue and the short end of the spectrum remains as an inherent characteristic of silver halide emulsions.

Photographic materials can be divided into four main groups according to whether this colour sensitizing has been done and (if it has been done) to which part of the spectrum the sensitivity of the emulsion has been extended. These groups are listed and considered below.

BLUE-SENSITIVE FILM

Some film materials do not have further sensitizing. They are used quite satisfactorily without response to wavelengths longer than the blue parts of the visible spectrum, and they are known as *blue-sensitive, ordinary,* or *non-colour sensitive* materials.

These films are used successfully for reproducing black-and-white subjects—for example documents, line drawings and diagrams—and even some coloured subjects where the colours are subdued and diluted. Films used in radiography are ordinary blue-sensitive materials except in certain special cases which are discussed in Chapter 17 and in Chapter 18.

ORTHOCHROMATIC FILM

Orthochromatic film has its sensitivy extended into the green part of the spectrum, and modern orthochromatic film is sometimes described as being 'fully orthochromatic'. These words like many others do not really mean what they seem to say. *Ortho* means 'correct, proper', and *chromatic* relates to colour, so the term implies that this material renders colours correctly. This is untrue, for it is still insensitive to the red part of the spectrum and will reproduce unsatisfactorily subjects in which there are many red tones. However, in photographic terminology the term orthochromatic film is fully understood to mean one which has had its sensitivity extended to the green part of the spectrum but no further (Fig. 2.11B). Photographers are neither deceived nor troubled by the exaggeration implicit in this name.

PANCHROMATIC FILM

Panchromatic film has its sensitivity extended to include the whole of the visible spectrum, and it responds to red as well as to green light. The name *panchromatic* implies sensitivity to all colours (Fig. 2.11C). If it is wished to reproduce a coloured subject in black-and-white so that there is correct representation of the various tones, panchromatic film must be used.

Photographers frequently modify colour rendering in black-and-white photography with the use of coloured light filters over the camera lens. These, together with panchromatic film, provide full control of the result and enable the photographers to achieve in black-and-white a faithful rendering of coloured subjects.

INFRA-RED FILM

Infra-red film has its sensitivity extended further than the red portion of the visible light spectrum, and its response includes reaction to wavelengths of the infra-red range (Fig. 2.12). Such material is used with a colour filter over the lens of the camera which prevents any ultra-violet and blue light from reaching the film. It is not intended for general photography in which the aim is to produce a faithful rendering of original tones, although infra-red film can be used in pictorial work for striking effects in certain cases. It has technical applications in aerial photography where the longer wavelength radiation used to make the picture penetrates haze, and a medical application in which use is made of the ability of infra-red rays to penetrate superficial tissue (Fig. 2.13).

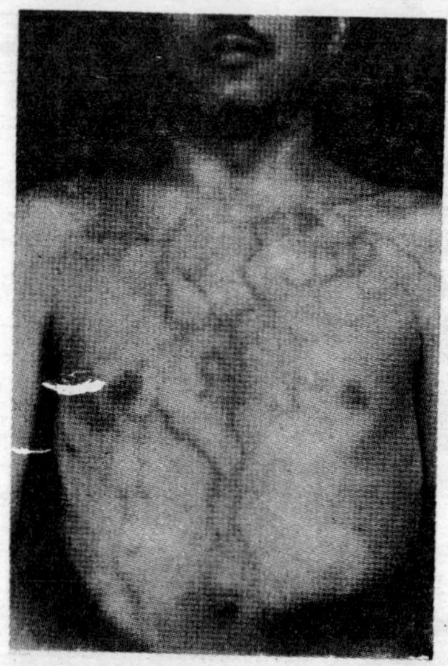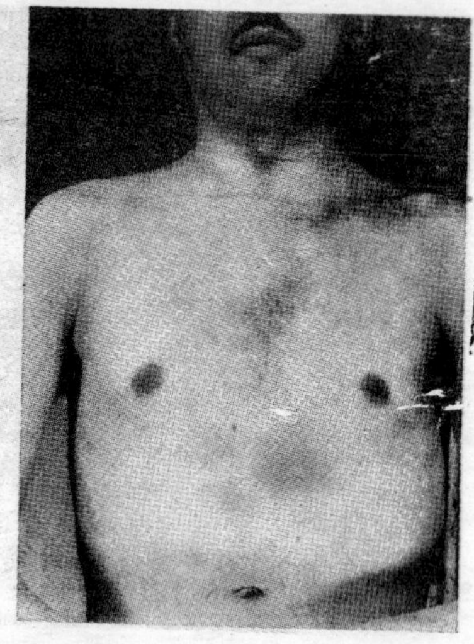

Fig. 2.13. Infra-red photography (a) reveals vessels beneath superficial tissue which are not shown by conventional photographic technique (b).

SPEED AND CONTRAST OF PHOTOGRAPHIC MATERIALS

Speed and contrast were mentioned in Chapter 1 as being significant to the photographer. They will be considered in more detail in Chapter 3 for it is important that these topics should be understood.

FILMS FOR RADIODIAGNOSIS

The manufacture and supply of medical X-ray film are undertaken by a number of commercial enterprises: many of their names must be already familiar to the student radiographer, because of associations with the photographic industry as a whole and from seeing boxes of their X-ray film in store rooms and processing areas in hospital.

In the United Kingdom, the Department of Health and Social Security issues a list of those firms which have a contract with the Department for the supply of X-ray film to the National Health Service.

This publication includes details of all the materials available and—because of their number—is quite a lengthy document.

In practice, in hospitals, no departmental head would attempt to stock all brands of X-ray film, or every variety of X-ray emulsion. Any such policy would diminish efficiency because of confusion among radiographers about the exact characteristics of a material employed: a consistent standard of radiography would become all the more difficult to maintain. Thus, student radiographers are likely to find, within the X-ray departments where they work, that the films in use perhaps may come from only one supplier and are of only a few kinds. The following paragraphs are concerned broadly with examples typifying radiodiagnostic film which may be encountered.

DUPLITISED X-RAY FILM

DIRECT EXPOSURE FILM

The descriptive terms *non-screen film* and *envelope wrapped film* are in common use for emulsions which dispense with the use of intensifying screens (see Chapter 5) and are intended for direct exposure to an X-ray beam. Each sheet of film is folder-wrapped in paper and pre-packed in a moisture-resistant paper envelope, the assembly being stiffened by the insertion of a piece of thin card in the envelope behind the wrapped film. A box containing 25 such sheets of film, ready for use in an X-ray room, is the usual package.

The availability of direct exposure film is limited to the smaller sizes (such as 18 cm × 24 cm and 24 cm × 30 cm), as it is not suitable for the examination of thick body parts, because of the large exposure doses which would be required and also the likelihood that movement-unsharpness of the image would occur. The film is particularly appropriate to radiography of the extremities and is often preferred, because of its excellent rendition of small bone detail (intensifying screens contribute to the intrinsic unsharpness of a radiographic image) and because contrast characteristics of the emulsion enable it better to record bone and surrounding soft tissue at one time. Direct exposure film has application also to the demonstration of intra-ocular foreign bodies: here it is important to exclude any possibility of imaging a small artifact—or several of them—which might be present within a cassette or upon an intensifying screen.

The emulsion layer of a direct exposure film is relatively thicker and contains more silver than is the case of X-ray films which are exposed not just to X rays, but to emissions of visible light and ultraviolet light from an intensifying screen (see Chapter 5). As X rays have a penetrative ability, images can be produced at depths in an emulsion layer which are inaccessible to light. Thus, an increased thickness of emulsion results in greater densities for any given X-ray exposure: the film is considerably faster than would be a 'screen-type' emulsion employed without intensifying screens. Direct exposure film has been desensitised to the light-emissions of intensifying screens and should not be used in association with them.

The limits to the thickness of an emulsion layer lie with several determinants, which include:

(i) the quantity of sensitive material which may be coated on a base;

(ii) the cost of the film;

(iii) the film's compatibility with the processing cycles of automatic machines in general use.

Since the emulsion layer is thicker and has a greater content of silver, direct exposure film often requires longer periods of processing, particularly for fixing the image. In the case of a 90-second processing cycle, a film manufacturer may advise that, where direct exposure film constitutes a high percentage of all film being processed, then it is desirable to increase the rate of fixer replenishment in order to assure the needed permanence of images. Table 1 indicates the order of such increases.

TABLE 1

% direct exposure film used	*% increase fixer replenishment rate*
10–20%	10%
20–30%	15%
30–40%	20%
40–50%	30%

Some direct exposure film available for medical applications is unsuitable for automatic processing where the processing cycle is as short as 90 seconds. It may have to be processed manually or processed in machines running on cycles of 3–8 minutes.

DENTAL FILMS

The small films required for intra-oral dental radiography are special examples of a prepared pack which is ready for direct exposure to an X-ray beam. Dental films and their packs have certain particular features to notice.

1 In order to identify the tube aspect of dental radiographs, each film carries an embossed dot upon one corner: the prominence of this

embossment appears on the surface which is nearer to the X-ray tube during the exposure; the concavity indicates the reverse aspect. The position of this little identifying device is apparent from the outside of the pack and careful dental radiographers usually place it towards the crowns of the teeth under examination: this is to avoid any possibility that its interruption of the emulsion's surface might impair radiographic detail near the apex of a tooth.

2   The pack includes a lead foil which is the same size as the film and is situated behind it. The foil's purpose is to protect the film from secondary X rays scattered towards it by irradiated intra-oral structures and tissues: thus, it improves radiographic contrast. The manufacturer's practice is to impress a chevron pattern on this lead foil, which becomes distinctive on the radiograph, should the user so place the pack in the patient's mouth that the incorrect aspect of the film faces the X-ray tube. Recognition of the error is then certain.

3   Dental films may be packed singly or in pairs, each film or pair of films being enclosed between pieces of black paper of a correspondent size. All the corners are well rounded, so that the package may be more acceptable in the mouth (especially of patients who have a particular sensitivity, hate swallowing tablet medications and frequently are caused to gag by dental gadgetry in situ). It is of obvious importance that the film pack's outer paper covering should be at least shower proof! The paired films will be required in a department where the practice is to send one set of radiographs to the referring dentist and retain another set for record purposes within the hospital.

4.   Dental films are available in two grades of speed and contrast. During processing, the slower emulsion may be safely handled by a competent technician in normal room lighting or even in subdued daylight. (This might be an appealing feature for those dentists who have X-ray equipment in their surgeries but whose darkrooms may be less nobly endowed, usually for lack of proper space on the premises; which might also be true of a small dental department in a hospital.) A yellow dye incorporated in the film results in a yellow tint to the radiographs. It is recommended that this 'daylight' emulsion should be manually processed in a particular X-ray developer.

5   Dental films are available in a number of sizes and styles to enable the material to be used for various techniques. The one known as an *occlusal film* from its position in the occlusal plane during radiography is 57 mm × 76 mm ($2\frac{1}{4}$ inches × 3 inches). (It is possible to obtain a screen-type film of the same dimensions for use in a special occlusal cassette.)

Films used intra-orally for examination of the dental apices and peri-apical tissues are categorised as *peri-apical film*. They are available in two sizes, broadly speaking, which may be expressed either metrically or in inches. The larger, standard film is 31 mm (or 32 mm) × 41 mm ($1\frac{1}{4}$ inches × $1\frac{5}{8}$ inches). The smaller film may be said to be substandard in size and its measurements are given in inches: they are $\frac{7}{8}$ inch × $1\frac{3}{8}$ inches but sometimes these films are described as 1 inch × $1\frac{1}{4}$ inches. No doubt, more important to radiographers than the knowledge of their exact dimensions is the fact that two sizes of periapical dental film are available, the smaller one being particularly useful for children and for examining incisor and canine regions in a narrow mouth.

Another type of pack and sizings is found in the dental films called *bitewing* which are used for investigation of the dental crowns: the pack carries a flap along the midline of its front surface and upon this the patient closes his jaws, for accurate positioning of the film and a simultaneous delineation of the coronal parts of teeth in the upper and lower jaws. Two sizes of bitewing film are available: $1\frac{1}{16}$ inches × $2\frac{1}{8}$ inches and $1\frac{1}{4}$ inches × $1\frac{5}{8}$ inches (the second corresponds to the dimensions of the standard peri-apical film).

SCREEN-TYPE X-RAY FILM

The terms *screen-type film* and *screen film* describe a duplitised X-ray emulsion which is to be used in conjunction with intensifying screens in a cassette (see Chapter 5). The image is produced mainly by light emitted from the intensifying screens when they are irradiated. Concomitant with its absorption by the intensifying screens, the X-ray beam naturally affects also the film, but the exposure from direct X rays is only a small proportion (2–7 per cent) of the total exposure: the great remainder of the density results from exposure to visible light.

Consideration of these facts must lead to a conclusion that the sensitivity of a screen-type emulsion to X rays is less important than its response to light. Following this argument a little further, we may agree that the emulsion should make its maximum response to those wavelengths (colours) of light which are emitted by the intensifying screen: for example, a screen of which the fluorescence is green cannot have its full effect on an emulsion which is relatively insensitive to that part of the visible spectrum (see p. 32).

The spectral emission of intensifying screens is more fully discussed in Chapter 5. At present we need merely note that a significant feature of screen-type films must be the emulsions' response to ultraviolet, violet and blue light and—in some instances—to green light.

A screen-type film has a thinner emulsion layer than has one which intended for direct exposure. There are two reasons for this.

1   The image is produced superficially within the emulsion, the screen's fluorescence not penetrating deeply, and thus a thick layer is unnecessary.
2   The usual arrangement in a cassette is to sandwich a film between a pair of intensifying screens. If the emulsion were very thick its absorption of the X-ray beam might significantly diminish the effectiveness of the distal intensifying screen.

SPEED AND CONTRAST CHARACTERISTICS. COLOUR SENSITIVITY

A close comparison of emulsion speeds and their contrast characteristics, made between the films of one manufacturer and those of another, may demonstrate some differences; but these differences are not usually significantly great. As a rule any manufacturer of X-ray film is likely to offer his screen-type product in two or more speed categories and possibly there will be differences of contrast as well, since these two emulsion characteristics are in close association with each other. For instance in the catalogue of a certain supplier we find three varieties of screen-type film to which the following descriptions apply.
1   A high speed medical X-ray film which is designed for blue-emitting intensifying screens and is suitable for manual or automatic processing. The qualities which are attributable to the emulsion include fine grain, balanced contrast and good exposure latitude.
2   Another high speed X-ray film which is appropriate to the use of blue-emitting intensifying screens and may be processed in either automatic or manually operated equipment. A significant difference between the two emulsions is seen in the contrast characteristics of the second, when these are compared by means of a characteristic curve (see p. 53) for each emulsion. Typical curves are depicted in Fig. 2.14. They show in a graphical form an emulsion's response to exposure.

A study of these characteristic curves shows that at low and medium densities the contrast of the two emulsions is virtually the same: we know this because the gradients of the curves are similar (see p. 59). However, at a density of about 1·5, the slopes of the curves begin to differ: the gradient for Film No. 2 becomes flatter, indicating that this emulsion exhibits less contrast in the case of high densities and has an extended latitude. Effectively, this means that the second emulsion has a capacity to record those small variations, in exposure dose to the film, for which soft tissue differences in a subject are responsible and which may need to be demonstrated if the information obtained from the radiograph is to be maximum. Thus many radiographers might prefer this type of emulsion for radiography of the chest and lung fields or the limbs, since in both subjects the parts to be X-rayed comprise bone and soft tissue together.

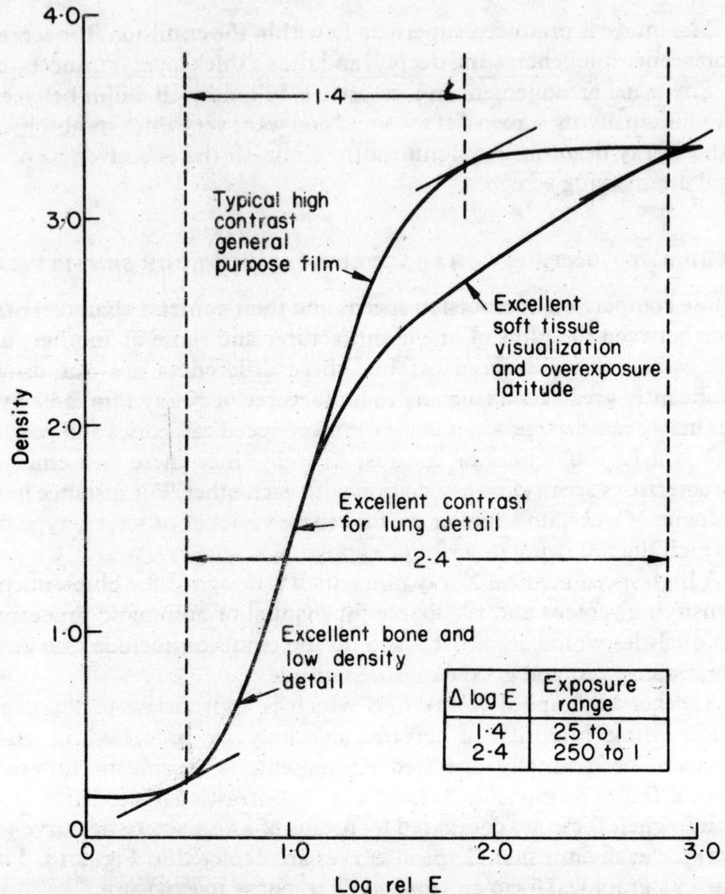

Δ log E	Exposure range
1·4	25 to 1
2·4	250 to 1

Fig. 2. 14. Two characteristic curves. Such curves depict the film blackening (Density) which results from a series of exposures (E). *By courtesy of Dupont (UK) Ltd.*

The provision in one emulsion of high contrast for the rendition of bone detail and lower contrast (a longer range of radiographic 'tones') for the rendition of other tissues is a favourable combination.

3   A third screen-type emulsion which is offered is again suitable for exposure to the emission of blue light from an intensifying screen and for both manual and automatic methods of processing. However, this is an emulsion of very fine grain and thus is fairly described as a high resolution material for medical radiography; it is often applied particularly to a partnership with rare earth intensifying screens or to barium fluoro-chloride screens. (See Chapter 5.) The high speed of such intensifying

screens annuls the relative slowness of this fine grain emulsion, so that its ability to record sharp detail may be utilised without exacting the familiar 'penalty' of long exposure times.

The three emulsions just considered were described as suitable for exposure to blue light. However, certain intensifying screens made from the rare earths (see p. 95) emit a green light when irradiated by X rays. To use these intensifying screens with a film which is insensitive to this colour of fluorescence is to obtain from them no significant speed advantage. A screen-type orthochromatic emulsion (one sensitive to green light) is available and should be used in conjunction with any green-emitting intensifying screen. It is to be noted in this connection that a darkroom which handles such orthochromatic material should have a red-brown illumination, rather than safe lighting of the pale amber colour which is adequate for blue-sensitive materials. (See Chapter 10).

SIZES OF SCREEN-TYPE X-RAY FILMS AND PACKING

Hospitals in the United Kingdom commonly use X-ray films in metricated sizes. The following are available:

    13 cm × 18 cm
    15 cm × 30 cm
    15 cm × 40 cm
    20 cm × 40 cm
    18 cm × 24 cm
    24 cm × 30 cm
    30 cm × 40 cm
    35 cm × 35 cm
    35 cm × 43 cm

In the above list, the last five sizes of film are the most frequently employed. A similar range of sizes, which more or less correspond to the metric ones but are stated in inches, is available if needed.

X-ray films intended for loading in a cassette are differently packed from their direct-exposure fellows. The usual box contains 100 sheets of screen-type film but a manufacturer may supply an 'economy' or 'thrift' pack of 500 films which sells at some financial saving to the purchaser. In this case, the presentation consists of a strong outer cardboard carton containing 4 or 5 separate light-tight boxes of 125 or 100 sheets of film. These boxes can be removed from the carton for storage purposes, if so wished, to save space and facilitate handling both in the store room and elsewhere in the X-ray department.

In some packs—but not the 'economy' variety—the sheets of films are interleaved or *folder wrapped* (FW). This description refers to the practice of inserting each film in a folded sheet of paper, of an appropriate size to cover the film on both sides and thus prevent it from rubbing shoulders with its immediate neighbours in the pack. The intention of this interleaving is to protect the film from damage, perhaps particularly from friction which might result in radiographic artifacts, such as those caused by the production of static electricity. Such wrapping is relatively expensive as the paper is of specially selected quality (it must be certain—for instance—not to contain any radioactive particle) and this is reflected in the greater price of interleaved film, compared with the *non-interleaved* (NIL) variety of pack.

The interleaving of sheets of film in this way is not an absolute need for their safe keeping and handling. In many departments the NIL packs are in general use without trouble. Films packed especially for daylight systems of dispensing and processing cannot be interleaved.

Student radiographers in the course of training have opportunities to open boxes of X-ray film, either in a darkroom prior to stocking a film hopper or in a daylight-processing area when a dispenser is to be reloaded. Within each box of 100 or 125 sheets, the films are found to be packed in a sealed bag of a material to combine lightness of weight with some degree of strength and impermeability (it must be impenetrable by light, as a first essential). This material might be a thick, silvered paper or—perhaps more commonly—a black plastic sheeting. In the case of a daylight system, it is this pack which is put in the dispenser. Loading or any other operation of a film dispenser should always follow strictly the instructions of the manufacturer on the use of the equipment.

Within their plastic or paper sacks, the sheets of film are usually protected by other materials. Even when there is no interleaving of the sheets, there will be thin cards or a stout folder-wrap to protect the surfaces of the first and last films in the pack and provide a more rigid assemblage.

It is not of importance for a radiographer to be familiar in detail with all types of film packaging but to open any of these presentations is to recognise that much attention and care—and indeed money—have been given to the matter of ensuring that X-ray film travels safely to its users in hospital. If it fails to do so, the technology applied to its manufacture will have been to little purpose.

SINGLE SIDED X-RAY FILM

Single sided emulsions employed in X-ray departments may be given the courtesy title of X-ray film but to a degree the description is misleading:

the exposure of the film is not to X rays but to light, during one or another of certain specialised radiographic techniques.

FILMS FOR FLUOROGRAPHY

Fluorography (photofluorography) is a process of recording on film, by means of a suitable camera, the fluorescent image which results from the stimulation of a phosphor by X rays: these effects occur during use of such equipments as image intensifiers or the Odelca camera, which employs a mirror lens system to obtain miniature radiographs, often of the chest.

Because of its association with image intensifiers and with fluoroscopic tables and their spot-film cameras, fluorographic film is sometimes listed as *spot film*; or it may be listed as film for mass miniature radiography (MMR).

ROLL FILM

Roll film in the photofluorographic category is of two varieties, depending upon whether it will be used with a cine camera (during cine fluorography), or with a single-shot camera or rapid-sequence camera: examples of the last two are the Odelca mirror camera and the spot-film cameras which appear on the serial changers of many fluoroscopic tables and give exposure rates of 1 to 6 shots per second.

Cine film—for reasons of increased speed—may be panchromatic (see p. 33) and consequently needs handling in total darkness. It has characteristics of medium to high speed and medium contrast, combined with fine grain. Cine film is available in 16 mm and 35 mm formats, with perforations along both edges. Typically, a roll of film may have a length of 30, 60 or 120 metres. The rolls are wound on a variety of cores or spools, appropriate to the cameras in use for cine fluorography.

Some of this material needs special processing but the rest may be put through a conventional automatic X-ray film processor, operating on a rapid—or other—dry-to-dry cycle.

Spot film generally is orthochromatic (see p. 33), so that its spectral sensitivity is matched to the colour of a screen's emission. It is likely to offer characteristics of medium to high speed and medium-high to high contrast. The following formats are available: 70 mm; 105 mm. Spot film may have perforated or unperforated edges. One roll contains usually about 45·7 metres (150 feet) and is wound on one or another variety of core or spool, depending upon the needs of the camera with which it is to associate; it is also the camera which determines whether a perforated or unperforated film is needed.

Spot film usually can be processed in a rapid-cycle machine but other processing cycles are equally appropriate. Because the film is orthochromatic, the safety of darkroom lighting may need to be particularly considered.

CUT OR SHEET FILM

Cut film for fluorography is supplied in a format which is 100 mm × 100 mm. The sheets are not interleaved and the usual pack contains 50.

Cameras utilising cut film cannot provide a rapid exposure rate and are for serial—rather than rapid sequence—radiography. The student is most likely to encounter this fluorographic film in association with an Odelca 100 mm mirror camera, used to provide a miniature radiograph of the chest (for groups such as out-patients and referrals from general practitioners and occupational health units).

In the interests of reducing radiation dose, the screen of the Odelca camera is usually green-emitting and the film used with it has an orthochromatic emulsion. (Darkroom safelight advisedly should be dark red, or fogging may result.)

Many automatic film processors may prove unhappy companions for 100 mm cut film. The small sheets tend to become wrapped round rollers and films 'get lost' in the processor. In the absence of special processing equipment, there is some advantage if these films are fed into a processor cornerwise, the diagonal of the film then appearing as the width to the processor; several films may be introduced simultaneously across the width of the feed tray. A careful selection of a suitable processor is necessary if these films are to be handled successfully, the advantage usually lying with the smaller models.

DUPLICATING FILM

Duplicating film is a single-sided, copy film which is particularly suitable for producing direct duplicates of radiographs by means of a printer : that is, the material produces a negative from a negative and it should be capable of copying the densities of the original faithfully. (See also Chapter 17.)

Radiographic duplicating film can be processed either manually (requiring the familiar 5 minutes development at 20 deg.C in an X-ray developer), or by means of any standard automatic X-ray film processor. A light red darkroom illumination is suitable.

The usual box of duplicating film contains 50 or 100 NIL sheets but the film is made in a restricted group of sizes; for example, 24 cm ×

30 cm, 30 cm × 40 cm and 35 cm × 43 cm. These are the commoner formats but 18 cm × 24 cm and 35 cm² are also available.

Some radiographic duplicating film is much slower than other copy films.

SUBTRACTION FILM

Special film materials are available for radiographic subtraction techniques (see Chapter 17). In some cases a distinction is made between the material (*subtraction film*) employed for making the positive radiograph, or mask, and the material (*subtraction print film*) which is used to obtain the final copy. Fine grain and low contrast are desirable features of emulsions to be used for making positive masks. The subtraction print emulsion, on the other hand, should be characterised by high maximum density and a steep gradation (high contrast). However, subtraction film itself is usually quite suitable for making the final copy, if desired.

Either of these materials may be processed manually or in an automatic X-ray film processor operating at any of the standard cycle times. All X-ray darkroom safelightings are appropriate. The film is available in boxes containing 50 or 100 sheets and in a limited number of formats: 24 cm × 30 cm; 35 cm²; 35 cm × 43 cm.

FILMS FOR SPECIAL PROCEDURES

MAMMOGRAPHY

Distinct from a xeroradiographic technique which records finally on paper, there are several film materials in use for mammography. Some are specific to the examination; others are emulsions having primarily an industrial application, their medical suitability being found in a limited group of procedures, such as mammography, beam localisation during radiotherapy and the radiography of morbid specimens.

Industrial film. Industrial film is duplitised and—in its medical role— is usually for direct exposure to the X-ray beam. It comes ready packed in envelopes (25 sheets in a box) and is available in a number of sizes: the two most often used for mammography are 18 cm × 24 cm and 24 cm × 30 cm.

In general, industrial film is characterised by fine grain and high contrast and is slower—in some cases very much slower—than a medical X-ray emulsion; this feature is bound to mean a higher—although not necessarily unjustified—radiation dose for a patient. When industrial film is employed for mammography it is common practice to combine perhaps three films of different speed and grain characteristics, for simultaneous exposure in one multi-pack.

Not all industrial radiographic film is suitable for rapid automatic processing and some is suitable only for manual processing; from these facts alone, its use may have a certain nuisance value in many radiodiagnostic departments.

Medical film. Medical film designated for mammography will be used in accordance with one or another of the following techniques:

1   direct exposure, either in a light-tight paper envelope, or in a polyethylene bag, or in a thin plastic cassette;

2   in a light-tight polyethylene bag, with one intensifying screen, which may be blue-emitting or green-emitting, depending on the system chosen;

3   in a light-tight polyethylene bag with one intensifying screen, the combination being then vacuum sealed to maintain an intensive film-screen contact.

Three types of mammography film are recognised:

1   a single-sided emulsion which is designated for use with one intensifying screen coated with a green-emitting rare earth phosphor;

2   a similar, single-sided emulsion designated for use with a single blue-emitting intensifying screen, having fine grain characteristics;

3   a duplitised emulsion containing more silver and having greater sensitivity to direct X radiation. (This film may be used without any intensifying screen or alternatively with a single intensifying screen, which may be either green-emitting or blue-emitting.)

All these films are offered in boxes of 100 NIL sheets in 24 cm × 30 cm and 18 cm × 24 cm formats. All are suitable for automatic processing on standard cycles of 90–110 seconds and 3·5 minutes. For the first emulsion, a red safelight filter gives the preferred darkroom illumination, but the other two are relatively insensitive to the usual amber safelights in a radiographic darkroom and consequently require no special handling.

RADIATION MONITORING FILM

Radiation monitoring by means of film badges requires special emulsions and packs. Two films are available, the appropriateness of one or the other being referable to the type of radiation to which it may be exposed during use.

1   *Radiation monitoring film*

Radiation monitoring film is a film designed for monitoring personnel, equipment and locations, where the exposure is to X rays or **gamma** rays. Thus, it is the film which student radiographers in a radiodiagnostic department will encounter in their film-badge dosimeters. The emulsion is double-sided and double-coated: this means that both sides of the base are coated with two emulsions, a fast one and a slow one. To measure small quantities of radiation, both emulsions are employed together. When large doses are to be measured, half the area of the fast emulsions is stripped from the base and the slow emulsion is used. In this way, the resultant densities on the film fall within an easily measurable range.

2 *Personal neutron monitoring film*

Personal neutron-monitoring film is a film designed for measuring—by means of a film badge—the dose received by a wearer, when the exposure is to fast or slow neutrons. (A neutron beam is the emission produced by certain equipment used for radiotherapy.)

The size of both these monitoring films and their packing are similar to those of dental film (31 mm × 41 mm, a box containing 150 packages). However, there is no lead foil in the pack and no identification of a 'tube aspect' of the film is necessary.

INDIRECT RECORDING

Indirect recording materials are those which have a special application to the records which must be made during use of a CT scanner (computerised tomography), a gamma camera (scanning with radionuclides), or a sonar scanner (ultrasound). In each case what is to be recorded is the image on the screen of a cathode ray tube (CRT).

In general it can truthfully be said that any orthochromatic or panchromatic emulsion can record the display from a CRT. However, there are several phosphors commonly used in cathode ray tubes: for example, one described as P 11 is blue-emitting and another (P 31) is green-emitting. Even more importantly, it should be noted that the three imaging systems with which we are concerned result in 'pictures' of diverse characteristics. On the one hand, the nuclear medical scan displays as a simple design of dots (often described as a 'hard dot' pattern); whilst the other extreme is found in medical ultrasound, as here the image may carry a full range of tones from light to dark (*grey scale imaging*).

An emulsion suitable for grey scale imaging preferably should have medium contrast and wide exposure latitude; whilst the other techniques require characteristics of high contrast, particularly at middle image densities. Consequently it is hardly surprising that special emulsions are needed for CRT recording and indeed that from one manufacturer two different films are obtainable: one of these is at its best with a CT scanner or a gamma camera, whilst the other has been planned particularly for ultrasonography.

CRT film has the emulsion coated on one side only of a blue-tinted polyester base. It possesses the expected feature of an anti-halation layer (see p. 21) of dyed gelatin, which minimises the spread of light in the emulsion and improves detail.

To assist in identifying the emulsion aspect, each sheet of film may be notched on one of the short sides. The emulsion surface is facing the operator when this notch can be seen or felt on the top edge on the right hand side.

A reader, who infers from the previous paragraph that CRT film should be processed either in darkness or in a dark red safelighting, has made an absolutely correct deduction. Conventional automatic X-ray processors handle CRT film without difficulty, though it is sometimes recommended that any single-sided film is better fed to an automatic processor with the emulsion aspect downwards: this facilitates even development of the film.

CRT film is available in boxes of 100 NIL sheets and in sizes appropriate to the equipments with which it will be used. Examples are: 10·2 cm × 12·7 cm or 4 inches × 5 inches; 20·3 cm × 25·4 cm or 8 inches × 10 inches; 27·9 cm × 35·6 cm or 11 inches × 4 inches.

In their different hospitals, student radiographers may encounter other materials than film in use for CRT recording: for example, there is the Polaroid imaging system, which yields an immediate print, and there is also available a bromide paper. Such paper is less expensive than film but this is really its only significant advantage. Film materials are much superior to papers and will be chosen whenever a high diagnostic quality in the record is the overriding consideration.

RADIOTHERAPY

Students of diagnostic radiography may be surprised to learn that X-ray films are needed in the radiotherapy department, in association with radiotherapeutic equipments. The circumstances under discussion are those in which the therapeutic beam itself is the source of exposure to the film. This may occur for either of two purposes:

1 in order to determine the position of a treatment field by means of a radiograph taken of it before a course of treatment is given;

2 as part of dosage estimations and as a verification of field orientation by means of a film placed beneath the patient, throughout the treatment period of a single-dose procedure.

Each of these situations requires an emulsion which is slow, is suitable for direct exposure to X or gamma radiation and has high contrast and fine grain.

The verification film, which is subject to exposures of relatively long duration (for example, one treatment period might be 2 minutes), has a very low speed indeed and is some 12 times slower than the localising film. Radiotherapy radiographers use high energy radiations and thus need slow radiographic emulsions; radiodiagnostic radiographers may have high energy patients (young children!) and thus need fast radiographic emulsions.

Both the radiotherapy films which have been described are available in a 'ready pack': this is a strong paper envelope, which is without any other stiffening and may be exposed from either aspect, There are 50 of these packs in a box. The sizes of the film are 25·4 cm × 30·5 cm (10 inches × 12 inches) and 35·6 cm × 43·2 cm (14 inches × 17 inches). The films are suitable for automatic processing under the usual X-ray darkroom safelighting (amber).

KIDNEY SURGERY

One manufacturer offers a highly specialised film pack, to enable a radiographic exposure of the kidney to be made extra-abdominally, during surgery for the removal of renal stones. The emulsion is of a direct-exposure type and the film is placed in position immediately beneath the kidney by the operating surgeon when he has gained access to the organ. Consequently, it is necessary for a film to be packed within a container which allows cold sterilisation of itself, without harm to the included film. This container is a specially designed polythene packet, which is light-tight, waterproof and flexible. Each packet in fact contains two films which are not a twin pair: the emulsions have different characteristics, in order to make the detection of small calculi of unknown radiopacity more certain; and perhaps also to provide a margin for error in choice of exposure factors, as well as eliminate confusion in the event of the occurrence of processing artifacts.

The packet size of these films for kidney surgery is approximately 11·5 cm × 13·6 cm and the usual box contains 5 film-pairs. They are equally suitable for manual or automatic processing and are tolerant of conventional X-ray darkroom safelighting (amber).

Chapter 3
Sensitometry

Certain aspects of photographic materials must now be discussed. It has been said previously that such materials have characteristics which are significant to the photographer who is to use them. Clearly it is possible to undertake some photography with a limited appreciation of the processes involved, but full understanding of the response of his materials to light is required of the photographer who is to use them most knowledgeably. Radiographers, using the photographic process in a technical application must be included within the group recognized as knowledgeable and they too should understand the response of films to radiation—both visible light and X rays.

The study of this response is known as *sensitometry*. The name suggests that it is a measurement of the sensitivity of the film. This is determined by giving known exposures to the film and measuring the results of the exposures when the film is developed.

For the sake of clarity this topic will be discussed in terms relating to photography. At the present stage it is unnecessary to differentiate between radiographic and photographic negative images, because we are concerned with the response of the film. This may be considered now to be the same both to visible light and to X radiation; in both cases the effect of the exposure is to deposit on the film black metallic silver when the film is chemically developed.

PHOTOGRAPHIC DENSITY

When a negative is held up to be viewed by the light passing through, it is obvious that the deposit of silver prevents the light passing to an extent which may be only partial or may appear to the eye to be complete. The deposit of silver may be said to have a light-stopping effect or a degree of blackness; this varies with the amount of silver present, which in turn varies with the exposure.

There are several ways in which this degree of blackness may be numerically expressed. All are based upon the fact that the intensity of the light falling on the film (the incident light) and the intensity of the light passing through a particular area of blackness (the transmitted light) can both be measured (Fig. 3.1).

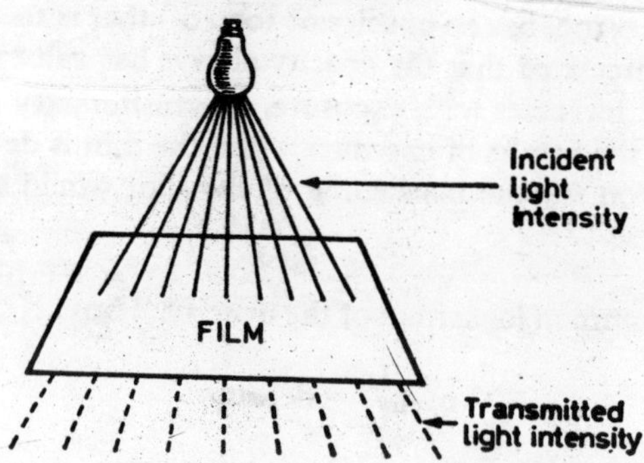

Fig. 3.1. Incident and transmitted light. *By courtesy of Kodak Ltd.*

Obviously greater blackening of the film allows less light to be transmitted. Thus the relationship between the separate intensities of incident light and transmitted light alters with the degree of blackness, and can be used as a measure of it. The relationship between the incident light (L_i) and the transmitted light (L_t) can be expressed in several ways, of which three will be considered now.

(i) Transmission

This is the ratio of the transmitted light to the incident light. Thus:

$$\frac{\text{Transmitted light}}{\text{Incident light}} = \frac{L_t}{L_i} = \text{transmission ratio}$$

It is often expressed as a percentage:

$$\frac{100 L_t}{L_i}$$

If 100 units of light fall on the film and 10 are transmitted, the transmission ratio is 10/100, and transmission is 10 per cent.

Since the incident light is bound to be greater than the transmitted light even for a slight deposit of silver, this value must always be a fraction less than unity and a percentage less than 100. This, together with the fact that transmission decreases with exposure, makes the expression less useful than those which now follow.

(ii) Opacity

This is the ratio of the incident light to the transmitted light; it is the reciprocal of the transmission. Thus:

$$\frac{\text{Incident light}}{\text{Transmitted light}} = \frac{L_i}{L_t} = \text{opacity}$$

The film considered in the previous paragraph which has a transmission of 10/100, has an opacity of 100/10—that is 10.

It can be appreciated that the opacity always has value greater than unity and that it increases with exposure. As sensitometry is concerned with measuring the results of exposure when the film is developed, this form of expression for the blackening of the film would seem to be a sensible one to use.

(iii) Density

This is the common logarithm of the opacity. Thus:

$$\text{Log}_{10}\frac{L_i}{L_t} = \text{density}$$

To take the film previously considered with a transmission of 10/100 and opacity 100/10, its density would be

$$\text{Log}\frac{100}{10} = \text{Log } 10 = 1$$

To give this some practical reality for the student radiographer, the range of densities most commonly encountered in the diagnostic areas of medical radiographs is 0·25–2·0. A radiograph of a chest has densities between 0·3 and 1·5 in those parts of the film where the rays have been absorbed by the subject. Areas of the film not covered by the subject have much greater densities, the range being of the order of 2·0–3·0. This looks to the eye so black that it is difficult to detect any difference between, say, 2·5 and 3, but a wide range of density differences can be measured by an instrument such as a densitometer. This device uses a photo-electric cell to measure the light intensity which falls on the density to be measured and the light intensity which is transmitted through it.

It can be appreciated from the foregoing description of these three terms that a density of 1 means a 10 per cent transmission; and a density of 2 (being a logarithmic value) means an opacity which is greater by 10 times, giving a 1 per cent transmission. A density of 3 is 0·1 per cent transmission, so it is hardly surprising that it seems completely opaque to the human eye, unless it is illuminated from behind by a very intense light and precautions are taken to prevent glare.

It has been explained that these three expressions—transmission, opacity, and density—give a numerical value to the degree of blackness in various parts of the exposed and processed negative. The last one—density—is most widely used in sensitometry, and is the most useful and important of the three. There are some reasons for this.

(i) Density increases with exposure.

(ii) Density is proportional to the amount of silver present. A density of 2 has twice the amount of silver present compared with a density of 1. These are approximate relationships.

(iii) In calculating the results of placing upon each other two areas of certain light-transmitting power, it is much simpler to add their densities (which are logarithmic values) than to multiply their percentage transmissions. This is obvious if the arithmetic required in both processes is considered for the following figures: $D = 0.5$ gives a per cent transmission of 32, $D = 0.9$ gives a per cent transmission of 12.5, $D = 1.2$ gives a per cent transmission of 6.3.

(iv) The eye seems to respond to differing tones in a way which is approximately logarithmic. If presented with a series in which density increases by equal steps, the eye accepts the increasing blackness as occurring in equal stages.

(v) The easiest way to appreciate the relationship between exposures and the results of the exposures is to make a graph. It is found that the most useful graph is obtained by plotting logarithmic values on both axes. Density, a logarithmic value as has been shown, is plotted on the vertical axis (the ordinate), and the logarithm of the exposure is plotted on the horizontal axis (the abscissa). Logarithmic scales enable a much wider range of values to be appreciated with understanding; also equal increments have the same ratio. The sensitometric graph which results is called a *characteristic curve* and will be considered now.

CHARACTERISTIC CURVES

A characteristic curve can be made for any photographic material. Here it will be considered in terms of negative material, since radiographers deal with X-ray film coming within this group. Such a curve is not characteristic of the material under every condition but is characteristic of the material under certain conditions of exposure and processing. The curve is a diagram which shows the results of exposure on the material, given certain conditions of exposure and processing; with these factors standardized, two different materials may be compared by study of their characteristic curves.

To make a curve a strip of the material to be tested is given a series of exposures which progress in steps. This could be done by adding a constant amount to the exposure as each section is exposed, or by multiplying the exposure by a constant factor for each step. A constant factor of multiplication is useful in practice: for example, the exposures might increase from step to step by a factor of × 2. Each step of the strip naturally has a different density as each receives a different exposure, and the series of densities can then be measured with a densitometer.

A graph is then made in which the densities are plotted on the vertical axis against *log* exposure values on the horizontal axis. The resultant curve has the same general shape for all photographic materials, and a typical one is seen on page 57 in Fig. 3.3. Such curves may be called Hurter and Driffield curves (sometimes abbreviated to H and D) after two pioneers in sensitometry; and sometimes D log E curves for the obvious reason that these are the values plotted on the axes.

MAKING A CHARACTERISTIC CURVE FOR X-RAY FILM

Characteristic curves can be made for X-ray film and can be used to compare the qualities of different films. A strip of the film for which a curve is to be drawn is given a series of exposures which proceed in steps. The progression of the steps is such that each exposure is related to the adjacent previous one by a constant known factor: this factor is called the wedge constant.

Twenty one different exposures are a number adequate for the making of a characteristic curve since it gives twenty differences and an acceptable number of exposure and density points for the plotting of the curve. We have already mentioned a factor relating the exposures (the wedge constant) which was the value 2. If this were selected, then the exposures would be plotted on the horizontal axis of the curve at 0·3 intervals: 0·3 is the log of 2 and the exposure values are recorded (as Fig. 3.4 shows) as Log Relative Exposure values.

The exposure points are brought closer together if the wedge constant is less than 2 and the curve may be more satisfactory if this is done. In conjunction with 21 exposures, the factor relating them may be $\sqrt{2}$ (that is, 1·414). If the wedge constant is 1·414, then the exposure axis has its values plotted at 0·15 intervals, for the log of $\sqrt{2}$ is 0·1492.

VARYING THE STEPPED EXPOSURES USING X-RAYS

As has been seen, what is needed to make a characteristic curve is a series of stepped exposures which are related to each other by a known factor. Using X-ray equipment available in the department there are two main ways of doing this.

First, there is the method of using variations along a time-scale. This involves giving a series of stepped exposures in which the only variation is the time interval, which is increased by a constant factor (the wedge constant). The tube kilovoltage and milliamperage, the focal spot setting and the focus-film distance used would not be changed.

Thus, for example, using lead shields over the cassette the film could be exposed in portions using a series of exposures which varied as follows:
(a) using a wedge constant of 2 and hence a multiplication factor of 2, the milliampereseconds would be 1·0, 2·0, 4·0, 8·0, 16·0, 32·0, 64·0 and so on;
(b) using a wedge constant of $\sqrt{2}$ and hence a multiplication factor of 1·4, the milliampereseconds would be 1·0, 1·4, 2·8, 3·9, 5·4, 7·6, 10·7 and so on.

The second method for achieving the stepped exposures is to use variations along an intensity scale. This is done by varying in a known way a set of radiation intensities transmitted to the film through a test object which is a stepped wedge of a material such as aluminium.

This in effect looks like a flight of metal stairs (Fig. 3.2). Clearly it

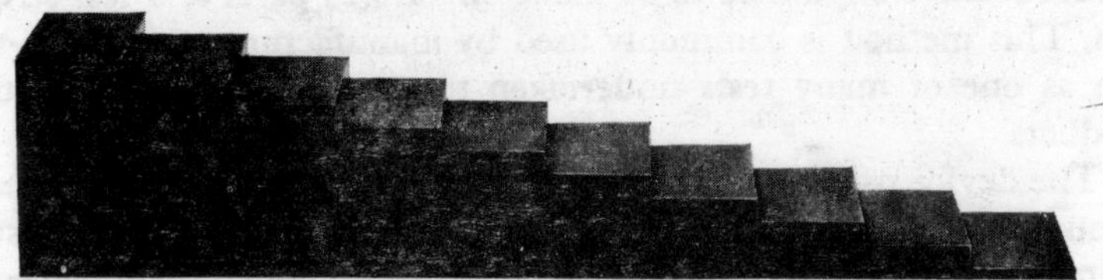

Fig. 3.2. An aluminium step-wedge.

allows varying amounts of radiation to reach the film resulting in a series of exposures with variation in intensity; this variation is from the least amount of radiation which is transmitted through the top step of the staircase to the greatest amount which is transmitted through the bottom step of the staircase. Step-wedges are made of aluminium or plastic if the beam of radiation is soft, and of steel if harder radiation is being used.

It must be realized, however, that there is an alteration in the quality of the radiation as it is filtered by the different steps of aluminium or other metal. If the steps have a constant increase in thickness going up the stairs, the intensity changes in the beam do not also proceed in a constant relationship; the change in intensity per step will be greater at the thin end of the wedge than at the thick end where the beam is more heavily filtered. This difficulty can be overcome by adjusting the thickness of the steps at the thin end of the wedge so that there is a constant change in intensity per step throughout the wedge. The addition of a thin copper filter at the underside of the wedge has been of help.

The use of such a step-wedge allows a single exposure from the X-ray set to give to the film a series of related exposures from the varied radiation intensities transmitted through the wedge: if the wedge has 21 steps it obviously gives 21 exposures. These related exposures from the steps can be plotted on the horizontal axis of the graph from the step numbers as the logarithms of the relative exposure values. If the relationship between the exposure steps (wedge constant) is a factor of times 2, then as we have explained the points on the log relative exposure axis are at 0·3 intervals (0·3 is the log of 2). If the wedge constant is √2 then the steps are plotted at 0·15 intervals (0·15 is the log of √2).

VARYING THE STEPPED EXPOSURES USING LIGHT

In testing the response of X-ray films to the fluorescence of intensifying screens.it is of course possible to avoid the use of X rays. The films can be exposed to a series of light intensities which are equivalent in spectral distribution (i.e. colour) to the light from the screens; it is arranged for correct relative exposures to be made on various parts of a test strip of film. This method is commonly used by manufacturers of screen-type film as one of many tests undertaken to control the quality of their products.

The device used is called a sensitometer and the exposures are made through a light-attenuator which gives a series of stepped exposures related by a wedge constant. There is more about sensitometers in Chapter 13 (p. 332).

An understanding of the main features of D log E curves is required of the radiographer. They are considered and explained in the following sections.

FEATURES OF THE CHARACTERISTIC CURVE

Fig. 3.3 shows a typical characteristic curve. It can be seen that the exposures are plotted logarithmically as relative exposures and not as absolute values of exposure. This is common practice and it does not alter the shape of the curve. Only when a curve is required to give information on absolute values of film speed is it necessary to plot logarithmically an absolute exposure scale.

The three main regions of the curve commonly described are as follows.

(i) The toe.

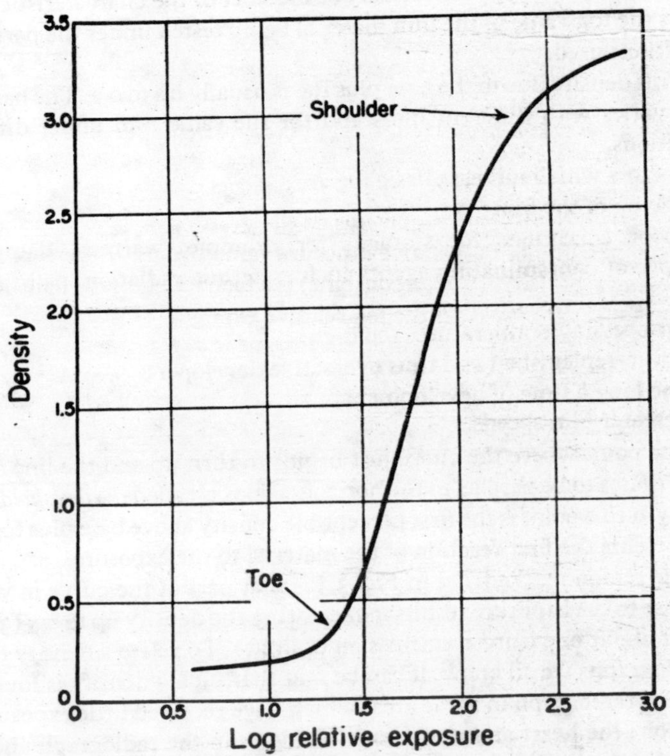

Fig. 3.3. Characteristic curve of a typical medical X-ray film, exposed with calcium tungstate intensifying screens.
By courtesy of X-ray Sales Division, Eastman Kodak Co., Rochester, New York.

(ii) The straight-line part.

(iii) The shoulder.

These three parts have also been described as regions of (i) under-exposure (ii) correct exposure and (iii) overexposure.

Density has a small value, even at the starting point although there has been no exposure or only a very small exposure. This density is produced by the development of silver halide grains which have not been exposed, or have received from the exposure such a small amount of energy that no latent image is produced. This low density is called *base plus fog*. All film materials have some fog, and this will tend to increase with age. It is also a function of the developer since failure by the developer to differentiate between exposed and unexposed grains (i.e. any tendency to treat unexposed grains as if they were exposed ones) results in fog. Fresh film materials and fresh developer correctly used should produce very low fog. The density at the start of the characteristic curve shows the fog value of the film material being tested under the particular conditions used.

This density due to the base plus fog is usually up to 0·2. The basic fog level varies with different films and for the same film under different conditions.

Factors which increase basic fog are:

(i) ageing of the film;

(ii) poor conditions for storage (for example, warmth, dampness, presence of contaminating agents such as actinic radiation, paint fumes etc.);

(iii) processing temperatures too high;

(iv) over-replenished and thus overactive developer;

(v) too long a time of development;

(vi) greater film speeds.

The point where the curve just begins to turn up and the line of the graph ceases to be parallel to the horizontal axis is called *the threshold*. The density at this point is the first perceptible density above base plus fog and it represents the first reaction of the material to the exposure.

The region marked *Toe* in Fig. 3.3 is that part of the curve in which response to the exposure results in increasing the density up to 0·5 (32 per cent or about one third transmission of light). To relate a density of 0·5 to radiographs we all know, it can be said that such a density is found in the chest radiograph in those areas which have received little exposure to radiation: the heart and mediastinal shadows in the radiograph and the region below the diaphragm.

The *shoulder* of the curve depicts the state where increasing exposure leads to decreasing differences in density. A horizontal line extended from the uppermost part of the curve at this point to cut the density axis as in Fig. 3.4 gives the maximum value of density which the material achieves in response to the exposure in the given development conditions. This maximum density is known as D max.

It can be seen from the bend of the graph in Fig. 3.4 that beyond D max. there is a part where increase in exposure results in decrease in density. This means that the material will become lighter as the exposure increases. Since this is a reversal of the normal response to light there will be as a result reversal of the image.

This region of reversal is known as the *region of solarization*, and different materials vary in the extent to which they can be solarized; the effect also varies with development. Exposures required to produce solarization are of the order of several thousand times greater than those in the region of correct exposure.

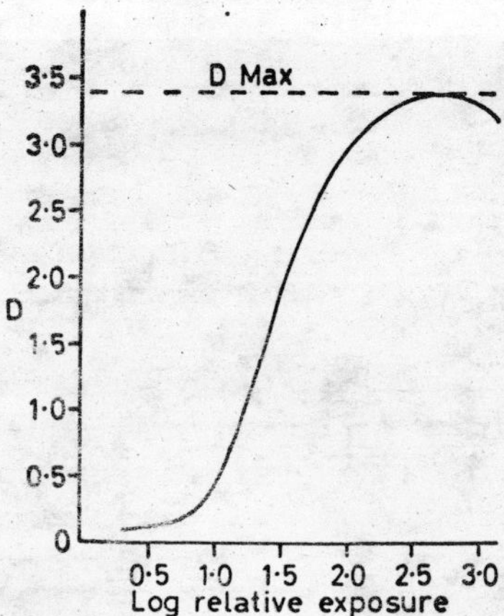

Fig. 3.4. A typical curve, showing D Max.

On page 11 in Chapter 1 a specially prepared emulsion was described to be used for obtaining positive images instead of negative ones. The material provided by the manufacturers has been previously solarized. On being developed without exposure it gives maximum density. On being photographically exposed before being developed it uses the solarization region of the characteristic curve, and yields a positive image from a positive subject, or (as described in Chapter 1) it results in a negative image copy from the negative image radiograph without need of an intermediate positive.

This is useful application of the reversal effect. Less happily radiographers can find themselves using solarized film unintentionally. If a film is accidentally fogged in the X-ray room or in the darkroom before or after being used for a radiographic exposure, partial or complete reversal of the image may result (Fig. 3.5).

The *straight-line* part of the curve has been called the region of correct exposure. In this part of the graph, if it is a straight line, the resultant densities increase linearly with the logarithms of the exposures causing them. One of the qualities on which this part of the curve provides information is the average contrast of the film material used.

CONTRAST AND THE CHARACTERISTIC CURVE

It was said in Chapter 1 that contrast is the way in which a material reacts to a certain exposure range. This can be considered in terms of photography by imagining a scene which contains both highlights and

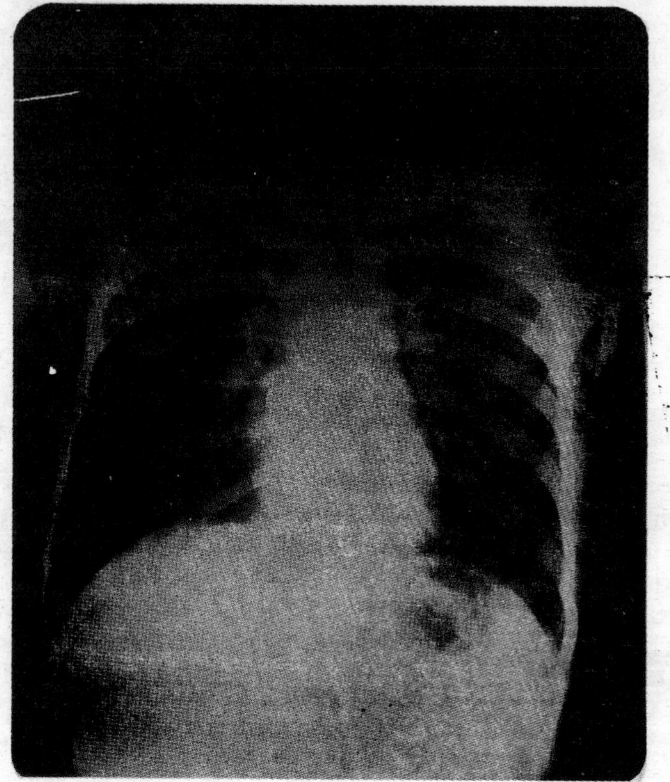

Fig. 3.5. Partial reversal in a radiographic image.

shadows—for example a white-sailed boat at a lakeside bordered with trees. The range of exposures to be accommodated on the film is between the small exposure reaching the film from the tree shade (the shadows of the image) to the relatively much greater exposure reaching the film from the white boat-sail (the highlights of the image). In the negative the highlights will be dark and the shadows light. A film material of high contrast will render the highlights black and the shadows white; a film material of low contrast renders both as tones of grey. The film material of higher contrast gives a greater density difference between the lightest and the darkest tones than does the one of low contrast.

This can be translated to radiographic terms by considering a subject such as a posteroanterior view of the chest. Here the range of exposures to be accommodated on the film is between the relatively little radiation transmitted to expose the film through the heart and the regions below the diaphragm; the much greater amount of radiation transmitted to expose the film through the air-containing lungs; and the maximum amount of radiation reaching the upper part of the film above the patient's shoulders, where his body has not been interposed as an absorber. Film material of high contrast will give maximum density differences in the radiograph from these radiation differences, which constitute exposure differences analogous to those of visible-light photography.

Radiographers require from their material much higher contrast than is needed in that used for conventional photography. It is important that small radiation differences should produce appreciable density differences in the image if various bodily structures are to be well seen. For this, high contrast in the film emulsion is required.

In a characteristic curve of any film material it has been seen that density on the vertical axis is plotted against log exposure on the horizontal axis. The film material of high contrast mentioned earlier (recording a white boat-sail and the shade of trees) will have a bigger density rise from shadow to highlight than the film of low contrast, though the range of exposures is the same in each case. It is clear that in the straightline part of the characteristic curve a material with a bigger density (vertical) rise for the same excursion along the horizontal axis *must* have a steeper slope to the straight line. This can be seen in Fig. 3.6.

The contrast of the material can therefore be measured by the slope

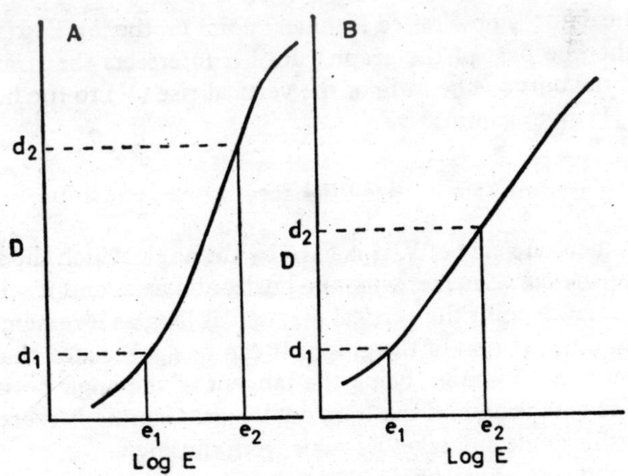

Fig. 3.6. Characteristic curves for two different film materials.

$e_1 e_2$ exposure range
$d_1 d_2$ density range

The curve under A shows higher contrast than the curve under B.

of the straight-line part of the curve, high contrast material showing a steeper slope. This slope of the straight line is called the *gamma* of the material; gamma is the third letter of the Greek alphabet and corresponds to our C.

Gamma can be measured and given a numerical value in this way: the straight-line part of the curve is continued until it intercepts the log E axis as in Fig. 3.7.

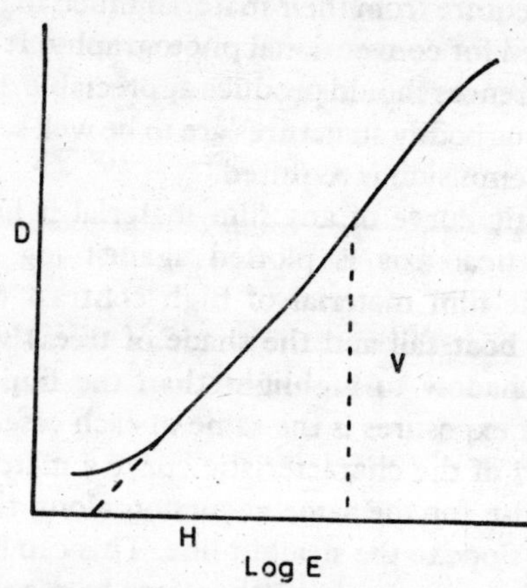

Fig. 3.7. Gamma = V/H.

A vertical line is now raised from any point on the log E axis (within the straight-line part of the graph) until it intersects the straight-line portion of the curve. The ratio of the vertical rise (V) to the horizontal distance (H) gives gamma.

$$\text{Gamma} = \frac{V}{H}$$

The numerical value of V/H is fixed by the angle which the straight-line part of the curve makes with the horizontal axis, and it will be the same at whatever point the vertical is raised as long as it remains within the straight-line portion of the graph. It can be appreciated that V/H is a trigonometrical function, being the tangent of the angle between the straight-line extension and the horizontal axis. Gamma is therefore the tangent of this angle and takes its value from the angle.

To the photographer gamma is important because it measures contrast and it tells him how truthfully the negative will reproduce the various tones of the original subject. If gamma is less than unity, the tones of the subject are compressed in the negative and the image will be 'flatter' than the original. If gamma is greater than unity, the image contrast is greater than that of the subject. Radiographic materials have gamma greater than unity so that small variations in the radiation transmitted through various parts of the subject may produce appreciable contrast in the image tones; the radiation contrasts (or differences in radiopacity) in the subject require to be amplified in the image. Although radiographers may not be concerned with values of gamma, an understanding of the significance of the steepness of slope of the straight-line part of the graph enables them to make comparison between the curves of different film materials.

It must now be said that characteristic curves for modern X-ray films do not show a 'straight line' region which is a true straight line throughout its length. Gamma as an expression of the contrast of these materials no longer applies. Instead another value is used which is called *average gradient* and this is explained on page 72.

In explaining gamma here we may be thought to have wasted our energy in explaining the obsolete but we make no apologies for it. We decided that the best way to bring our perhaps reluctant readers to some understanding of the importance of the angle of slope in this part of the curve was to consider the simple true straight line and the unelusive trigonometrically-based value which is called gamma. Once you understand this and its determination by the slope of the line, a line which changes in slope should not confuse you.

SPEED AND THE CHARACTERISTIC CURVE

In general the term *speed* in relation to a photographic material refers to whether it requires more or less exposure in relation to another material in order to produce a comparable negative. The material which requires less exposure is said to have higher speed than the other or to be faster.

In regard to the characteristic curve it can be said simply that the speed of the material determines the location of the curve along the D log E axis. In Fig. 3.8 are shown characteristic curves of two materials—Film C and Film D. From the curves it can be seen that Film C requires less exposure than Film D to produce say, a density of 1. Film C has therefore greater speed than Film D. Faster materials thus have their curves located further to the left along the horizontal axis since exposure increases to the right along this axis.

A quick perception that there is a difference in speed between the two films shown in Fig. 3.8 is gained by looking at the separation of the curves along the horizontal line from D 1.0. If there were no difference in speed at D 1.0, there would be no separation at that point; the greater the horizontal separation, the faster is Film C in relation to Film D.

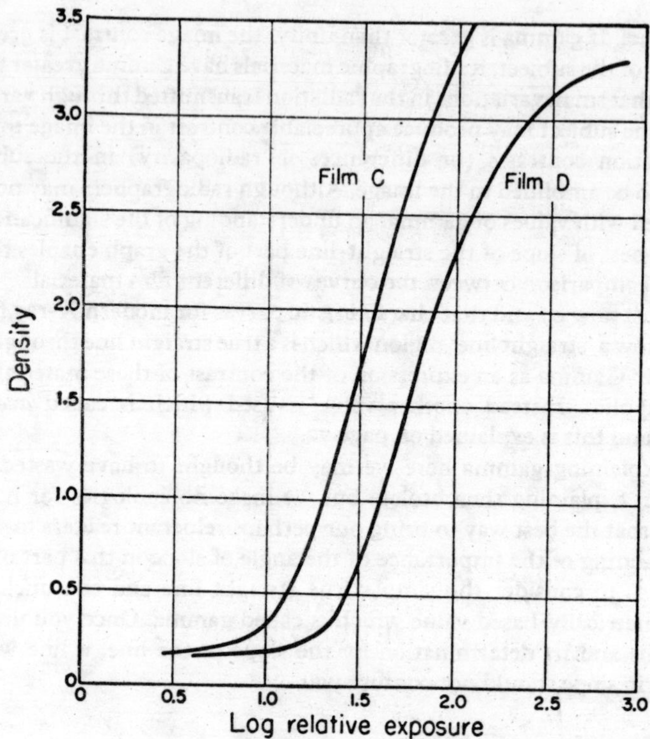

Fig. 3.8. Characteristic curves of two typical medical X-ray films, one (C) being faster than the other (D). Exposures made with calcium tungstate intensifying screens.
By courtesy of X-ray Sales Division, Eastman Kodak Company, Rochester, New York

Fig. 3.8 also shows the knowledgeable observer whether the two films maintain their speed relationship throughout the range of useful densities (taken as 0·25 to 2·0). Readers who make the effort to compare the horizontal separation along lines from D values 0·25, 0·5, 1·0, 1·5 and 2·0 will see that it stays constant: the speed difference is maintained. This could be a useful piece of information if you were planning to use the faster film for radiography.

If you are curious enough to pursue your measurement of the horizontal separation to the D value 3·0, you will find that the horizontal separation along that line is somewhat greater than it was before: Film C has become still faster in relation to Film D and it is at once obvious to a glance that this increase in relative speeds progresses until the curves stop. As a practising radiographer you are now in possession of a piece of useless information since it relates to densities too high to be differentiated by the eye and so valueless in a radiographic image.

To go back to the difference in speed between the two films within the useful density range, from the D log E curves shown in Fig. 3.8, the relative speeds of the two films C and D can be calculated, as follows.

For a density of 1·0, the points corresponding on the exposure axis are about 1·6 for Film D and 1·3 for Film C. So we can calculate the difference between the logarithms of the relative exposures as

$$1·6 - 1·3 = 0·3$$

Now when we establish a difference between logarithms by subtracting one from another, what we are doing to the actual values which the logarithms represent is to establish a ratio: in this case the ratio established is that for the relative exposures required by these two films to give a density of 1·0.

Our calculation above gave us a logarithmic value of 0·3 and the figure of which this is the logarithm is 2. So we now have the information that these exposures are related by a factor of 2. In other words, Film C is twice as fast as Film D.

VARIATIONS IN THE CHARACTERISTIC CURVE WITH DEVELOPMENT

It was said earlier that a characteristic curve is not characteristic of an emulsion in every condition, and it is affected by conditions of exposure and processing. The curve alters with degree of development. This effect can be seen if a family of characteristic curves is made for one emulsion, the development time being varied and other conditions remaining constant. The result is seen in Fig. 3.9.

What changes have been made in the characteristic curve as a result of increasing the development times over the range shown?

THE BASE PLUS FOG DENSITY

It can be seen from the levels on the density axis at which the curves begin that increasing the development time raises the fog level. This is insignificant up to 5 minutes but at 15 minutes the fog has markedly increased to a value that would unacceptably deteriorate the image.

THE CONTRAST OF THE FILM

If the slope of the straight line part of each of the four curves is examined it will be found that the angle increases noticeably between 1½ minutes and 5 minutes: after that it hardly changes. This shows that increasing

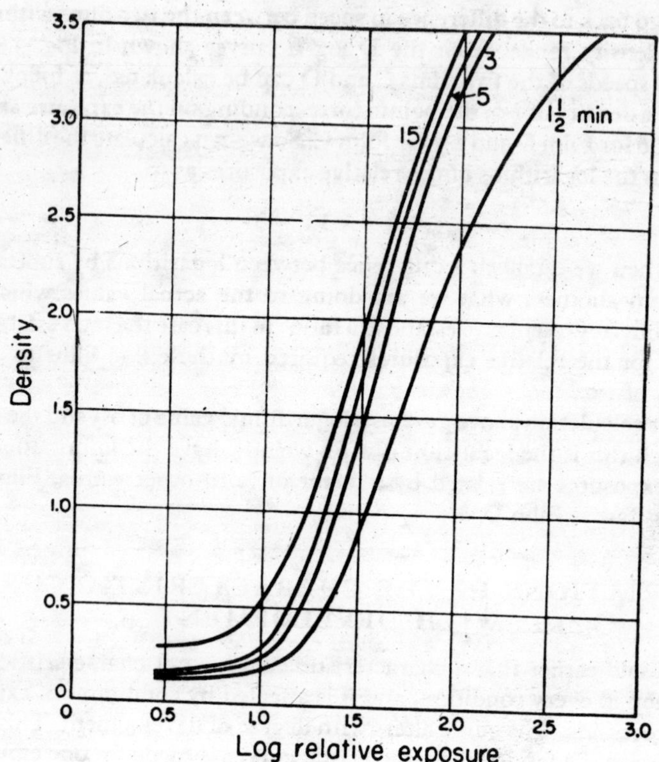

Fig. 3.9. Characteristic curves of a typical screen-type X-ray film, developed for a series of times at 68°F.
By courtesy of X-ray Sales Division, Eastman Kodak Company, Rochester, New York.

the development time increases the inherent contrast of the film material up to a certain point. Beyond that point, extending the development time does not increase the contrast.

If the time is prolonged further (this is not apparent from the curves shown in Fig. 3.9) the developer begins to act on the unexposed as well as the exposed silver halide grains. This increases fog and the contrast deteriorates as a result.

THE SPEED OF THE FILM

It can be seen from the family of curves for differing development times shown in Fig. 3.9 that, in addition to a change in slope of the curve, there is shift of the curve to the left as development time is increased. This corresponds to an increase in speed of the material, and as can be seen it does not take place at a uniform rate, being greatest in the early stages of development.

Prolonging the development time is not a useful technique in radiographic processing in order to increase both the contrast and speed of the film used. The material should reach maximum contrast and, if it has been correctly exposed, maximum usable density in that time of development which is standard for the method of processing which is in use. Any attempt to depart from the standard may impair the quality of the resultant image.

COMPARISONS OF EMULSIONS BY THEIR CHARACTERISTIC CURVES

In Fig. 3.10 are shown the characteristic curves of two emulsions used for radiography. With an understanding of the features of the graphs certain

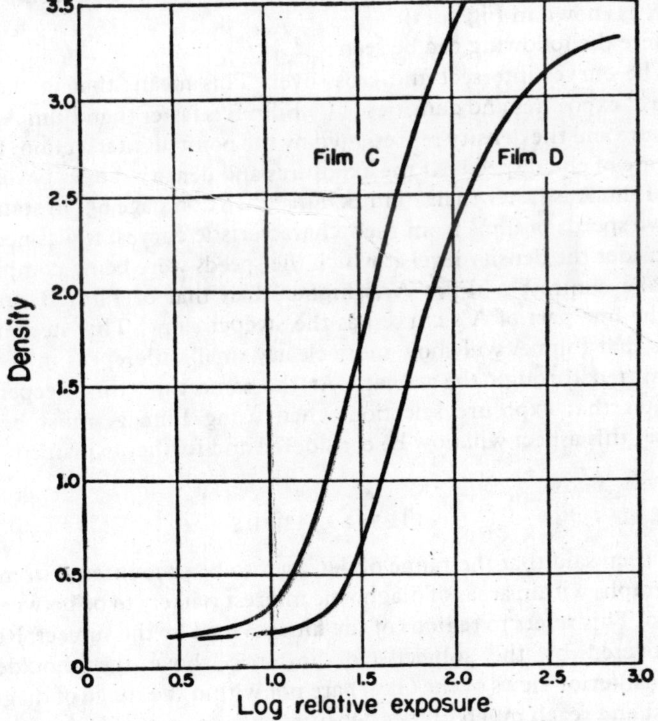

Fig. 3.10. Characteristic curves of two typical medical X-ray films, one (C) being faster than the other (D). Exposures made with calcium tungstate intensifying screens.
By courtesy of X-ray Sales Division, Eastman Kodak Company, Rochester, New York.

comparisons can be made between the emulsions from study of these curves. The conclusions to be drawn are as follows:

(i) Film C is faster than Film D since the whole of its curve is further to the left on the horizontal axis. The amount of their separation is a measure of the speed difference between the emulsions.

(ii) Film C begins to react to the exposure before Film D, since the threshold (the point where the graph begins to turn upwards) of C is further to the left on the horizontal axis.

(iii) Their contrast is not markedly different over the range of densities 0·25—2·0 (commonly encountered in diagnostic fields). This is deduced since the slope of the straight-line parts of the two curves looks the same.

(iv) Film C has slightly greater fog level than Film D since the start of its curve is placed slightly higher on the vertical axis.

(v) Film D has a lower shoulder than Film C. The maximum density achieved by Film C is not accommodated within the range shown on the vertical axis. (It reaches its maximum density above a density of 3·5.)

The curves of two emulsions may show a different relationship to each other, as shown in Fig. 3.11.

Here the following can be seen:

(i) The curves intersect and cross over. This means that in the lower range of exposures and densities (D_1) Film B is faster than Film A. At the exposure and the density represented by the point of intersection, the two films are of equal speed. At the exposures and density ranges beyond this (D_2) Film A is faster than Film B. This is why on page 65, in stating the relative speeds of films from their characteristic curves, it was necessary to consider the density level at which the speeds were being compared.

(ii) The contrast of Film A is higher than that of Film B since the straight-line part of A's curve has the steeper slope. This steeper slope means that Film A will show more clearly small differences in radiation transmitted through the subject. At the same time this steeper slope indicates that exposure selection when using Film A must be more precise; this aspect will now be considered and further explained.

FILM LATITUDE

It has been said that the range of densities to be encountered in medical radiographs within areas of diagnostic interest is likely to be between 0·25 and 2·0. This refers to regions of the film covered by the subject. Regions not covered by the subject (for instance above the shoulders in posteroanterior views of the chest) are not within the range of diagnostic interest and reach much higher densities.

The reasons why densities greater than 2·0 are not useful in medical

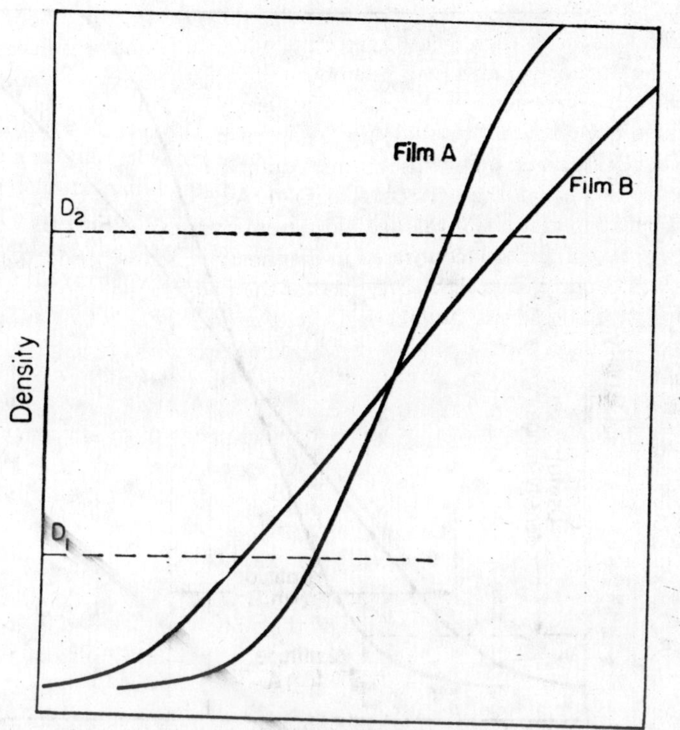

Fig. 3.11. Characteristic curves of a hypothetical high contrast film (A) and a low contrast film (B). The relative speeds of the two films depend upon the density at which they are measured.
By courtesy of X-ray Sales Division, Eastman Kodak Company, Rochester, New York.

radiographs is that most X-ray illuminators are not bright enough for viewing higher densities; even if they were to be made bright enough, the eye would be so dazzled by the light transmitted by regions of low density (behind the heart in a posteroanterior view of the chest), that it could not perceive details in the high density range. The student should keep in mind the meaning of density 2; 1/100 part of the light falling on this density is transmitted through it.

The range of densities 0·25 to 2·0 may be described as the *useful density range*. In Fig. 3.12 horizontal lines have been drawn from the vertical density axis at the extremes of the useful density range. From the points at which they meet the curves, verticals are dropped to meet the log E axis.

It can be seen that in the case of Film B these verticals occur further

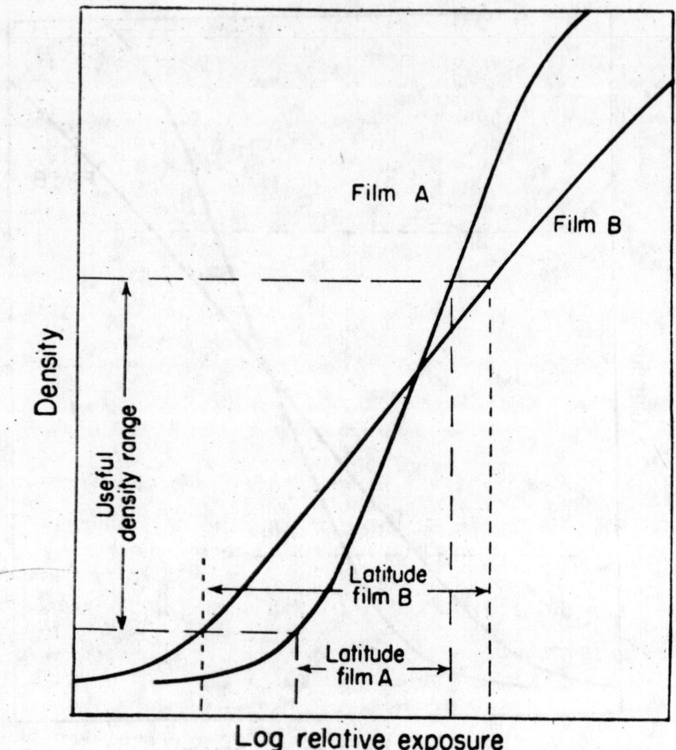

Fig. 3.12. Characteristic curves of two hypothetical radiographic films. (A, high contrast film; B, low contrast film). The range of exposures that can be covered within the useful density range (i.e. the latitude of the film) depends upon the average gradient.
By courtesy of X-ray Sales Division, Eastman Kodak Company, Rochester, New York.

apart on the log E axis than they do for Film A. Film B is therefore said to have greater *latitude* than Film A (latitude being defined as the exposure range covered within the useful density range).

It is clear that films with curves of lower slope must always show more latitude than films with curves of steeper slope; high contrast material always has less film latitude than low contrast material. The importance of film latitude to the radiographer is this: a wider range of exposures can be accepted by Film B and the resultant densities will be within the useful density range and the radiograph will be acceptable for viewing. This wider range of usable exposures means that for a given kilovoltage the radiographer can select over a wider milliamperesecond range and still achieve an acceptable result. The selection of exposure conditions must be more precise when using high contrast material with little film latitude if the range of densities in the resultant radiograph is to be placed within the useful range acceptable for viewing.

Latitude may be considered also in relation to another range of exposures—those produced by the different radiation intensities transmitted through the subject being radiographed. Some subjects transmit a long scale of radiation intensities. Examples are the dorsal spine in an anteroposterior view, and the pregnant abdomen in a lateral projection. The region of the upper thoracic spine transmits very much more radiation than that of the lower, where the overlying heart and diaphragm absorb X rays heavily. In the pregnant abdomen there is a marked difference in absorption of the beam by the region of the posterior uterine wall close to the spine, where absorption is heavy, and by the region of the anterior uterine wall, where transmission is much greater. Some subjects—for example the fifth lumbar vertebra in a coned view—transmit a short scale of radiation intensities.

If a long scale of intensities (or exposures transmitted to the film) is to be recorded with the resultant densities all placed within the useful density range, a film material of little latitude requires this range of exposures to be most precisely placed on the log E axis: this requires careful selection of exposure factors by the radiographer. If the latitude is too small in extent it may be in fact impossible to place the range of transmitted exposures or intensities so that *all* the resultant densities come within the useful density range. A film material with extensive latitude will record a long scale of radiation intensities, and allows this long scale to be moved about on the log E axis (or less precise selection of exposure factors by the radiographer) without placing the resultant densities outside the useful density range.

It can therefore further be said of the two emulsions in Fig. 3.12 that: (iii) Film B will transmit a longer scale of radiation differences than Film A and will allow greater range for exposure choice. If correctly exposed, Film A will show the radiation differences more clearly as it has the higher contrast and it will therefore render more distinct from each other structures which show little difference in radiopacity. The maximum differentiation of detail will be obtained in the ideal condition when the log E range is adjusted so that the whole of the useful density range is utilized. The exposure, however, would need to be accurately determined.

INFORMATION FROM THE CHARACTERISTIC CURVE

It may be useful to sum up the characteristic curve simply with a list of the points on which it can provide information about a film material.

(i) Fog level—from the point where the curve begins.

(ii) Contrast—from the slope of the straight-line portion.

(iii) Extent of film latitude—by consideration of the useful density range and the corresponding range on the log E axis.

(iv) The maximum density which the material will give in the conditions of exposure and development used to make the curve—from the shoulder of the curve.

(v) The solarization region (if the material will solarize)—from the region of the curve beyond D max.

(vi) The speed of the material—from the location of the curve on the horizontal axis.

(vii) The comparative performances of different emulsions over the same exposure and density range in the same conditions of development.

In radiography characteristic curves can be used for:

(a) The comparison of films.

(b) The comparison of intensifying screens.

(c) The determination of the added speed gained by the use of intensifying screens.

(d) The testing of developer solutions to check their performance.

MODERN EMULSIONS AND AVERAGE GRADIENT

So far in this chapter characteristic curves have been discussed mainly in terms of the classic curve, with its toe, its straight-line portion and a region of solarization. However, many X-ray films and films used for fluorography have a shape like a flattened, elongated 'S' and the straight-line portion is not really a straight line at all, even though to the casual glance it may look very like one. The curve shown in Fig. 3.13 is an example.

Where there is no true straight-line part of the characteristic curve, gamma (the slope of the straight-line part of the characteristic curve) ceases to be useful as a number to indicate the contrast of the film material. Another consideration which makes gamma not very useful is that when films are being employed for radiography the densities may not fall within the straight-line parts of characteristic curves. The reader should remember that the useful range of densities in a medical radiograph is between 0·25–2·0. To look at Fig. 3.13 with this in mind is to see that this range of densities relates to parts of the curve which are at different slopes. The minimum end of the range is on the toe of the curve and not on the straight-line part at all; the maximum end of the range comes on a portion of the curve which is approaching the shoulder. In this case gamma as a statement of the contrast of the material would not

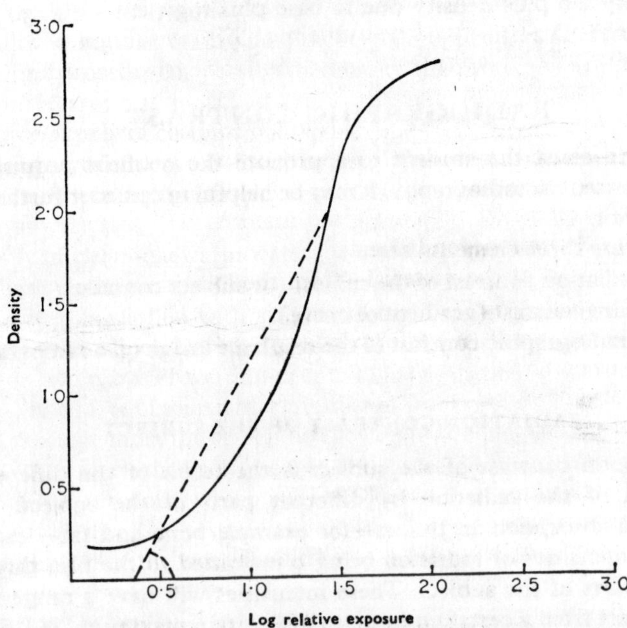

Fig. 3.13.

tell us anything about the contrast in some parts of the curve which were in fact being used.

There remains a need for a number to indicate the contrast of the material, and the number used in this case is the *average gradient*. Where there is no straight-line it is necessary to invent one and average gradient is the slope of a straight line joining two points of density on the characteristic curve. In Fig. 3.13, the two points $D = 0.25$ and $D = 2.0$ have been joined by a dotted line; these two points are the minimum and maximum densities occurring in general radiographic use and it is usual to take two such points in order to specify average gradient. The slope of the dotted line joining these points is the average gradient of the parts of the curve being used. The useful numerical value for contrast is the tangent of the angle which this line makes with the exposure axis when it is extended to intersect the exposure axis of the graph.

In practice it is usual to take account of the density due to base plus fog and to measure average gradient between the two density points which are:

(i) density 0·25 plus density due to base plus fog (in Fig. 3.13 density base plus fog is about 0·2, so the lower point for taking average gradient is D 0·45);

(ii) density 2·0 plus density due to base plus fog (so in Fig. 3.13 this upper point is D 2·2).

RADIOGRAPHIC CONTRAST

In order to assist the student to appreciate the qualities required in emulsions used for radiography, it may be helpful to consider further the term *contrast*.

There are three elements here.

(i) The radiation contrast of the subject (or subject contrast).

(ii) The film contrast (gradient of curve).

(iii) The radiographic contrast of the resultant image on a radiograph.

RADIATION CONTRAST OF THE SUBJECT

The radiation contrast of the subject is the result of the differential absorption of the radiation by different parts of the subject. This differential absorption in tissues—for example bone and fat—leads to different intensities of radiation being transmitted to the film through different parts of the subject. These intensities will have a range for a given subject from a certain minimum to a certain maximum. If I_1 is the greatest and I_2 is the least intensity transmitted, the subject contrast can be expressed as the ratio I_1/I_2. It can be expressed logarithmically as the difference between the logarithms of these intensities.

For any given subject this ratio is reduced by increasing the tube kilovoltage. Fig. 3.14(a) depicts two structures, one composed of fatty tissue and the other of bone, irradiated by means of a beam produced at a relatively low kilovoltage. The fatty tissue does not absorb the radiation very much and a high intensity (I_1) is transmitted through this part of the subject; beneath this area the film is black. The bone absorbs the radiation very heavily and a low intensity (I_2) is transmitted through this part of the subject; beneath the area the film is white-grey. There is a big difference between I_1 and I_2 and the ratio I_1/I_2 is high.

In Fig. 3.14(b) the fatty tissue and the bone are irradiated by means of a beam produced at a higher kilovoltage. The fatty tissue again transmits a high intensity (I_1) and the film beneath this part of the subject is black. The more penetrating radiation produced at the higher kilovoltage is now absorbed less heavily by the bone than the previous radiation was. So more radiation is transmitted through the bony structure (I_2) than before; the film beneath this part of the subject is black-grey. I_1 and I_2 have come closer together and the ratio I_1/I_2 is reduced.

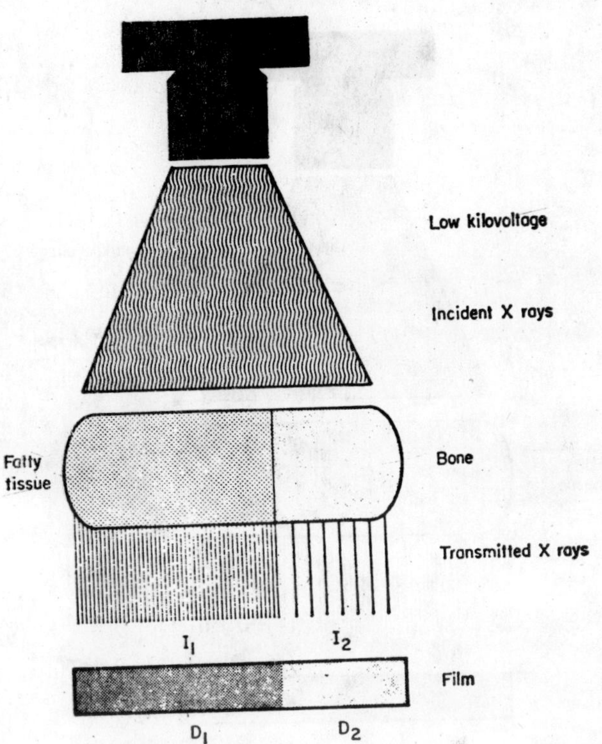

Fig. 3.14.
(a) Radiography at low kilovoltage.
Radiation contrast in the subject = I_1/I_2.
Radiographic contrast in the image = $D_1 - D_2$.

In the image the contrast is obviously reduced since the difference in density is in (a) between black and white-grey and in (b) between black and black-grey.

Higher kilovoltage thus 'levels out' differential absorption and makes different tissues transmit intensities which are more nearly the same. So the radiation contrast of the subject depends on the kilovoltage.

It also depends on the nature of the tissue traversed.

For example in a barium meal study taken erect the barium-filled stomach will absorb radiation heavily and transmit none; the 'gas bubble' in the stomach will transmit a great deal. Thus the ratio I_1/I_2 is high. In a plain radiograph of the abdomen there will be little difference between the intensities transmitted by each kidney and its surroundings, and the radiation contrast ratio (I_1/I_2) will be low. In the absence of a contrast

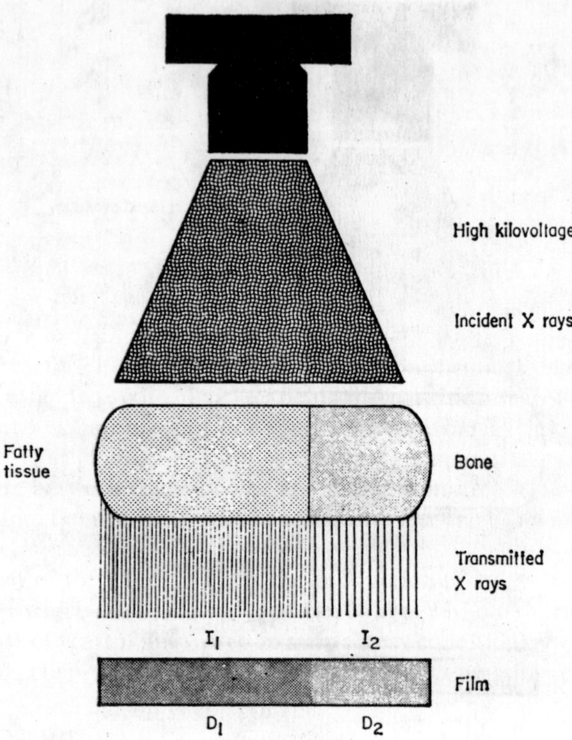

Fig. 3.14.
(b) Radiography at higher kilovoltage.
Radiation contrast in the subject $= I_1/I_2$.
Radiographic contrast in the image $= D_1 - D_2$.

agent, there will be no difference in the intensity of radiation transmitted by the normal gall bladder and its surroundings; no image of the gall bladder is obtained. If, however, the gall bladder is filled with contrast agent, there will be an appreciable difference in the transmitted intensities from the organ and from its surrounding tissue and the ratio I_1/I_2 will be relatively higher. Fig. 3.15(a) (b) and (c) indicates these differences.

FILM CONTRAST

Film contrast has been already explained in terms of the characteristic curve and its slope. It depends on the type of film and the conditions of exposure and development.

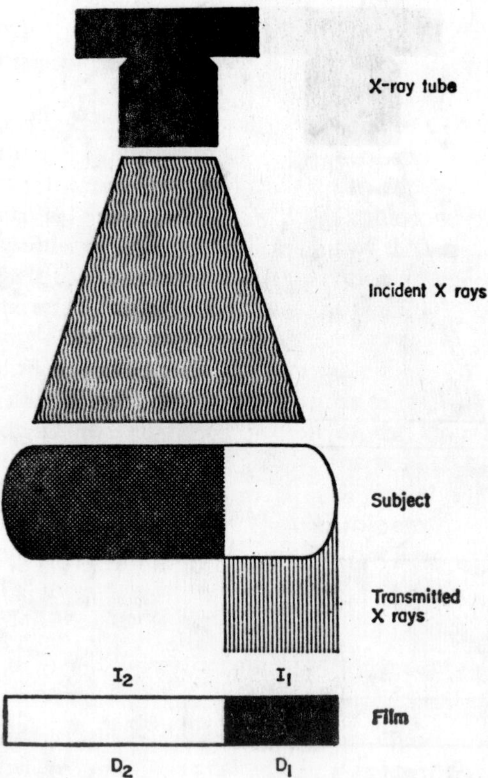

Fig. 3.15.
(a) Radiation contrast in a barium meal.
Radiation contrast in the subject $= I_1/I_2$.
Radiographic contrast in the image $= D_1 - D_2$.

RADIOGRAPHIC CONTRAST

Radiographic contrast is a function of the previous two. Radiographic contrast is altered by (i) altering the contrast of the film and (ii) altering radiation contrast in the subject as shown in Figs 3.14 and 3.15. In practice film contrast is not altered by the radiographer, since it is an inherent characteristic of the material in given conditions of exposure and development. The radiation contrast of the subject can be altered by the radiographer in selection of tube kilovoltage, being for a given subject greater at low kilovoltages than at high. From what has been said, it can be understood that the use of contrast agents in radiography is designed

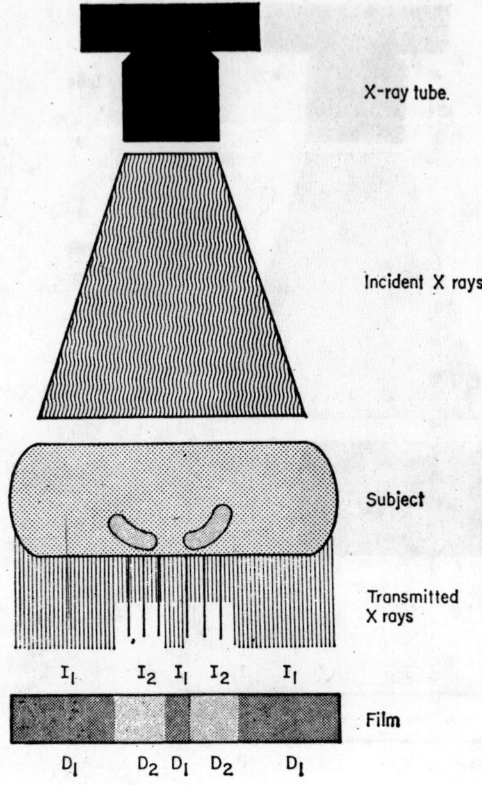

Fig. 3.15.
(b) Radiation contrast between the kidneys and their surrounding soft tissues.
Radiation contrast in the subject = I_1/I_2.
Radiographic contrast in the image = $D_1 - D$

to extend the radiation contrast of various body parts beyond that given them by nature in order to make them demonstrable upon film.

The contrast of the material, it is clear, is in the knowledgeable hands of the manufacturer. The radiation contrasts of the subject (which in many cases may be slight) require to be amplified by the film. It is found that satisfactory results may be obtained when the contrast of the material can give a radiographic contrast which rather more than doubles the radiation contrast of most subjects. Radiographic contrast is discussed again in Chapter 12.

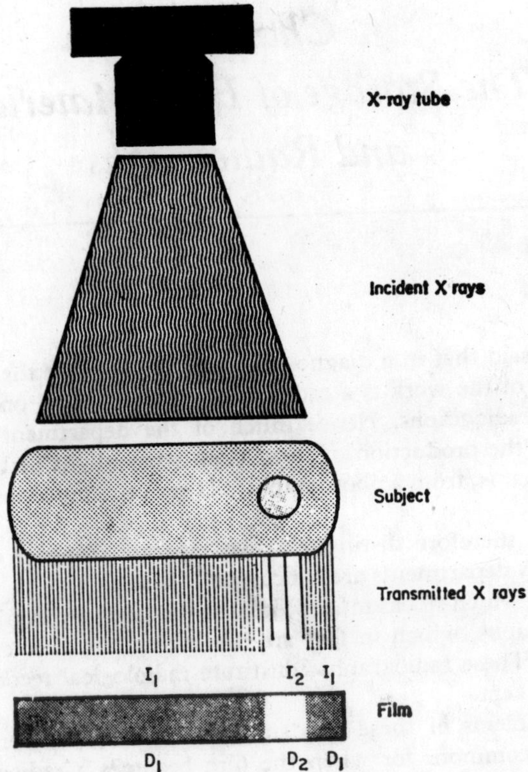

Fig. 3.15.
(c) Radiation contrast in a cholecystogram.
Radiation contrast in the subject $= I_1/I_2$.
Radiographic contrast in the image $= D_1 - D_2$.

Chapter 4
The Storage of Film Materials
and Radiographs

It may be said that in a diagnostic X-ray department the end product from most of the work is a radiological opinion based on appearances shown in radiographs. Hence much of the department's activity is directed to the production of these from what might be termed a raw material: that is, from a photographically sensitive emulsion coated on a film base.

We can therefore distinguish two separate material entities with which X-ray departments are concerned. These are:

(i) films, of which stocks must be kept so that they are available for use;

(ii) radiographs, which in fact are the same films after exposure and processing. These radiographs constitute radiological records and they too must be kept.

The problems of these two storages are very different and have nothing in common, for when the film becomes a radiograph it has indeed changed its nature. So in this chapter we consider the storages separately from each other.

THE STORAGE OF UNPROCESSED FILMS

In regard to the storage of film materials prior to radiographic exposure so that they may be kept available and in good condition, we can differentiate between those stocks which must be to hand for immediate use and those which are kept in reserve, ready to bring forward for immediate use as supplies are consumed.

Films to hand for immediate use will be kept either in a film hopper in a darkroom (see page 265) or, if a daylight system operates in which packs are loaded into dispensers without the need for safelights, then the packs will be kept at points near the dispensers so that the charging of the dispensers can readily be done. The reserve stocks from which such points of use as the darkroom and the film dispensers are ultimately supplied are kept in a film store which may be remote from the X-ray rooms in which the films are to be used.

In all these situations, the most significant considerations for keeping films in good condition come from their susceptibilities. They are sensitive to light and ionizing radiation and to contaminating agents of various types.

In production they are handled with care so that they remain in the first class condition for which the manufacturer aims. It follows that when these materials reach the user they must be stored with the same degree of attention if all the previous care is not to be in vain. Even in the best conditions of storage, material will deteriorate inevitably with keeping, and the period for which it may safely be kept before use has been called its 'shelf-life'. Fast film materials have shorter shelf-life than slow ones.

KEEPING FILMS IN A STORE

Much care, time, and money are spent by the manufacturer in devising film wrappings, and these clearly cannot be bettered by the less knowledgeable. Films should be stored therefore in their original wrappings intact for as great a part of the keeping period as is possible; only when it is close to the time of use should they be taken to the darkroom and unwrapped. Screen-type film kept in the darkroom hopper for immediate use is best left with each film in its wrapper if any. This separates the films, and makes easy the removal of each one for loading into a cassette. The folder and film can be taken from the hopper and the film slid from its folder into the cassette as the folder is withdrawn. The film itself is thus not touched at any stage with the hands, and finger marks can be avoided.

When ordering film stocks for their departments, radiographers should adjust the intake to the rate of use and keep a stock sufficient to meet week-to-week needs without a large reserve supply. In this way no batch of films need stay too long upon the shelf, and spoil simply with keeping. When the boxes of film reach the department they should be checked to see that they are sound, and they should be date-stamped on arrival so that the oldest stock can be detected. The boxes should be stored so that they can be used readily in order of arrival, the oldest first.

The boxes should stand vertically upon the shelves not laid horizontally like a pile of pancakes. Film in quantity is not light in weight and the lower boxes in such a pile would be under pressure liable to produce artefacts upon the films. A further reason for vertical storage is that it is more easily arranged to enable the oldest stock to be used first.

Dampness and high temperatures have a most damaging effect on photographic materials: probably moisture is the more severely ravaging and the more difficult to exclude. The ideal store is one in which the temperature is in the region of 50°F (10°C) and does not rise above 65°F (18°C), the relative humidity being in the region of 50 per cent. Rooms with damp walls and floor, and rooms prone to sudden changes of temperature and the probability of condensation are to be avoided.

The store should be well ventilated, and the storage shelves arranged with adequate air-space above and below them. They should not run past heating pipes or any pipes from which water may leak. Films must be stored away from the effects of ionizing radiations. The store should be at a sufficient distance from diagnostic and treatment rooms. If it is close at hand then it may be necessary to pay special attention to this aspect, and ascertain that walls, ceiling, and floor as may be necessary have full protection incorporated in them. Some manufacturers have included in film boxes a strip of lead foil running round the upper part of each box. If the film should be fogged by radiation while in the box an image of the strip on the films gives the clue to what has happened.

Storing films so that they are kept safe from radiation might be simple if the only sources were the controllable ones used in diagnostic X-ray and radiotherapy departments. The problem is complicated by the presence of background radiation. This is radiation which occurs in our environment. It includes cosmic rays and the radioactive emanations from certain natural materials in the earth and from certain building materials (for example, light concretes) which could well be used in the construction of a film store. The level of background radiation should be no higher than 10 μR per hour for a good store and the highest level for acceptability is 15 μR per hour.

How does a level of 10 μR per hour affect the films in store which are subjected to it? The result of course is fogging so that the fog level of the film material rises above its basic value. Higher dose rates from the background radiation result in a given figure for the fog level being reached in a shorter time and more sensitive film materials subject to a given dose rate reach a given fog level in a shorter time.

Thus if the background radiation in a film store had a count of 10 μR per hour, an ordinary X-ray film for fast-cycle processing would have its fog level raised to 0·3 above the original basic value after about two years on a shelf in the store. If the background count were as high as 40 μR per hour, the same fog level would be reached in the same film at six months storage and in a more sensitive direct-exposure (non-screen) film at three months storage.

As well as being sensitive to heat, moisture, light, and other actinic radiations, film material can be damaged by various chemical fumes, and even by emanations from some paint. The best possible storage conditions are therefore not easy to achieve or maintain, and storage has such an influence on the length of time a material will satisfactorily keep that no manufacturer will commit himself and say dogmatically that a certain film will keep for so long. All materials begin to deteriorate from the time of manufacture, and poor storage hastens this. With good storage, deterioration before use is not noticeable. Film has given reasonable results in some single cases after a very long period of time.

On keeping film *after* exposure and *before* processing, it can be said that this seldom comes within the practice of the radiographer since it is usual to process radiographs almost immediately after they are exposed. It is a fact, however, that the latent image regresses if the film is kept for a long time before being developed. This process is more rapid than the loss of sensitivity shown by unexposed materials during the time they are kept, although there have been instances of film successfully developed years after it had been exposed.

STORING RADIOGRAPHS

Radiographs are part of a patient's medical records. They provide permanent evidence of findings when the X-ray examination was made and they display facts about a bodily state which existed at that time. As records, radiographs must be kept and under law in the United Kingdom there is a statutory requirement that they be kept for a specified number of years.

If an X-ray department undertakes 50 thousand examinations in a year, then at the end of the year there may be 150 thousand or more radiographs to be stored. If these radiographs are to be kept for as short a time as 5 years and the same rate of production is maintained, then at the end of 5 years the hospital has 750 thousand radiographs in its hands; at the end of 10 years (if the records are to be kept for that period) the number of radiographs to be held is 1·5 million. This is certainly a collection that it is daunting to contemplate.

The significant facts on the keeping of so many radiographs are:
(i) a great deal of valuable space will be occupied;
(ii) the weight of such a number of radiographs is considerable;
(iii) running the system (filing and retrieving from the files) requires increasingly the time and attention of numerous filing staff;
(iv) storage is expensive to provide.

These facts are pertinent wherever the store is to be. It may be in the

X-ray department; it may be within the medical records section of the hospital; or it may be in both, the X-ray department holding the more recent radiographs so that they are readily available for radiologists who wish to assess a patient's progress by comparing the latest radiographs with those previously taken.

REQUIREMENTS OF A STORE FOR RADIOGRAPHS

It is possible to state some general requirements which should be met by a store where full-size radiographs are to be kept and from which they must be retrieved for consultation. These requirements are as follows.

(i) The store must be spacious, for filing and retrieval in cramped conditions are intolerably tiresome and certain to be inefficiently performed by human beings.

(ii) The store must be big enough to hold those numbers of radiographs which accumulate over the period of years during which they are to be kept.

(iii) The store must be well ventilated and well lit, free from dust and dampness and regulated in temperature to provide surroundings in which the radiographs will not spoil and the staff will find it acceptable to work.

(iv) The shelving must be strong and made of metal. It must be of sufficient height and depth to hold the large envelopes in which radiographs are usually stored. The shelf space must be compartmented with stout partitions.

(v) The flooring must be strong, especially if the store is on a level above the ground floor of the hospital.

(vi) Access must be easy and the location must be such that those who visit the store to file and retrieve radiographs do not spend much time and effort in going and returning.

FIRE HAZARDS IN FILM STORES

There are fire risks to be considered in the storage both of films before use and of full-size radiographs in large numbers. Modern film-base material has been said to be comparable with paper in the degree of its associated fire risk. The authors have seen a hospital fire-officer as a test deliberately ignite two envelopes containing radiographs and it seemed that the film material burned somewhat more easily than the paper, the flame spreading with readiness. Furthermore, the film became molten and sticky. It was easy to imagine the dissemination of fire in a store both upwards in the common way that flames spread and downwards as the molten particles fell from shelf to shelf.

All papers and obviously films too burn less readily when laid flat than when standing vertically on one edge: if you have ever tried to burn a mass of paper, you will know this! The reason is that to maintain itself any outbreak of fire needs fuel (combustible material), high temperature and air: paper laid flat in piles does not readily admit air to surface areas in the inner regions of the pile. It is unfortunate that film stocks for reasons that we have seen and radiographs for easy access must be stored vertical and not laid flat. This required way of storing them aids the spread of fire.

Because of the fire risk, steel cabinets with metal shelving are the most suitable containers and the best form of heating is a low-temperature one. Electric heaters should be enclosed convectors installed at a high level and under thermostatic control. Electric wiring must be permanently installed in metal-sheathed cable or steel trunking: that is, it should not be in the type of insulated lead which trails over the floor and is used in a domestic setting for portable electrical devices. Flammable materials should not be used in the finishes of ceilings, walls and floors of these storerooms.

When the storerooms are not occupied by staff, especially in the night-hours, all the doors should be closed. If a fire breaks out, the doors must be closed and it should be possible to shut down easily any air-conditioning and ventilating systems in the store: in some cases automatic shut-down may be available. Automatic fire-detectors connected to the hospital fire-alarm system should be provided.

MINIATURIZATION OF RADIOGRAPHS

In an earlier section of this chapter the problems of storing radiographs were indicated and it is clear that several of these exist because of the physical size and weight of the records which are to be kept. Reducing the dimensions of the radiographs is an obvious way of making the same amount of overall space hold many more and the reduced weight lowers the criteria for specifications on shelving and floor-strength.

If the radiographs are made small enough to be placed in a patient's hospital folder with notes and other records, it may be thought unnecessary to provide for them any separate store. Such procedures clearly save money. Some hospitals therefore use a system which miniaturizes the full-size radiographs which are originally taken.

THE SIZES OF MINIATURES

In selecting a method to be used for making smaller copies of conventional radiographs, a question to be discussed is: how small are the miniatures to be? The basic process is to use a camera unit to photograph the radiographs and clearly the size of the reproduction depends on the size of the film which is in the camera.

Roll films of 35 mm (or less) size are widely used for storing many kinds of documentary record. Reproductions of radiographs within 35 mm frames are sufficiently clear for such copies, with a radiological report on the appearances, to be legally acceptable in the place of originals. There are, however, certain problems to regard to using 35 mm film for radiographic records. These are as follows:

(i) naked-eye viewing is unsatisfactory and suitable viewers must be provided in every situation where the 35 mm radiographs are to be used;

(ii) 35 mm rolls of film are not easily handled;

(iii) such small images make it difficult to include identifying information as to the patient and the X-ray examination so that it can be read with ease and certainty and speed.

So the conclusion reached is that 35 mm copies are too small for keeping as radiographic records. So what about making copies on films which provide a larger frame than 35 mm?

A copying system using 100 mm sheet film is available and this size eliminates the dissatisfactions which we noted with the 35 mm roll film.

For the 100 mm system it can be said as follows.

(i) The copies can be viewed with the naked eye or by means of an ordinary magnifying glass.

(ii) The copies are a convenient size for storing or for putting into patients' folders of hospital notes.

(iii) The sheet films are easy to handle.

(iv) The reproduction of detail in the image is satisfactory.

(v) The copies are small enough to constitute a great saving of storage space: for example a chest radiograph on 100 mm film has an area of 100 cm^2 and on a 35 cm by 43 cm film has an area of 1505 cm^2.

(vi) A thousand radiographs stored together weigh very much less when each is on 100 mm film than when each is on a conventional full-size X-ray film. The silver content of developed photographic emulsions makes up most of the total weight of a radiograph. The film used for the 100 mm copies has emulsion coated on one side of the base only and thus before use has 100 cm^2 of emulsion on one film. A conventional X-ray film has emulsion coated on both sides of the base and thus a film which is 35 cm by 43 cm has (before use) 3010 cm^2 of emulsion on its surfaces.

Furthermore, the copying film has a lower coating weight for each square centimetre of area to be coated.

METHODS IN MINIATURIZATION

Copies of full-size radiographs on 100 mm film are made by means of a special copying machine. This embodies a light-source, a camera with a lens which is automatically focussed, a copying surface where the large radiograph is placed and two cassettes to hold up to 50 cut sheets of

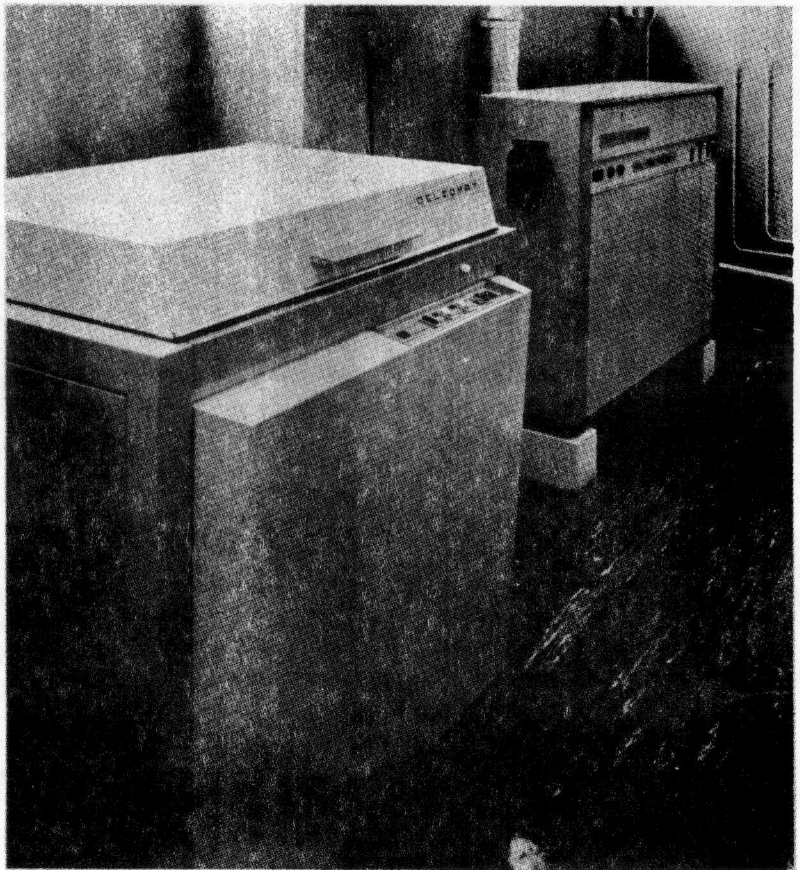

Fig. 4.1. The Oldelft Delcomat Copier for the miniaturization of radiographs with its associated Odelcomatic processor. (*Illustration by courtesy of Oldelft England Ltd.*)

100 mm copying film. One of these cassettes is a supply cassette which is loaded with unexposed copying film before the machine is used. The other is a take-up cassette which receives each sheet of 100 mm film after it has been exposed to the light source through the lens of the camera in making the copy.

The copy is made by placing the large radiograph on the copying surface of the machine and closing a lid on it. The closure of the lid initiates the exposure which lasts for a pre-selected time and ends automatically at the end of the chosen period. The take-up cassette with its exposed films must be removed from the machine for processing to be done. When all the films in the supply cassette have been exposed, the machine is re-loaded with a full cassette for further use.

For processing the copies, one possibility is to use a purpose-built dedicated automatic processor. Into this the films are automatically fed from the receiving cassette of the copying machine when it is taken from the machine and attached to the entry of the processor. This method allows the copying machine and the processor to be close to each other in a room or area with ordinary white-light illumination and no safelights. The other possibility is to take the receiving cassette into a darkroom and unload it by hand. The films are then passed into an automatic processor which may be in general use for large films and can take (or readily be adapted to take) 100 mm sheets. After reporting and copying (the order of events in practice might just as well be copying and reporting) the large radiographs may be discarded at once or may be kept for a brief interval (say, 3 or 6 months). Whether immediate or delayed, the discards are sent for the recovery of their silver content. This ensures that they are not a total waste of a valuable and scarce material.

CONSERVING SILVER

Silver is valuable and is diminishingly available. X-ray departments, busily exposing many metres of silver halide photographic materials, are heavy consumers over a period of years. So what may be done within the usual practices of such departments to ensure that silver is not wasted and is not casually used? The following are important points in the conservation of silver.

(i) Radiographers should unfailingly pay attention to detail and use their techniques with such ability that no radiographs are repeated because of preventable errors.

(ii) The sizes of films used should be the smallest to cover the regions under examination.

(iii) In any radiographic procedure, the number of films exposed should be the smallest to constitute a fully satisfactory examination and to meet the radiologist's requirements for a diagnosis.

(iv) Equipment should be well-maintained and carefully used so that it is unnecessary to repeat radiographs because of failure either in the operation of the equipment or in the judgement and practice of the operator.

(v) Automatic processors should be well-maintained and correctly functioning so that radiographs are not repeated because of processing errors.

(vi) All film materials should be carefully stored and handled so that they are not wasted by the occurrence of preventable artefacts.

(vii) An efficient system for recovering silver from used fixing solutions should be operated in good order.

(viii) Regular tests should be undertaken in the department to ensure that the quality of the finished product (the radiograph) is maintained. Such control of quality (see Chapter 13) also ensures that the number of repeat radiographs and doubtful examinations which fail to yield a diagnosis is minimized.

(ix) Discarded radiographs should be sent to a silver refiner so that silver may be recovered from them.

It may be of some interest for the student to think for a while about the recovery of silver from an X-ray film in which the metal is embodied in a silver halide photographic emulsion. This emulsion is uniformly spread over the surface area of the film. In what ways will the silver subsequently be recovered? When the film has been exposed and processed, in those areas which have received exposure the silver halide has been converted to black metallic silver. This forms the permanent radiographic image. The silver in it can be recovered eventually but not until the radiograph is discarded to be submitted to the attentions of a silver refiner and destroyed.

In those areas of the film which have received no exposure, the silver halide emulsion is unchanged when the film comes out of the developer in its processing. In the fixing solution, the agents act on the silver halide and there is conversion to soluble silver complexes. These silver complexes dissolve in the water of the fixing bath and the silver may be recovered from there by processes applied to the used fixer solution.

Thus from all parts of the film, the exposed and the unexposed, the areas which are to be developed and the areas which are to be fixed, the silver content is potentially recoverable.

Chapter 5
Intensifying Screens and Cassettes

When X rays fall upon certain substances light is emitted. The physical principles involved in this phenomenon should be familiar to the student radiographer and are outside the scope of the present work. They are summarized in the statement that energy changes have occurred in the irradiated material which result in the production of characteristic radiation of wavelengths within the visible spectrum.

The emission of light from a substance bombarded by radiation is termed *luminescence*. This includes two effects, *fluorescence* and *phosphorescence*. The first means that luminescence is excited only during the period of irradiation and will die upon termination of the X-ray exposure. Phosphorescence is afterglow; that is the irradiated material continues to emit light for a time after cessation of exposure. Afterglow in any appreciable degree is not acceptable in luminescent materials. Its occurrence blurs detail in moving images when these are viewed fluoroscopically; and in the case of intensifying screens, if it is sufficiently prolonged, afterglow may transfer a radiographic image from one examination to the next film with which the cassette in question is loaded.

It can be said that the property of X rays of exciting luminescence played a part in their discovery. It was the fluorescence of a card coated with barium platino-cyanide for some other purpose which drew Röntgen's attention to the presence of this invisible penetrating radiation.

The luminescent effect is used radiologically in two ways.

1   To obtain on a fluorescent screen an image which may be observed by the eye, as in the procedure of fluoroscopy, or may be recorded by a camera, as in miniature radiography of the chest (fluorography).

2   To increase the photographic response of a silver halide emulsion. In this case the fluorescing material in a practical form is referred to as an *intensifying screen* and is placed in direct contact with the film during exposure. Its function is to reinforce the action of X rays by subjecting the sensitive emulsion to the effects of light as well as X radiation.

In this chapter we are concerned with intensifying screens rather than with those designed for fluoroscopy or fluorography.

CONSTRUCTION OF AN INTENSIFYING SCREEN

It has been established that a silver halide emulsion changes on exposure to X rays in a manner similar to its reaction when exposed to light. However, when such an emulsion is exposed to X rays it absorbs very little of the incident radiation. An intensifying screen exposed to the same radiation absorbs the beam much more heavily and the effects of this absorption are seen in the emission of light. The use of the intensifying screen provides a method of converting X rays to another actinic radiation to which the photographic emulsion is responsive and thus obtaining after processing a comparable degree of blackening for a shorter interval of exposure or at a reduced level of intensity.

In practice an intensifying screen consists of a base which may be polyester or cellulose acetate. This base must be radioparent and chemically inert. It must combine characteristics of toughness and flexibility and should not either curl or discolour with age. The base is coated first with a smooth white pigment and then with a uniform homogeneous layer of the fluorescent material. This in turn receives a thin transparent supercoat. The purpose of the latter is protective but for reasons explained later it must be very thin and care is always required in handling intensifying screens to avoid any kind of abrasion.

In some instances the flexibility of the material is significant in order to allow the screen to be bent in a small radius without fear of cracking. This will be necessary whenever a curved cassette is used in association with intensifying screens. Such cassettes are available for general radiography, being applicable to some X-ray examinations of the shoulder and knee and they are required accessories to pantomographic dental equipment.

Since X-ray films are coated on both sides intensifying screens are commonly employed in pairs. Each emulsion surface is placed in close contact with the effective surface of one intensifying screen. When this sandwich of screen-film-screen is exposed to X rays both screens fluoresce, the light from each activating the emulsion surface which is its immediate neighbour.

Though used as a pair the intensifying screens may not in fact be twins. It is accepted practice to try to obtain equal blackening on both emulsion surfaces of the film as theoretically this arrangement results in maximum speed. Radiation which has passed successively through the first screen, the first emulsion, the film base and the second emulsion is necessarily attenuated. The lessened intensity of radiation in turn produces decreased fluorescence in the second screen. It is clear that this sequence of events will result in unequal blackening of the two film surfaces, that remote from the X-ray tube being lighter than the one proximal to it.

To overcome this, the two screens may not be identical in structure. In this case the first or front screen is only thinly coated with fluorescent material, since a deep layer will increase the attenuation of the X-ray beam. The second screen is more thickly coated; increasing the density of the luminescent substance leads to greater fluorescence if stimuli are equal and here operates to maintain the same level of brightness from a diminished stimulus. There is naturally an optimum thickness for both screens, in which the need to match the blackening of the two emulsions is not the only factor. There is also the consideration that light produced in the deep layers of a thick screen may fail to reach the film because of absorption in the superficial layers and thus will be ineffective.

The difference in thickness of such paired intensifying screens makes it important not to interchange them in their relationship to the X-ray source. If the thicker screen faces the tube aspect of the film and thus functions as a front screen considerable attenuation of the beam will occur from absorption. The thinly coated, less active front screen—now behind the film—no doubt will fluoresce from the action of such X rays as reach it but the intensifying effect from a practical point of view will be plainly inadequate. Due to both factors the resultant radiograph is found to be seriously underexposed.

In practice this source of underexposure can be troublesome to determine as other agents are usually blamed first: the X-ray tube current is thought to fluctuate mysteriously, no one having observed the behaviour of the milliampere meter, or processing techniques become suspect. Care should be exercised in the use of unequally-coated intensifying screens to ensure that this error does not occur.

Not all intensifying screens are thus differentiated, however. At present a manufacturer may put equal coating weights on both of a pair of screens and either screen can be used in the front or the back position in a cassette. The economic advantages of this and the elimination of errors outweigh in many instances the very slight gains in obtaining equal blackening of both emulsions.

THE FLUORESCENT MATERIAL

Materials which convert invisible radiation into luminous radiation are known as phosphors. A number of such substances exist though we are concerned in radiography with only a few of them. They are used in crystalline form, since their luminescent characteristics are virtually absent in any other, and their correct chemical preparation is a delicate and exacting procedure. Even small traces of impurity—of the order in some instances of one part in a million—will diminish the efficiency of many phosphors. Such imperfections can be considered as minute islands of inactive material and in the case of intensifying screens will lead to an appearance of mottle (structure mottle) on the image. It is obvious that the standards of purity and cleanliness required for the manufacture of these phosphors are extremely high and could scarcely be more demanding even in a laboratory employed in bacteriology. Perhaps it is not surprising that intensifying screens are expensive pieces of equipment: they deserve respectful handling.

THE COLOUR OF LUMINESCENCE

All phosphors do not luminesce with the same colour. This is clearly of importance in their radiographic applications. The colour of light emitted by a fluoroscopic screen should be that to which the human eye is most readily receptive: in fact this is in the yellow-green region of the spectrum. On the other hand the fluorescent colour of phosphors employed for the manufacture of intensifying screens or of those designed for fluorography has an obvious relation to the spectral sensitivity of the film with which they will be used. A screen which is emitting green light can be fully effective only if the associated film is either orthochromatic or panchromatic. (Chapter 2.)

In many phosphors the production of any appreciable luminescence requires the presence of an *activator*, a small quantity of some foreign element. This activator is significant not only in increasing the fluorescent powers of the material but because it affects the colour of the resultant light.

X-RAY PHOSPHORS

To achieve its purpose, a phosphor which is to intensify the effect of an X-ray beam on a photographic emulsion must possess two characteristics:
(a) it must absorb X rays (the absorption coefficient);
(b) it must efficiently convert the absorbed X-ray energy to light to which the photographic emulsion is sensitive (brightness gain).
It must also be transparent to its own luminescence and must allow the luminescent radiation easily to leave the affected crystal.

Phosphors in use for intensifying screens at the present time are:
(i) calcium tungstate
(ii) barium fluorochloride
(iii) gadolinium oxysulphide

(iv) lanthanum oxysulphide
(v) lanthanum oxybromide
(vi) yttrium oxysulphide.

The last four of these substances constitute a group denoted as rare earths because they are difficult to isolate and costly to prepare. Rare earth intensifying screens—a relatively recent innovation in screen technology—are many times more expensive to purchase than others. Few diagnostic X-ray departments in the United Kingdom are found at present to employ them exclusively.

With these phosphors the following rare earth elements are used as activators:

terbium;

thulium;

europium.

In the paragraphs which follow, the X-ray phosphors are considered individually.

CALCIUM TUNGSTATE

Calcium tungstate was the first substance to be used in the commercial preparation of intensifying screens and remained the most commonly used for many years. Even now, in X-ray departments in the United Kingdom there are probably more intensifying screens of calcium tungstate than of any other phosphor.

Unlike other X-ray phosphors, calcium tungstate luminesces in the pure state and requires no activator.

The spectrum of the fluorescence of calcium tungstate extends from the ultra-violet to the yellow-green bands of the spectrum. However, the region of maximum fluorescence is about 420 nanometres, i.e. the colour of the emitted light is violet or violet-blue. The student radiographer may easily prove this by exposing an open cassette to a beam of X rays. The demonstration will be more impressive if the room lighting can be temporarily subdued, in which case the violet-blue luminescence of the screens appears very brilliant. The experiment, if repeated at a different value of tube current, will also show that the brightness of luminescence is dependent on the intensity of radiation reaching the screen surface.

Under present day conditions the colour of fluorescence produced by a calcium tungstate screen is independent in practice of the wavelength (i.e. kilovoltage) of the exciting radiation, at least over a very wide range of tube tensions. The blue fluorescence of these screens results in a maximum photographic response, since the majority of X-ray film is most sensitive to this region and also to ultra-violet light which comes within the luminescent spectrum of calcium tungstate. This means that comparable blackening of the film is produced for much shorter intervals of exposure or at markedly decreased levels of radiation output. The reductions which occur may be expressed as an intensification factor for the screens in question (see page 97).

BARIUM FLUOROCHLORIDE

Relative to calcium tungstate, barium fluorochloride
(i) absorbs much more of the X rays in the energy range employed for medical diagnosis (that is, it has a higher absorption coefficient);
(ii) more efficiently converts X-ray energy to light (greater brightness gain). These properties mean that the intensifying effect of barium fluorochloride is much increased relative to calcium tungstate.

Activated by europium, barium fluorochloride emits ultraviolet and blue light in a rather narrow band, the region of maximum emission being about 380 nanometres. Some intensifying screens made from barium fluorochloride include a substance similar to the optical brightening agents which are found in washing powders. This constituent absorbs some of the ultraviolet light emitted by the phosphor and re-emits blue light. The effects of this are to broaden the emission spectrum of the screens and move the peak emission to a longer wavelength (about 400 nanometres). To obtain similar densities on a radiograph, barium fluorochloride screens require about half the exposure necessary for screens made from calcium tungstate.

The question of the speed of intensifying screens is further discussed on page 102.

THE RARE EARTHS

If the rare earths lead to an unrare confusion in the student reader, it is understandable: in fact, the variety of intensifying screen/film combinations which are now available may generate an uncertainty in choosing them wisely, even among experienced radiographers.

The screens to which is given the collective description of *rare earth* consist essentially of four phosphors:
(i) gadolinium oxysulphide, activated by terbium;
(ii) lanthanum oxysulphide, activated by terbium;
(iii) lanthanum oxybromide, activated by thulium and terbium;
(iv) yttrium oxysulphide, activated by terbium.
The rare earth phosphors based on lanthanum and gadolinium (the first

three in our list) exhibit the desired much greater efficiency in absorbing the X-ray beams usually employed for medical radiography and in converting the absorbed energy to light. The luminescence of the rare earths is concentrated in a number of narrow bands of wavelengths, the 'colour' differing for the several phosphors and activators.

Although gadolinium oxysulphide (with terbium at the most usual concentrations) has about as much blue emission as a fast calcium tungstate screen, when this rare earth is combined with terbium-activated lanthanum oxysulphide a green light is produced (about 540 nanometres). These phosphors nearly always are used together. Lanthanum oxybromide with thulium fluoresces in the ultraviolet and blue bands of the spectrum; and with terbium mainly in the blue region.

Yttrium oxysulphide requires separate consideration. Yttrium is much lighter than the other rare-earth elements and its X-ray absorption consequently lower: indeed at the energies used during most medical radiography, it is no better a performer in this respect than calcium tungstate. On the other hand, its conversion efficiency is high and this makes screens of yttrium oxysulphide as fast as other rare-earth intensifying screens. However, they are 'noisy' (see page 106) and are not in use for general radiography. The emission from yttrium oxysulphide (with terbium) is 'white' blue.

The colour of the emitted light has an important implication for film emulsions employed with rare earth intensifying screens. Very little advantage will be obtained from associating the oxysulphides of gadolinium and lanthanum in a partnership with emulsions which make their peak response to ultraviolet and blue light. These rare earths need a film which has been sensitised to green light (orthochromatic film) if they are to exhibit their maximum intensifying effects. Manufacturers and suppliers of such intensifying screens usually recommend and provide a special X-ray film, the sensitivity of which is matched to the emission from the screen.

This advisable and necessary practice can translate to a few—perhaps relatively insignificant—disadvantages for an X-ray department:

(i) radiographers are more restricted in their choice of film;

(ii) darkroom safelights may require changing, from the usual amber or green, to filters which give red light, orthochromatic film being relatively insensitive to this end of the visible spectrum. Appropriate filters are, of course, easy to obtain but the dark red illumination which they provide reduces detail perception and usually is considered a less acceptable working environment. However, recent improvements in the design of safelight filters may reduce or eliminate these problems.

THE INTENSIFICATION FACTOR

The intensification factor of a pair of screens can be simply stated. It is the figure by which we should have to multiply the exposure if we were to use the film without intensifying screens. Putting it differently, we can say that it is the ratio of the energy (which we will express in milliampere seconds) necessary to produce a certain blackening on a film exposed alone, relative to that required by the *same* film in conjunction with intensifying screens.

Referring to an imaginary numerical example, we might know that a certain pair of screens has an intensification factor of 15. If 3 sec., 50 mA and 60 kVp were technical factors applicable to a certain subject without the use of screens, then we could alter these to 0·2 sec (3 divided by 15), 50mA and 60 kVp if we used the same film with the screens in question.

In practice, the intensification factor for any variety of intensifying screen is a quantity which radiographers seldom employ and do not ordinarily know. There are a number of reasons why a statement of this factor as a single absolute value is hardly helpful information: the more important of these are explained below.

1   The intensification factor is derived from the performance of the *same* emulsion in each of the two situations of exposure without intensifying screens and of exposure with them. In radiographic practice, emulsions intended for direct exposure have different characteristics from those which are designed to be used with intensifying screens: radiographers do not usually subject one type of film to the two techniques.

2   Strictly speaking, the intensification factor for a pair of screens is not a constant for all intervals of exposure. This is due to reciprocity failure (see p. 386) of the film emulsion when it is exposed to light. Absence of reciprocity means that film-blackening may be less than some predicted value when a weak stimulation of the screens occurs during a long exposure; and again when strong activation is present during a very brief interval of time. When the exposure is to X rays alone, the radiation intensity and the exposure interval correlate inversely to produce the same density.

3   The intensification factor is not a constant at all densities. Characteristic curves, drawn for a screen-type emulsion exposed first between screens and then exposed without intensifying screens, have different slopes. They show that the intensifying effect of the screens becomes greater as density increases within the diagnostically useful range (from $D = 0·25$ to $D = 2·5$).

4   The intensification factor is influenced by the length of the period of development given to the image. An image produced on an emulsion by

X rays alone is distributed almost uniformly through the whole depth of the emulsion. If light is the activating radiation—as it is very largely, whenever a radiographer employs intensifying screens—then the image tends to be concentrated in the superficial layers of the emulsion. Once the film is immersed in the developing solution, the developer necessarily begins its action on the surface and—provided that the developing time is short—a film exposed between screens will show greater blackening relative to its fellow which has been exposed to X rays alone. Longer times of development give the latter a chance 'to catch up', as the solution permeates the emulsion more deeply and the difference in blackening between the two films becomes less.

From these points we can appreciate how difficult it is to give to the intensification factor a numerical value which has either reality or signficance for the practising radiographer. It is doubtful if any of us know or have ever been told such a figure for any of the screens we habitually employ.

Nevertheless, the student radiographer will commonly hear in the X-ray department comments or instructions to the effect that a certain pair of screens is 'slow' or that another pair will need 50 per cent less exposure because the screens are 'fast'.

Let us think what these statements really mean. We may ask ourselves, if these screens require a reduction to half the normal exposure, with what are they being compared? The answer then is obvious. We are certainly not talking about the intensification factor which relates the screens to the performance of the same film without screens. Instead we are balancing the effect of the 'fast' screens against the same film and some other pair of screens which we regard as requiring 'normal' exposure. A student radiographer who reads the pamphlets and data sheets on intensifying screens, issued by suppliers as customer information, will notice that a statement of an intensification factor as such is not included.

The information provided in these and other similar publications usually will relate the performance of the new or test screens to some standard type already familiar in radiographic practice. Exposure ratios between different varieties of intensifying screen are frequently stated in technical publications and are used by radiographers as a realistic and helpful assessment of the intensifying effect.

THE INFLUENCE OF KILOVOLTAGE

The response of a pair of intensifying screens to a beam of X rays is influenced by the mean energy of the beam; that is, by kilovoltage and filtration. For the present, as we are concerned with the use of intensifying screens by radiographers in clinical situations, we propose to omit discussion of the effects of filtration, which we may assume to be about 2 mm aluminium. While diagnostic radiographers seldom change the filter in a beam between examinations (other than the filter which is the patient himself), they commonly alter kilovoltage: any significant effect on the performance of intensifying screens consequently is of concern.

CALCIUM TUNGSTATE

In the radiographic use of calcium tungstate intensifying screens, it is usually assumed that the screens' response to the beam is more or less the same, at whatever kilovoltage the exposure is made. During the general run of diagnostic X-ray examinations these kilovoltages are likely to lie between 60 kVp and 100 kVp, with an upper limit of perhaps 120 kVp for some procedures. The assumption of a constant response (that is, a constant light output per unit incident dose) from the screens to all kilovoltages within the medical range has a certain practical validity, although objective physical measurements would not sustain its strict truth; light output **does** increase with kilovoltage, although arguably—in diagnostic X-ray rooms—not to an effective extent.

A graphical depiction of the performance of calcium tungstate screens, in which their intensifying effect (effectively their speed) is plotted against increasing kilovoltage, would show a line which is almost—but not quite—horizontal. The general form of such a graph is sketched in Fig. 5.1 and indicates that calcium tungstate screens become faster in performance with increasing kilovoltage, but only slightly faster. Many generations of radiographers have shown, in the course of professional practice, that speed changes which occur in calcium tungstate screens, through the kilovoltage range in medical use, are negligible: they do not affect the diagnostic acceptability of any resultant radiograph.

BARIUM FLUOROCHLORIDE

The response of barium fluorochloride to increasing kilovoltage is arguably similar to that of calcium tungstate. Fig. 5.2 sketches the general shape of a curve obtained for screens of this material when increasing kilovoltage is plotted against speed (here expressed in relation to the performance of fast calcium tungstate screens).

Between 70 kVp and 120 kVp, the response of barium fluorochloride is again almost a horizontal line. It is seen that radiographers act reasonably who take the performance of barium fluorochloride screens to

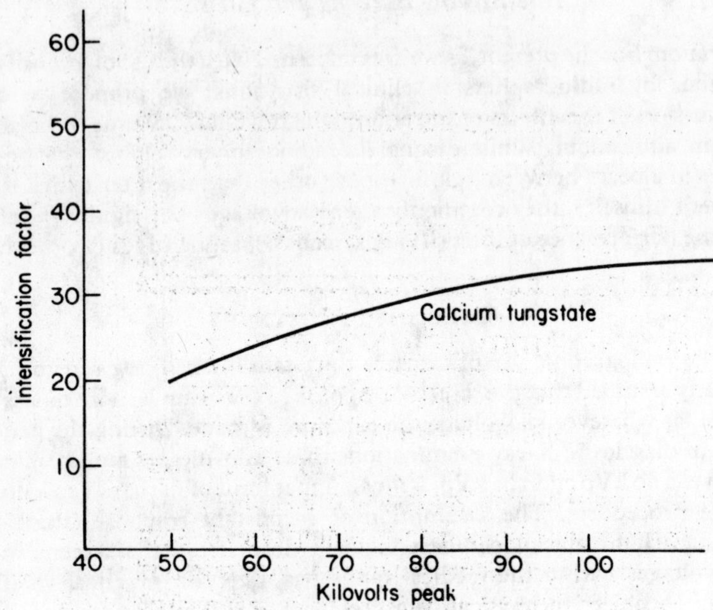

Fig. 5.1. A curve to illustrate the intensifying effect of calcium tungstate over a kilovoltage range applicable to medical diagnostic radiography.

be without significant change, no matter the kilovoltage which is selected. In strict accuracy, the graph tells us that barium fluorochloride screens gain some speed at 70 kVp compared with 60 kVp and begin to lose a little beyond about 115 kVp.

THE RARE EARTHS

So far as the rare earths are concerned, response to kilovoltage is not the same for all of them and their relative speed (compared with calcium tungstate) is more strongly dependant on the kilovoltage across the X-ray generator.

Up to the present, a number of authors have reported tests which they have made of certain intensifying screen/film combinations and the interested reader is referred to their publications in various professional journals. Generalizations are apt to prove misleading, particularly here in the absence of a detailed statement of experimental conditions and because manufacturers seldom precisely describe the constituent phosphors of the intensifying screens which they supply.

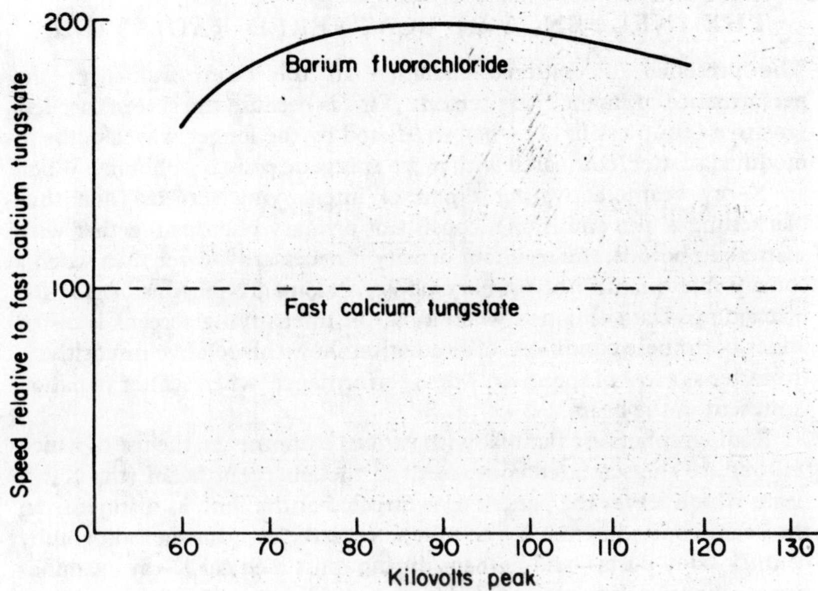

Fig. 5.2. A curve to show the emission of barium fluorochloride with increasing kilovoltage.

Lanthanum is close to barium in the periodic table. Intensifying screens based solely or largely on this rare earth element exhibit a speed/kilovoltage relationship which is akin to that of barium fluorochloride. Gadolinium, however, is dissimilar and the speed of gadolinium oxysulphide increases steadily up to 100 kVp or so. Commercially available green-emitting screens all contain more gadolinium oxysulphide than lanthanum oxysulphide; effectively, therefore, these intensifying screens become rather faster as kilovoltage rises, reaching their maximum speed at about 100–120 kVp.

Because the speed of the rare earth systems to a greater extent is dependant on beam energy, it may not be easy to find an exact and simple formula which allows the user satisfactorily to convert exposure factors from calcium tungstate screens to the lower values suitable for the rare earths. In general, acceptable clinical results should be obtained from speed factors varying between 2 and 5 for different rare-earth screens and film combinations. Higher factors are sometimes quoted by manufacturers (for example, a speed gain of 8, relative to fast calcium tungstate screens) but may be less acceptable. The reasons for this are further discussed on page 106.

THE INFLUENCE OF SCATTERED RADIATION

The presence of scattered radiation in the beam influences the performance of intensifying screens. This is because the screens are less sensitive (emit less light) when irradiated by the longer wavelengths in modified scatter, compared with more energetic primary photons. When an X-ray beam, activating a pair of intensifying screens (and thus blackening a film emulsion), consists of primary photons together with scattered photons, the resultant density is necessarily lower than when a comparable quantity of primary photons alone are responsible for the blackening. Data obtained when a pair of intensifying screens is tested under both these conditions of irradiation show this relative insensitivity to scatter as a loss of speed, or 'worse performance' when scatter radiation is present in the beam.

Radiographers are familiar with various equipments, the use of which will reduce the scattered component in the emergent beam (the X-ray beam which leaves the patient or is directed at the film, as distinct from the beam emitted by the X-ray tube). Nevertheless, during radiography of thick body parts—and perhaps during most medical X-ray examinations—the emergent beam includes scatter radiation and any intensifying screens employed will be subject to its influence. The effect is more marked for rare earth screens than for calcium tungstate.

However, let us consider this effect from another aspect, which offers radiographers a bonus, in trade-off for a dimunition of speed. If the intensifying screens are relatively less sensitive to scatter radiation, they are in some degree protecting the film from it, as does a secondary radiation grid. Consequently their use increases radiographic contrast. The less responsive are the screens to scatter radiation, the higher is the contrast obtained from them. In some circumstances, there is the possibility that the increased contrast provided by rare earth screens might allow secondary radiation grids of lower ratio—and therefore less expensive grids—to be employed in an X-ray department.

DETAIL SHARPNESS AND SPEED

RESOLVING POWER

In earlier Chapter 2 the resolving power of film materials was explained and discussed and we saw that when we speak of the resolution of a photographic system we refer to its ability to render the separate parts of an image distinguishable by the eye; that is, to show fine details of structure. It was said that the capacity of an emulsion to resolve detail was influenced by grain size, contrast and the extent to which it may absorb or scatter light.

In the crystalline form of calcium tungstate or other salt intensifying screen we have a composition analogous to the silver halide grains of a film emulsion. It must be evident that when such an intensifying screen is used in medical radiography the same features of crystal size and dispersion of light are significant in the production of resolution. Indeed the resolving power of the intensifying screens may be the limiting factor in the production of detail by a radiographic system.

In theory we cannot record radiographically details of the subject which are smaller than the salt particles composing the screen. However, in medical radiography this is not a practical consideration. The dimensions of these crystals are expressed in microns, a micron being a thousandth part of a millimetre: even the smallest lesion which could be observed on a radiograph is many, many times larger and its size is normally expressed in terms of one millimetre or more.

In a later chapter (Chapter 12) the several sources of unsharpness in a radiograph will be further discussed, particularly their relationships to each other and their combined effect upon the X-ray image. They are of three kinds.

1 Geometric unsharpness, dependent upon the size of tube focus and anode-film and subject-film distances.

2 Motional unsharpness which arises from voluntary or involuntary movements of the subject during the exposure.

3 Intrinsic or photographic unsharpness due to the characteristic structure of the luminescent screen and film material.

All of them are important. They can be added together arithmetically and in any particular case the one which makes the largest contribution will dominate the radiograph, however the others may be diminished. Consequently it is ineffectual technique to attempt to reduce any of these factors at the marked expense of another.

At the present time it is only intrinsic unsharpness which we shall consider. The presence of intensifying screens increases intrinsic unsharpness in the radiographic image, although not necessarily to an unacceptable level. We can appreciate that it does so if we compare the radiograph of an extremity taken on direct exposure film with another for which intensifying screens were used.

The unsharpness introduced to a radiograph by the use of intensifying screens is difficult to measure. Such assessments do not come within the experience of practising medical radiographers, who should regard warily and accept only cautiously numerical quantities which profess to be a statement of the resolving power of intensifying screens. They are of value only when the conditions of measurement are fully specified and have little practical meaning to the radiographer using the screens for clinical work.

The explanation of the unsharpness inherent in all intensifying screens is to be found in the fact that light diverges.

DIFFUSION OF LIGHT

From simple experience we are all familiar with the fact that light spreads outwards in all directions from its source. We may visualize the fluorescing particles of an intensifying screen as a number of sources of light.

Theoretically if there were no divergence of the radiant beam there would be no spread of image detail in the radiograph. In practice this state of affairs cannot exist. Even from crystals considered to be in contact with the film there would be a spread of light in other directions and this light could be bent towards the film by remote crystals: even crystals at the surface of the screen are not in contact with the film owing to the supercoat and this is a reason why the transparent supercoat is made as thin as possible. The further away each source of fluorescence is from the film the greater will be the degree of image spread and the worse the obtainable radiographic definition.

SPEED

Reference has been made earlier to differences in the speed of intensifying screens. It was stated that increasing the density of the phosphor, that is the thickness of the fluorescent layer, must increase also the amount of light activating the film. Consequently a thick screen has a greater intensifying effect and it is said to be faster than a thin one of the same material.

However, if the screen is thick the average distance between its particles and the photographic emulsion must be greater. We have already seen that this means that radiographic resolution will be worse because of wider divergence of the light.

The speed of an intensifying screen can be increased if the size of the crystals is large because this again leads to a higher emission. However, large flat crystals provide an unrestricted pathway for light travelling obliquely through them. This situation is depicted diagramatically in Fig. 5.3 in which the lines L_1, L_2 and L_3 represent variously diverging rays of light.

When light is spread in this way over a wide area, radiographic

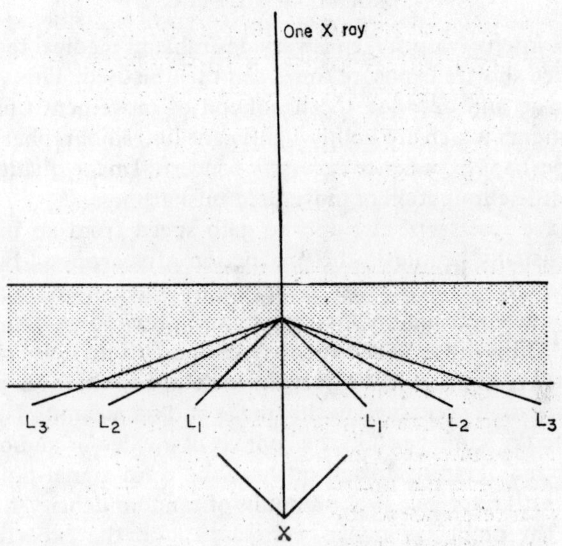

Fig. 5.3. Diagram to illustrate how light spreads over a wide area from an X-ray beam passing through an intensifying screen composed of large flat crystals. This effect deteriorates image sharpness.

sharpness inevitably is poor. These effects can be overcome on the principle of providing 'obstacles' which hinder the passage of the light. In Fig. 5.3 the rays represented by L_2 and L_3 are more influenced by the presence of obstructing devices than are the rays L_1 because their track to the film is longer. In this way the cone of light reaching the film is made narrow and detail sharpness in the image improved.

In the manufacture of intensifying screens two methods are available for obstructing the sideways spread of light and have been widely used in screens of calcium tungstate.

1 The use of crystal powder which causes light to be scattered by the surfaces of the many small crystals in its path.

2 The use of dyes—usually yellow or red—in the fluorescent layer to absorb light. Both these measures—because they decrease the quantity of actinic radiation reaching the film—also reduce the speed of the intensifying screen; while at the same time, they improve detail because of their greater effect on obliquely travelling light. These characteristics are irreconcilable: intensifying screens which have a fine crystal structure give sharp images but lack speed; those which are composed of large crystals have greater speed but their use results in poorer detail.

QUANTUM MOTTLE

Speed in an intensifying screen is very desirable in medical radiographic practice since shorter exposure times can then be used. This will reduce patient dosage and decrease the likelihood of movement unsharpness, two components which are highly significant for radiographers and with which we perhaps experience excessive concern. Image quality does not lie solely in the elimination of movement unsharpness.

As we have just seen, attempts to gain speed from an intensifying screen are usually hostile to the production of sharpness; but there is another reason, as well, why a very fast intensifying screen may deteriorate our appreciation of an image and prove to be 'too much of a good thing'. This is due to the appearance of quantum noise or mottle.

'Noise' in a radiographic image refers to densities which are extraneous to the information contained in the image and its meaning here may be compared to the same word in the context of a video or audio signal. In analyses of radiographic image quality, the term signal-noise ratio is often used with reference to the amount of random density-fluctuations present in the processed image, compared with the expected density variations which comprise the informative parts of the image. Quantum mottle is an example of the fortuitous irregularities in density which constitute image noise.

Quantum mottle is found on a radiograph when the number of X-ray quanta used to create the image is too small. Thus, it is a product of—and a risk associated with—any very fast radiographic system. In such a system, nearly all image noise is quantum mottle, which should be distinguished from structural mottle, caused by lack of uniformity in the size and packing of the grains composing the intensifying screens. Structural mottle in an appreciable degree should not occur in contemporary, well made intensifying screens.

Perhaps the best way of understanding the occurrence of quantum mottle is to think of the irradiated area—in this case the intensifying screen, but sometimes the film, directly—as a paved court consisting of a great number of separate flag stones. During the exposure a shower of X-ray quanta fall on the cassette and we can picture the early stages of this process as a thin shower of raindrops just beginning to fall on the paved area of our imagination. Examination of the paving stones at such a moment would show a few drops of water on each, which would vary in number and distribution and present a dotted or mottled pattern to the overseeing eye. Only when there are enough raindrops to cover each paving stone entirely, do we lose the impression of 'dottiness' and see instead a continuous dark tone.

Densities produced on a radiograph by X-ray quanta may be considered to behave similarly. If there are very few quanta (that is, when the exposure time is short and the milliamperes low), then our appreciation of image detail may be overcome by visual sensations of mottle, which becomes intrusive.

On p. 93 it was stated that the suitability of a phosphor for use in an intensifying screen depended on two characteristics:
(i) its efficiency as an absorber of X rays;
(ii) its efficiency in converting absorbed X rays to light (brightness gain).
To augment either of these alone would increase the response of the screen but the effect of each is different in respect of quantum mottle. If the sensitivity of an intensifying screen were to be enhanced solely by improving its ability to absorb photons, the total number of photons in the beam could be reduced without affecting the number which formed the image, this number being then merely a larger proportion of the beam. In these circumstances quantum mottle would remain unchanged, however 'fast' the intensifying screen became.

On the other hand, when the sensitivity of a screen is increased by means of greater brightness gain from the phosphor, then equivalent film densities will be obtained from fewer X-ray quanta; greater quantum mottle in the image will directly result.

Quantum noise present in a radiographic image is not a function only of the intensifying screens: it originates outside the film/screen system and consequently the resolution of the system influences its appearance. A film/screen combination, which offers high sharpness of detail in the imaged subject, makes the same offer in respect of quantum mottle! The mottle will be clearly depicted, too.

DIAGNOSTIC QUALITY

Practitioners of medical radiology must judge radiographs by their diagnostic quality. A radiograph is created only so that someone ultimately will look at it and form a clinical opinion from the evidence provided by the image. Assessments of radiographic quality which physically measure such photographic characteristics of the image as have just been discussed do not tell the whole story about the diagnostic value of that image: this must include not only objective, physical factors but physiological and psychological components involved with vision and the recognition of images from previous knowledge. These subjective, rather than objective, elements mean that the effects of noise upon image quality are influenced finally—for the observer in the reporting room—by the nature of the subject examined.

It has been shown that we find the presence of mottle more distracting when we look at images from objects which are low in contrast and unsharp in detail. Correspondingly, we find mottle less disturbing in images made from objects of high contrast and fine detail. Both these types of 'objects' are commonly subjected to radiography: in the first variety we may recognise the gall bladder; in the second, any part of the skeleton or the recorded image of a metallic foreign body, such as a needle in the tissues. Let us consider the practical significance of these facts.

Radiographers, when X-raying the gall bladder and using a fast system in order to limit movement unsharpness, should pay attention to:
(i) reducing quantum mottle in the image;
(ii) suppressing the visibility of that mottle.
The best way of reducing the mottle in the system would be to use a slow film. The best way to suppress its appearance is to associate the film with a fast intensifying screen, whilst accepting that some small detail may thereby be lost. The gall bladder is a 'bad' subject for radiography because it is very likely to move during the exposure; but the radiographer who employs simply the fastest screen-film combination available does not necessarily obtain for an observer easy recognition of the gall stones which may be present. On the other hand, if noise is present on a skeletal radiograph, our appreciation of the detail of the image is less likely to be unfavourably influenced by it: we may confidently use a high-detail intensifying screen for such an examination.

TYPES OF INTENSIFYING SCREENS

From what we have already said of the different characteristics of an intensifying screen, and from readers' experience during practical radiography in their own X-ray departments, it is clear that several varieties are available. Even if the products of one manufacturer alone are considered, the number of different grades of intensifying screen which a catalogue may offer are great enough perhaps to confuse the inexperienced; four and six varieties are two typical instances. These— alongside different categories of X-ray film—can result in very numerous screen-film combinations, nineteen being one example which is seen.

It is unnecessary and disadvantageous for any single department to include in its working armamentarium all possible permutations of intensifying screen and X-ray film: a plague of doubt and errors among staff radiographers would ensue. It is more likely that a superintendent radiographer will limit the number of screen-film combinations in use in a department, or in a discrete section of a department. A choice can be made which is based upon knowledge of both the department's work and the characteristics of the available materials and will result in no more than two—or perhaps three—grades of intensifying screen being to hand. A clear indication of the nature of the contained intensifying screens must be provided on the outside of any cassette: labels to this effect should be renewed as soon as they become too worn to be easily legible.

Their accounts of the differing characteristics of several intensifying screens make trade catalogues quite useful revision reading for student radiographers. The following generalisations are offered as a preliminary guide.

A STANDARD INTENSIFYING SCREEN

A screen which is described as being 'standard' or 'regular' or 'par speed' is a medium fast, calcium tungstate, intensifying screen which aims to give the user the best of both worlds (adequate speed with satisfactory rendition of detail). Suitable for many general radiographic applications, it often provides the base from which, in practice, the speeds of other intensifying screens, and the entailed changes in exposure factors, are computed.

HIGH SPEED INTENSIFYING SCREENS

Calcium tungstate intensifying screens which make a special feature of their speed are variously described as 'fast' or 'high speed' or by variations which suggest the same idea. These screens, which inevitably sacrifice some degree of detail sharpness, will be chosen for radiographic examinations where the risk of unsharpness from movement—particularly involuntary movement—is high: radiography of the gastrointestinal tract is one example; and another is a chest examination with a portable X-ray unit (maximum output perhaps 20 mA).

More than one grade of 'fast' intensifying screen may be available from the one supplier: for example, Du Pont's Hi-Plus screen requires half the exposure dose of their Par-Speed version and their Lightning Plus is content with approximately one third of the dosage relative to the Hi-Plus.

HIGH DEFINITION INTENSIFYING SCREENS

The terms 'high definition' and 'detail' are applied to intensifying screens which offer the positive characteristic of fine detail sharpness. These intensifying screens necessarily are 'slower' than other calcium tungstate screens and may entail exposure doses at least two or three times greater than those required in the case of a regular screen. They are applicable to those radiographic subjects which contain small detail and may be effectively immobilised during a relatively 'long' exposure interval: examples are found in the small bones of the skull and in the extremities.

GRADUATED INTENSIFYING SCREENS

Intensifying screens are available which have a progressively decreasing intensification factor across the screen's surface. In a pair of screens, both may be graduated longitudinally; or the front screen may be longitudinal in progression and the other have a crescentic area of reduced speed at one long edge. The variation in intensifying effect is obtained by variation in either the coating weight of the phosphor or the density of a dye incorporated in the fluorescent layer. Usually these intensifying screens are available only in the larger sizes, such as 20 cm × 40 cm and 35 cm × 43 cm.

Graduated intensifying screens are intended for the examination of regions characterised by the transmission of a long scale of radiation intensities. Examples of such regions are the leg, if its full length is considered from upper thigh to ankle, and the lumbar vertebrae in the lateral projection, from bodies to spinous processes.

OTHER INTENSIFYING SCREENS

Intensifying screens manufactured from the rare earths are fully discussed earlier in this chapter. Briefly, it is to be said that their outstanding characteristic is greatly increased speed, with maintained detail sharpness. Rare earth screens may be offered in more than one grade of speed, with consequent reductions of exposure dose to quantities which vary approximately from one half to one sixth of the dose required in the case of a standard calcium tungstate screen. (We should note, however, that to obtain their maximum performance it is usually necessary to combine particular types of rare earth screen with particular film emulsions.)

Radiographic situations which call for rare earth screens are those where radiation risks to the patient may be a significant feature, or where exposure doses are restricted for technical reasons. In the first category we find many X-ray examinations of young children, especially those entailing serial exposure, such as intravenous urography. Another example occurs in minimising irradiation of the foetus when X-raying pregnant women.

In the technical category are X-ray examinations of thick body parts made with low powered equipment and also certain angiographic procedures, during which the duration of an exposure interval may be severely restricted because of a high exposure-repetition rate; this makes rare earth intensifying screens probable partners of a rapid film changer.

Much of what has just been said about the rare earths similarly applies to those intensifying screens in which barium fluorochloride is the active phosphor. However, to achieve conditions of maximum 'speed', these screens do not require coupling with a particular emulsion and this may be regarded as an administrative convenience of their use.

CASSETTE DESIGN

A cassette by definition is a small flat box used for transporting a film— but it is doubtful if anyone who has carried a couple having dimensions 35 cm × 43 cm, from the department to a distant ward in order to X-ray a patient's chest, would consider that 'small' is an operative term.

The general appearance of an X-ray cassette is no doubt quite familiar to student radiographers once they have begun to give practical assistance in a radiological department (Fig. 5.4). Cassettes are used in association with intensifying screens and they have three related purposes:

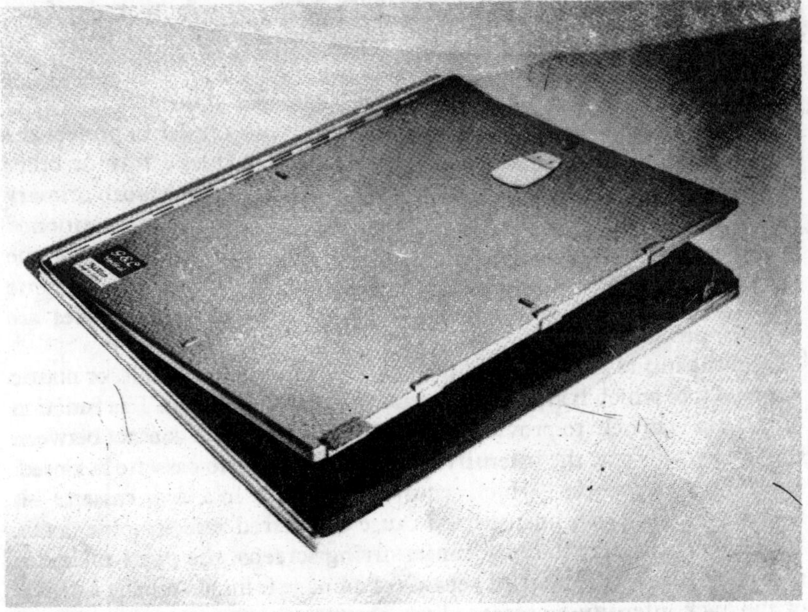

Fig. 5.4 A typical cassette for medical radiography. No intensifying screens are fitted. *By courtesy of Pickering International Ltd*

1　to maintain the film in close uniform contact with each of the screens during exposure;

2　to exclude light;

3　to protect the intensifying screens from physical damage.

Apart from some cassettes for daylight film-handling the structure of a cassette suggests perhaps a book rather than a box, as it consists of two flat rectangular plates hinged at one long edge. It is conventional to describe one of these as the front of the cassette; that is, it is that aspect which will face the X-ray tube. The other is the back of the cassette; it is the side turned away from the X-ray tube during the exposure.

Cassettes are available from various suppliers and have many minor differences of feature. These perhaps reflect the difficulties of producing the ideal model.

In the construction of a typical cassette, a steel or aluminium frame supports a tray-shaped front which forms a shallow container for one intensifying screen and an X-ray film. The front of the cassette naturally must be transradiant. For example, it might be made from aluminium of 1·2 mm gauge, in which case the cassette is sometimes described as being all metal in structure; alternatively the substance of the front might be a plastic laminate. The front is often riveted to the frame but, even so, a commonly occurring deterioration with heavy use is that the front imperceptibly becomes loose; film edges are consequently fogged by admitted light.

Almost always the back of the cassette is metal—for instance, a heavier gauge aluminium—and usually is lined with lead in order to protect the film from radiation scattered backwards from a Bucky tray or other surface. However, there is not sufficient filtering effect to absorb primary radiation totally, as anyone knows who has ever inadvertently positioned a cassette with the wrong aspect facing the X-ray tube during the exposure. This usually occurs in the operating theatre when the cassette is surgically draped and some curious radiographic appearances are thereby produced.

On the inside of the back of the cassette is fixed a black felt, or plastic foam pad, to which is attached the back intensifying screen. The function of the pad is to help to provide permanent and complete contact between the X-ray film and the intensifying screens when the cassette is closed. Loss of screen contact—which occurs more readily in a large cassette—is a common and often unsuspected cause of blurred radiographic detail. When it is necessary to replace intensifying screens, the pad's efficiency sometimes becomes impaired because of damage inflicted during removal of the back intensifying screen; little chunks of material may pull away with the screen, unless the operator is careful.

The internal parts of a cassette, including the frame, are usually anodised black. The front and back surfaces of a metal cassette may be clad with vinyl, which is easy to clean and is warm to the touch, should it be placed—as cassettes often are—in contact with a patient's skin. Usually there is a colour difference—for example, blue PVC on the front and black on the back of a cassette—in order to simplify recognition of the cassette's tube aspect by hurrying radiographers.

It is useful if the back of the cassette carries a clip which can hold a card or chit conveying a patient's identification data. Such a clip may be seen towards the top of the cassette depicted in Figure 5.4.

Fastenings for X-ray cassettes, which should be rapid and positive in action, come in several varieties. Any of the following may be encountered.

1   A sliding locking bar on the long 'opening' edge of the frame. This is operated by a small lever in the upper right-hand corner of the cassette.

2   Two stainless steel 'turn-over' catches, one in the lower half and the other in the upper half of the long edge of the frame, on the 'open' side.

3   Two press latches on the front of the cassette near the top and bottom of the long 'opening' edge. Usually these are of a synthetic material, such as Du Pont's Delrin acetal resin.

4   A pair of flat springs or compression straps of stainless steel. These are mounted on the front of the cassette one above the other, either vertically or horizontally; each usually moves in a guide and provides a latch-type fastening.

Radiographers, darkroom technicians and others who regularly unload and reload X-ray cassettes tend to have individualistic and subjective reactions to cassette fastenings. Some people find one variety easier to operate and another kind much more tricky; but there appears to be no universality of choice and doubtless readers of this book will form, or will have formed already, their own preferences from their experience.

Criteria of a good practical cassette relate to the following points.

1   Weight. It should not be so heavy as to be a constant source of distress in handling.

2   Robust structure. Cassettes are in continuous daily use and even assuming that no one actually drops one—this is to be avoided for the sake of the cassette and the radiographer's toes—nevertheless, thrust into darkroom hatches, loaded into serial changers or edged under heavy patients, they are subject to considerable stress and wear in a busy department. A damaged cassette is likely to be impaired in function: screens may fail to maintain contact with the film or leakage of light at the edges may occur. Cassettes deserve and should have stringent care in

handling. They are themselves expensive and harm to them tends to spoil other costly materials—the screens and the film. A very light cassette is pleasant to use but, while acceptable in a small department, may prove flimsy for the hard work of a large general centre. A compromise between weight and strength must usually be accepted.

3   Ease of operation. Whatever its form of fastening the cassette should not be troublesome to open and close, particularly as this act is necessarily performed in diminished visibility in the darkroom. It should have smooth outlines and rounded corners to avoid abrasion of either patient or radiographer.

Cassettes are provided in sizes appropriate to those in which X-ray film is supplied. The latter are given in the previous chapter and, as the student radiographer will know, it is common to refer to cassettes in these terms, though their actual dimensions are necessarily a little larger. Any other nomenclature would be inconvenient. Certain specialized X-ray cassettes deserve notice for some particular features. Some of these are described below.

CURVED CASSETTES

These have the front convexly curved in a shallow arc. Their object is to maintain a parallel near relationship between subject and film in anatomical regions where a plane surface may be difficult to accommodate: for example to obtain an acceptable anteroposterior view of the knee when extension of the joint is limited. They are used in the smaller sizes, for instance 18 cm × 24 cm.

CASSETTES IN A FILM CHANGER

In certain film changers designed for angiography cassettes may be stacked in a group of three to five, one behind the other. The topmost cassette in the pile is exposed and withdrawn in series. For this type of succession it is of course essential that the back of each cassette should completely absorb primary radiation, otherwise fogging of the film in each of the underlying cassettes will occur every time an X-ray exposure is made. It is possible to back each cassette with a sufficient thickness of lead. However, in preference to modifying individual cassettes, perhaps the more economical and usual practice is to place the standard cassette in a lead-lined tray for the purpose, especially as this tray can include a handle to facilitate rapid withdrawal of the cassette from the apparatus.

CASSETTES AND PHOTO-TIMERS

The student radiographer will no doubt be familiar with the principle of controlling X-ray exposure by means of devices capable of switching the circuit when the film has received an acceptable exposure. The radio-sensitive element may be a photo-electric cell or an ionization chamber. In the case of the photo cell its position is behind the X-ray film, that is behind the cassette. These cassettes then require the reverse feature of those in the angiographic cassette changer: not only their fronts but their backs also must be fully radioparent in order not to attenuate further the radiation transmitted by the subject. Automatic exposure timers now available more usually depend on the operation of an ionisation chamber placed behind a secondary radiation grid and in front of the cassette. In these circumstances the characteristics of the back of the cassette have lesser relevance.

GRIDDED CASSETTES

Cassettes can be supplied in most of the usual sizes which have incorporated in the front a secondary radiation grid as an integral component of the cassette. They are a little deeper, slightly heavier and commensurately much more expensive than the standard cassette. However, they have marked practical advantages when radiography is undertaken with a mobile unit or when horizontal projection of the X-ray beam is mandatory. Centring is more easily determined accurately when film and grid remain aligned as a single unit; film and grid are maintained in close contact and are easy to handle; the grid is automatically protected from the kind of damage which often occurs when a cassette is placed under a grid larger than itself and a heavy patient placed on top of them both. These cassettes advisedly should carry some external indication that they contain a grid or mistakes in exposure technique are likely to occur. One manufacturer obligingly colours them red but a robust labelling system would also serve.

FLEXIBLE CASSETTES

Like the curved cassette, the flexible type is designed for adaptation to rounded surfaces but in this case the arc can be of surprisingly small radius. Their applications in industry, for example to girders and pipelines, are evident and numerous. In medical use they may be necessary for certain specialized equipment associated with rotational tomography of the jaws, when the film must be bent to a shape correspondent to the right and left halves of the maxilla considered simultaneously. Either a flexible cassette or a curved cassette is applicable.

The flexible cassette is a simple envelope of plastic material, folded at one end and fastened with press buttons of conventional design. It is an uncomplicated and practical piece of equipment.

MULTISECTION CASSETTES

Intended for simultaneous multisection radiography these cassettes must be deep enough to hold at any one time a group of films varying in number from 3 to 7. In order to obtain a useful variety of level in the tomographic planes there should be a distance between the films of about 1 cm for most examinations, although in some cases a separation of 0·5 cm or less is requisite.

This cassette is in fact a box some 3 inches deep which contains the appropriate number of intensifying screens separated by spacers of some suitable material. The nature of the spacing substance is important since it must not be of a character to absorb or scatter X rays to an appreciable extent. At present it is usually a plastic polyfoam material, although balsa wood has been employed.

If simultaneous multisection tomography is to be a practicable and useful procedure, it is evident that every film in the group must be comparably exposed. To ensure this, special measures are necessary because of two factors.

(a) The film at the bottom of the cassette is further from the source of X rays than is the film at the top. Consequently the intensity of radiation which reaches it will be diminished in accordance with the operation of the inverse square law.

(b) Each succeeding screen absorbs some radiation, thus diminishing again the quantity reaching the last film.

Of these two effects, (a) is comparatively insignificant since the depth of the cassette is small compared with the distance between it and the X-ray source. It is (b) which is responsible for most of the attenuation of the beam during its passage from the first to the last film. To offset this a combination of intensifying screens should be employed which becomes progressively faster. For example in the simultaneous exposure of 5 layers, uniform radiographic density could be obtained by the following arrangement.

1st film (nearest to the X-ray tube)	1 high definition front screen only.
2nd film	1 standard back screen only.
3rd film	Conventional pair of high definition screens.

4th film   2 standard front screens, one in front of and the other behind the film.

5th film   Conventional pair of fast screens

If three layers only are to be exposed at one time the top film might have a single fast front screen, and the other two successively a pair of high definition and a pair of standard screens.

To avoid the increased hazards of damage when screens are loose and particularly the risk of placing these in incorrect sequence, it is usual to attach the screens and spacers together in the form of a book between the leaves of which the appropriate number of films can be placed. The whole arrangement is then inserted into the cassette, a little care being required to ensure that the correct aspect is uppermost.

Other multiple arrangements of screens are sometimes used in special cassettes, either to obtain radiographs in duplicate or triplicate or to record different densities (for example bone and soft tissue) during a single radiographic exposure of the subject. The principle again is the balancing of the speeds of several different screens in one cassette.

CARE OF CASSETTES

Treated with kindness X-ray cassettes are good for years of hard work. Their general care is aimed at the avoidance of rough handling by all who use them. It may be helpful to mark each cassette, perhaps at a corner or along one edge, with identifying numerals which are inconspicuously apparent on each film. In a department where there are many this makes it easy to eliminate the innocent cassettes and screens, if radiographic faults are observed ascribable to damage of some kind to one or the other. Such numbering can be done with a pencil inside the cassette but it must be a small brief legend and graphite dust can sometimes be a source of artificial appearances on radiographs. If metal or other opaque characters are used, room for their insertion must be made by cutting away part of the intensifying screens, otherwise there will be loss of contact at this and adjacent areas. Some manufacturers save the X-ray department the trouble of this exacting little task by serially numbering their screens at source.

The following further points should be noted.

REGULAR INSPECTION

Cassettes should be inspected at regular intervals to maintain them in serviceable condition. Hinges and clips are subject to stress and their proper functioning should be checked frequently to ensure that wear has not occurred.

Intensifying screens may become adrift and should be re-fixed immediately. Loose screens are an invitation to error in the darkroom for even with the best of intentions it is very easy indeed, when loading a cassette, to slip the film on top of both screens if these are unattached.

The felt pad in the back of the cassette may have become insecure or worn. This can result in failure of the intensifying screens to maintain uniform contact with the film and this in turn produces on the radiograph a localized area of unsharpness, due to the spread of fluorescent light between the screens and the emulsion. If this appearance is detected a test can be made of the suspect cassette.

TESTING PROCEDURES

In Chapter 13 two tests are described which a radiographer may use to check a cassette's efficiency. These refer to its abilities to maintain film-screen contact and to exclude light.

MOUNTING INTENSIFYING SCREENS

It was stated earlier that loose intensifying screens are a source of errors in manipulation in the darkroom. The film may not be in correct relation to the screens or the positions of the front and back screen may be accidentally reversed in the cassette. In addition to these mistakes, unattached screens are much more susceptible to damage from handling. From every point of view it is sound practice to mount the screens in permanent position within the cassette.

No attempt should be made to fasten intensifying screens into a cassette with any adhesive which may be handy in the department. Considerable attention has been given to the selection of a fixative to ensure that no chemical inter-reaction is likely to occur between this and the screens. It is not unknown for a small degree of radioactivity to be present in such an adhesive and this has resulted in bands of fog along the edges of radiographs, particularly of course if the film has lain idle for some time in the cassette.

Intensifying screens are commonly provided by their manufacturers with special adhesive tape, usually already in position on the back surface of each screen, ready for mounting. A protective layer of paper or thin plastic material must first be stripped off before the screens are positioned.

Throughout the procedure the screens should be handled gently, being held by pressure from the palms of the hands along their edges. This will avoid possible finger marks on the active surface of the screen.

The front screen is mounted first. It may be specifically named FRONT and deliberate attention should be given to its identification: usually differentiated screens are marked clearly on the reverse aspect. The protective ribbon is removed from each strip of adhesive tape and the screen is then dropped carefully into the well of the cassette with its active surface facing the operator. No pressure from the hands or from anything else should be put upon the screen at this stage.

The back screen is then identified in the same way as its fellow and adhesive tape prepared as before. This screen is then laid carefully on top of its partner, active surface towards active surface. The back of the back screen now faces the operator. That edge of the screen which is adjacent to the hinge should not be placed too close to it or it will foul the edge and become damaged when the cassette is in use.

The last part of the procedure is simply to close the cassette, fasten it and to leave it thus for some little time, preferably overnight. This is the only pressure necessary to give the adhesive adequate hold.

CARE OF INTENSIFYING SCREENS

An intensifying screen damaged in any way is irreparably damaged. The only remedy is a new pair of screens. As they are sold in pairs, there is little to be done except replace both screens in the cassette, otherwise the odd screen must be kept in storage. Like one glove on its own, it may subsequently never have a match.

Screens are very exposed to the possibility of minor lesions. Their fluorescent emission will be affected if the active surface is even only soiled; for example by finger marks or the presence of dust or other foreign fragments such as particles of metal from the cassette itself. This makes constant attention to their cleanliness a first rule in the care of intensifying screens.

In the darkroom cassettes should not be stored or opened and reloaded in the vicinity of chemicals. From this point of view automatic processing offers reduced hazards to intensifying screens compared with manually operated units. There is no means of removing the contamination of chemical splashes. On inspection in white light they are apparent on the screen's surface as faint brown or yellow stains and they are faithfully reproduced on every radiograph as areas of reduced density, owing to inhibition of the normal fluorescence in these areas.

Another likely source of damage to screens in the darkroom are processing hangers. If these are stored above the loading bench, as frequently they are, and the racks are insufficient for the numbers put upon them hangers may easily fall, particularly when the technician is pulling one free to use it. An open cassette lying on the bench below almost certainly will be victim to their passage, whatever may happen to the unwary technician. It is good practice always to leave cassettes closed, on a bench or anywhere else. Physical defects on the screen surface prevent fluorescence and again appear radiographically as areas of reduced density.

Heat is another agent which can diminish the efficiency of intensifying screens. Cassettes should not be left lying close to radiators or stored near hot pipes. It may be noted that film emulsions gain speed with increased temperature but screens lose it: this occurs to a greater extent and the overall effect is of loss. Furthermore when heated the screens may absorb moisture which will condense on cooling and cause the film to adhere to them. If the cassette has a plastic front this may warp and spoil the contact of the front screen.

Chemical splashes have been mentioned as a common risk to intensifying screens but there is another if technicians or radiographers are talking while putting films into cassettes. A fleck of saliva may fall on the film or on the screen during loading. It will soften the gelatin and stick the film to the supercoat of the screen. Subsequently removal of this film is likely to leave a blister on the active surface of the phosphor.

Summarizing the care of intensifying screens we can say that three good rules apply.

1　Give regular attention to their cleanliness.
2　Finger them as little as possible.
3　Protect them from exposure to damaging agents such as chemicals or physical assault of any kind.

METHOD OF CLEANING SCREENS

Intensifying screens should be dusted frequently with a soft brush: those sold for use on camera lenses are suitable for the purpose. During the operation the cassette should be held vertically so that loosened particles of dirt fall out of it. Dust and grit remaining in a cassette over a long period of time may become embedded in the supercoat of the screens.

Careful inspection of intensifying screens at regular intervals in a white light should be made in order to observe possible marks or defects. Screens which are old can be seen to have a faintly mottled appearance and this will be reproduced on radiographs taken with them. When this is noticed it is time to discard the screens.

In addition to dusting, the screens require washing from time to time.

This should be regular darkroom practice, though on a less frequent schedule. The procedure is possible because of the protective supercoat. Items required are:

1 An ample supply of cotton wool swabs.

2 Good quality scentless toilet soap or a liquid detergent, such as one of the proprietary wetting agents. Never use an organic solvent, for instance ether soap.

3 A supply of clean lukewarm water.

4 A dry soft cloth.

Each screen is washed with a figure of eight motion, using a damp cotton wool swab which has been lightly rubbed with soap or moistened with one or two drops of wetting agent. This pad is then discarded and the screen wiped free of soap with a number of wool swabs soaked in clean water. At no stage must the screen be allowed to become excessively wet nor must water reach the back or edges of the screen. The surface is then mopped with a soft cloth, which is free of loose fibres, and left to dry by exposure to the air. The cassette should stand upright for this purpose and as far as possible the work should be done in a dust-free, draughtless atmosphere.

Grease may be removed from intensifying screens by the careful local application of carbon tetrachloride. This chemical should not be used in a confined space owing to the risk of inhaling its fumes.

LOADING AND UNLOADING A CASSETTE

Not least in the care of intensifying screens is the technique by which cassettes are unloaded and reloaded for further use. The following method is neat and trouble-free and if faithfully observed will assist in prolonging the life of intensifying screens. Unloading is described first as this is the sequence usually met by student radiographers working in the darkroom for the first time.

UNLOADING

The cassette is placed face downwards and opened from the back. It is then turned over and the front of the cassette tipped so that the film falls from the well of the cassette away from the front screen. This is illustrated in Fig. 5.5. The film is removed with the free hand and the cassette closed.

If a pencilled legend has to be put on the film the cassette should *not* be used as a desk for the purpose. Repeated pressure from this source may eventually distort the cassette and spoil screen contact. Furthermore

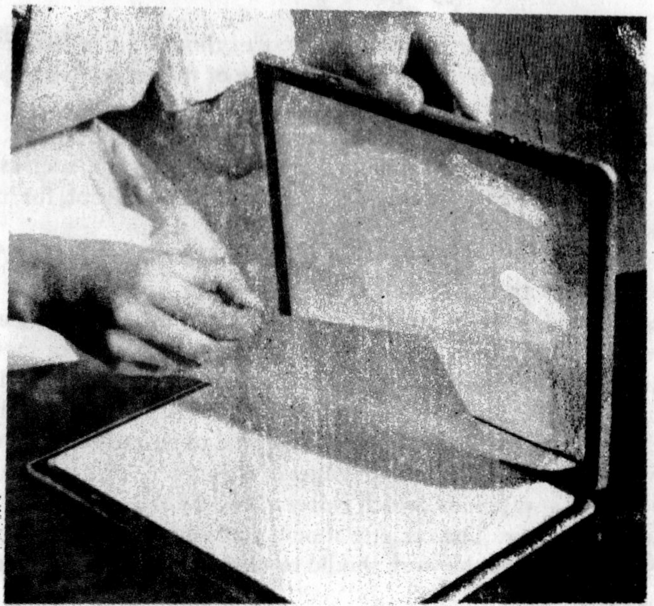

Fig. 5.5. Unloading a cassette. *By courtesy of Ilford Ltd*

graphite dust may be thus introduced. The screens themselves may be accidentally marked by the pencil lead or indented by transmitted pressure.

LOADING

The cassette is placed face downwards on the bench and opened from the back. A film in its paper folder is removed from the box or hopper and held vertically at the folded margin. On the side nearer the operator the paper is drawn away from the film which can then be lowered gently into the well of the cassette and in smooth contact with the front screen. These two manoeuvres are illustrated in Figs. 5.6 and 5.7. The cassette is closed by bringing over the back and then locking the clips or bars.

For reasons of saving both money and space, many departments at present prefer to use film which is packed without interleaving paper between the sheets. In this case the above account must be modified in certain obvious repects. The guiding principle is still to avoid handling the surface of the film to any extent.

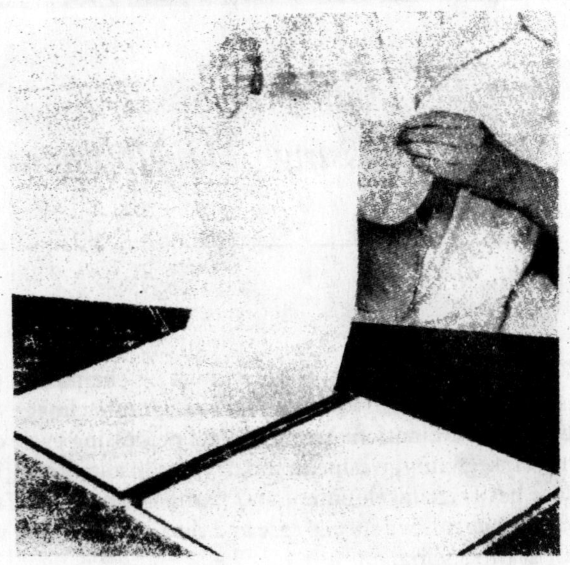

Fig. 5.6. The first stage of loading a cassette with a folder wrapped film.
By courtesy of Ilford Ltd

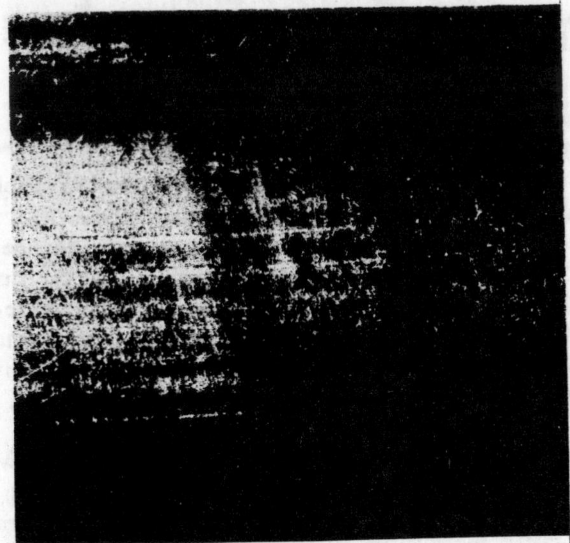

Fig. 5.7. The second stage of loading a cassette. The film has been lowered from the folder to the well of the cassette.
By courtesy of Ilford Ltd

Chapter 6
Film Processing : Development

After an X-ray film has been exposed, it must be chemically treated or processed in order to produce a permanent radiographic image which can be viewed by transillumination. The complete processing cycle comprises development, rinse, fixing, washing, and drying; in automatic processing units the rinse between development and fixing is omitted in favour of a squeegee action, but this is a special case and the rinse can be an important part of efficient processing.

The object of the whole cycle is the production of a dry radiograph with an image which can be viewed, and can be kept without deterioration over a number of years if it is stored in satisfactory conditions. In this and the following chapters, the several stages of the processing cycle are considered.

THE NATURE OF DEVELOPMENT

Development is the first stage. This is the production of a visible metallic silver image from the latent one which exists in the sensitive material after exposure to light or X radiation. The fundamental change that takes place as a result of exposure and development is that the silver halide grains in the emulsion which have been exposed to light become converted to metallic silver, while those which have not received light remain largely unchanged. The conversion to black metallic silver accounts for the blackening of those parts of the film upon which light or X rays have acted.

In practice, the developer is not completely selective between those silver halide grains which have been exposed and those which have not. In time the developer will blacken *all* the silver halide grains. It is therefore more accurate to say that the function of a developer is to reduce to metallic silver the exposed grains of silver halide very much more quickly than the unexposed ones. Silver resulting from the development of unexposed grains is called *fog*. A good developer in this respect is one which shows the biggest difference in its action upon exposed and unexposed grains, and produces a radiograph with minimum fog.

A silver photographic image can be produced by the action of light alone without the aid of a developer. A piece of sensitive material left exposed without protection from light is seen to darken eventually, but the process is relatively slow. In most photographic materials the image produced by exposure to light *plus* the action of the developer is many times denser than that produced by the action of light alone. The developer may be said to amplify the action of the light and the result is that the sensitivity of the process is multiplied by a factor of about 1,000 million times; if the developer were not available the exposures required would be 1,000 million times greater than those in use. The developer is producing almost all the effect, the action of the light being one of initiation. This action is truly remarkable, for it can be produced by minute amounts of light; it is so important in beginning the formation of the image, but so slight that it produces no visible or measurable change after short periods of exposure. Photography is not possible without light or other activating radiation, but it is the use of a developer which makes it a practical proposition.

THE LATENT IMAGE

The silver bromide crystals of a photographic emulsion consist of positive silver and negative bromine ions arranged in a geometric pattern known as a crystal lattice. When a silver bromide grain is exposed to light (or X radiation) the first occurrence is that some of the bromine ions in the lattice emit electrons. These electrons are able to travel through the crystal with great mobility (remaining within the boundaries of the crystal), and their extremely rapid movement carries them into what are known as electron-traps existing in the crystals.

An electron-trap is a region in the crystal of low energy called a *sensitivity speck*. These sensitivity specks are produced in the silver halide crystals during various stages of manufacture. Electrons tend to collect at a sensitivity speck in the crystal, and they confer on the speck a negative charge; this grouping of electric charges at the sensitivity specks is a stage in the formation of the latent image.

The silver ions in the crystal have a positive charge. Not all the silver ions in the crystal are held in the lattice, some being free to move. Those that are able to travel are attracted to the negatively charged electrons in a sensitivity speck. The negative charge on the electrons neutralizes the positive charge on the silver ions, and when this happens silver atoms are formed. The silver atoms at the sensitivity specks increase in number. We recapitulate what has happened as follows.

(i) Electrons (released by light from the bromine ions) are trapped by sensitivity specks.

(ii) Positive silver ions are trapped at the sensitivity specks by the negative charges on the electrons.

(iii) Positive charges on the silver ions are neutralized by the negative charges on the electrons and silver atoms form.

The sequence repeats itself and soon the sensitivity speck has a number of atoms of silver and is part of a photographic latent image.

This cycle of events takes place extremely quickly (one electron can travel to an electron-trap in 10^{-11} seconds), and even in a very short photographic exposure the sequence repeats itself many times. Nevertheless, unless exposure is greatly prolonged, the number of atoms of silver at each sensitivity speck is not enough for the presence of silver to be detected by ordinary tests. It is the action of the developer which most clearly reveals a difference between the exposed crystals which contain metallic silver atoms, and the unexposed crystals which do not.

THE ACTION OF THE DEVELOPER

The basic action of the developer is to reduce to metallic silver the exposed silver halide grains in preference to unexposed grains. This reduction is achieved by the developer donating electrons to silver ions in the grains, thus neutralizing their positive charges and converting them to metallic silver.

As just explained an exposed silver halide crystal has sensitivity specks which contain atoms of silver. When the developer makes contact with this silver, it donates electrons to neutralize positive silver ions. This allows further silver ions to attach to the speck, and these in their turn are neutralized to metallic silver until eventually the whole crystal has become metallic silver. The negative bromine ions which formed the crystal lattice with the positive silver ions disperse into the developer solution as free bromine ions, for they have no silver ions to keep them in place.

The function of the silver atoms in the sensitivity specks seems to be to make it possible for electrons from the developer to combine with silver ions, and also to accelerate the process. Each silver bromide crystal in the emulsion is surrounded by a negatively charged barrier of bromine ions, and this of course will tend to repel electrons from the developer and keep them out. An exposed crystal however has a gap in its complete electron barrier where the latent image speck of silver has formed. This allows the negative developer ions to penetrate at points where the barrier of bromine ions is weak.

This explanation makes understandable the developer's ability to select between exposed and unexposed grains. Only the exposed grains have sensitivity centres which constitute weakness in the bromine ion barrier; only the exposed grains have a combination of silver atoms and attached silver ions. These facts increase greatly the speed with which a developer can attack an exposed crystal and reduce the whole to metallic silver, giving a black visible image.

The theory of the latent image and the action of the developer is recapitulated below in general elementary terms in the hope that this may be of help to the student.

Basic photographic action :

Conversion of silver bromide $\rightarrow$ metallic silver.

(a) Initiated by light or X rays :

Silver bromide = Bromine ions (negative) and silver ions (positive).

Bromine ions + light $\rightarrow$ electrons emitted.
Electrons + silver ions $\rightarrow$ silver atoms.

These silver atoms begin to form the latent image.

(b) Continued by the action the developer :

Developer $\rightarrow$ gives electrons to silver ions.
Electrons + silver ions $\rightarrow$ silver atoms.

Developer finds it easier to give electrons to *exposed* silver bromide crystals; these have some silver atoms already as result of light action and there are breaks in the negative charge round crystals containing these silver atoms. Electrons from developer gain easier access and reduce whole exposed crystal to metallic silver.

THE pH SCALE

The pH scale is used to express the degree of acidity or alkalinity of a solution, and the student is likely to encounter it since pH values in processing solutions are relatively critical. It will be considered before proceeding with an explanation of the constituents of developing solutions.

Probably even those of us with the scantiest chemical knowledge recognize that water is a neutral solution and that its chemical formula is H_2O. Water contains hydroxyl ions (OH) which are negative and hydrogen ions (H) which are positive. In pure water these two ions are present in equal concentrations. The concentration of each is 10^{-7} gramme ions per litre. This is the state of affairs in a neutral solution.

If the solution is made acid, the hydrogen ions are present in greater concentration than the hydroxyl ions; if the solution is made alkaline, the hydrogen ions are present in less concentration than the hydroxyl ions. A scale of acidity can be made based on the hydrogen ion concentration, and such a scale is the pH scale.

In a neutral solution, the hydrogen ion concentration is 10^{-7} gramme ions per litre, and the pH of a neutral solution is 7. So 7 is the neutral point of the scale, with the acids ranged on one side of it, and the alkalis on the other; for any given solution, the further away from 7 its pH lies on the scale, the more acid or alkaline it is. Thus:

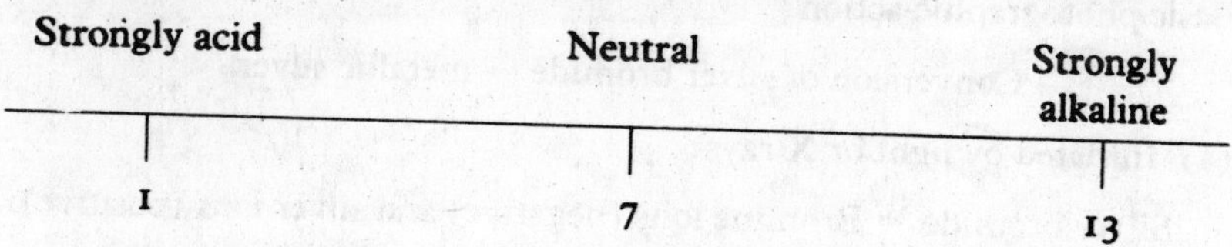

A pH 1 means that the hydrogen ion concentration is 10^{-1} gramme ions per litre; that is there are many more hydrogen ions than hydroxyl ions. A pH 13 means that the hydrogen ion concentration is 10^{-13} gramme ions per litre; that is, there are very much fewer hydrogen ions and many more hydroxyl ions. pH numbers below 7 mean greater hydrogen ion concentration, and pH numbers above 7 mean reduced hydrogen ion concentration as compared with a neutral solution.

The addition of an acid to an alkali lowers the pH towards the neutral 7; the addition of an alkali to an acid raises the pH towards the neutral 7. These therefore neutralize each other. In photographic processing, developers lie on the alkaline side of 7, and fixers are on the acid side of 7. Thus:

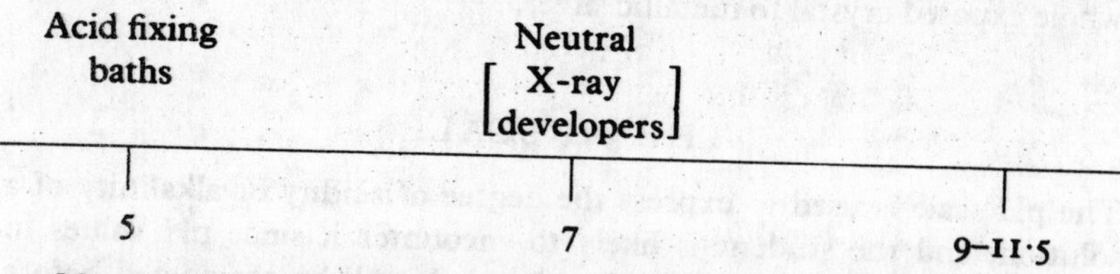

Most radiographic developers function at a pH above 9, and require to be kept constant within 0·1 and 0·2 on the scale. Fixers are contaminated by developer carried into them, and in use their pH rises as the alkaline developer reduces their acidity.

The pH scale is logarithmic and small changes in pH mean large changes in acidity. On a logarithmic scale a change from 1 to 2 indicates an alteration which is ten-fold. In a developer this could mean a difference in activity between no development action at all, and an energy which fogged every film immersed in the solution.

THE CONSTITUTION OF DEVELOPING SOLUTIONS

DEVELOPING AGENTS

A developing agent is a substance able to change silver halide into metallic silver. The conversion of a salt or oxide of a metal to the metal is described as chemical reduction; the conversion of metals to their oxides or salts is described as oxidation. When reduction occurs atoms or molecules gain electrons; when oxidation occurs atoms or molecules lose electrons. From this it follows that when one substance is reduced by gaining electrons, another must be oxidized by giving electrons to it.

Photographic developing agents are thus chemical reducing agents. As explained in a foregoing section they neutralize silver ions in the silver bromide by donating electrons to them. Since the developing agents lose electrons in this transaction, they become oxidized in carrying out their function. An important characteristic in the reducing agents used in photographic developers is their ability to differentiate between exposed and unexposed grains of silver halide; lack of this ability would make a reducing agent totally unsuitable for use in a developing solution.

The activity of a reducing agent in donating electrons can be measured, and comparisons can be made between agents on this basis. They do not all donate electrons with equal freedom; those that do it readily are said to have a high reduction potential; those which do it less readily have a low reduction potential.

During the action of development bromine ions are released into the solution, and developing agents differ in their susceptibility to this increased bromine concentration. It has greater restraining action on some developers than on others; those which are readily restrained by it quickly become weaker in use as the bromine concentration becomes greater.

Numerous substances have been used as developing agents, and varieties of solution have been compounded for use in general photography. The properties of various solutions differ, though their basic components may remain much the same. It is the proportions in which these components are present which alter the results obtained. For student radiographers, however, there is no difficulty since the number of developing agents used for radiographic processing is very small.

METOL-HYDROQUINONE COMBINATIONS

For many years two particular reducing agents have been used together in one solution for the development of X-ray films (and also for general photography). These two agents (which are still in use) are Metol and hydroquinone, and solutions in which they are combined are known as MQ developers.

Metol and hydroquinone both achieve the same basic function common to all developing agents; they reduce silver halides to metallic silver. Yet they act in different ways.

Metol. As a developing agent Metol begins reduction readily, and will develop all exposed grains, including those which have received only slight exposure. Once the reduction is initiated, the process continues rather more slowly. Being susceptible to increased concentration of bromine, Metol becomes weak with use relatively quickly. In the absence of any bromide to act as a restrainer, Metol tends to fog—that is it becomes unselective between exposed and unexposed silver halide grains in the emulsion.

Hydroquinone. As a developing agent, hydroquinone requires a strongly alkaline solution in which to act. It does not begin development so rapidly as Metol, and it has less effect on grains which have had little exposure. It functions to give high contrast. Once hydroquinone has begun to act on the exposed grains, development proceeds vigorously.

Since these two agents produce different effects it may be easily understood that when they are used in combination the solution could be expected to combine the characteristics of the two; and that alterations in the amount of each agent present could affect the result obtained. In practice there is a hidden bonus in using Metol and hydroquinone together, for the combination has photographic properties which are an improvement on the sum of those of each agent. Developers which contain Metol *and* hydroquinone produce a photographic density which is greater than the sum of two densities obtained by Metol and hydroquinone acting apart in separate solutions.

This phenomenon whereby we appear to get something for nothing— a combined effect which is better than the sum of individual effects—is known by the awkward name *superadditivity*. Not every combination of developing agents can form a superadditive system, but Metol and hydroquinone most certainly do. This is one of the reasons why MQ developers have been so extensively used in photographic practice.

The mechanism of superadditivity is that hydroquinone regenerates the Metol in part at least, reacting with the Metol which has been oxidized in the action with silver bromide to reform Metol and itself becoming oxidized in the process.

PHENIDONE-HYDROQUINONE COMBINATIONS

There is another developing agent which was first made useful by the laboratories of Ilford Ltd and has the brand name Phenidone. It shows many of the properties of Metol. It functions to give high speed and low contrast, and it tends to fog. It is markedly affected by increased concentration of bromine in the used developer particularly at pH values below 9·4.

Phenidone is combined with hydroquinone in various types of developer. Such a combination is known as a PQ developer, and it shows certain advantages over the MQ type.

Phenidone and hydroquinone are superadditive together, but the bonus is even bigger and better than that given by MQ combinations, the Phenidone being from 10 to 15 times more effective. This means that smaller quantities of Phenidone can be used to achieve a given result. Because only a little Phenidone in comparison with Metol is required, it is easier to prepare highly concentrated solutions. PQ combinations are the basis of developers provided in concentrated liquid form.

Phenidone is regenerated by hydroquinone with greater efficiency than Metol is, and this prolongs the working life of the solution. Phenidone is much less susceptible than Metol to the restraining influence of the increased bromide concentration which inevitably occurs as the developer acts, and therefore PQ developers do not exhaust as quickly as their MQ counterparts.

The developing solution needs more constituents than simply combinations of reducing agents if it is to act efficiently. These additional components will be considered now.

THE ACCELERATOR

In an earlier paragraph it was said that developing solutions must be alkaline. The pH of the developer has a significant effect on its activity, and variations in alkalinity alter the rate at which development takes place. Too little alkali results in the developer being sluggish in action; too much makes it over-active and uncontrolled so that it develops unexposed crystals and produces fog. A wide range of developers of varying activity can be compounded by adjustments in pH to the required level. The pH range of X-ray developers is 10–11·5.

Developing solutions therefore include an alkali so that they may react at the desired rate, and this alkali is called the *accelerator*. Certain developing agents need high alkalinity if they are to be active at all.

The alkalis used in solutions for radiographic developers are sodium carbonate, sodium hydroxide, potassium carbonate, and potassium hydroxide. The hydroxides are strongly alkaline, and used in conjunction with the developing agent hydroquinone they result in a developer of high activity and contrast. Small amounts of the hydroxides are often added to the carbonates. The sole advantage of the potassium salts over the sodium salts is that their higher solubility allows them to be used in higher concentrations.

THE RESTRAINER

To include a *restrainer* such as potassium bromide in the developing solution as well as an alkali to increase developer activity may sound like trying to drive a car with one foot on the accelerator, and the other just as firmly on the brake. However the manufacturers of these solutions can be expected to be more sensible than this, and there is in fact reason underlying the practice of including a restrainer.

One of the qualities of a good developing agent is its ability to act on the exposed silver halide grains very much more rapidly than it acts on the unexposed ones. The function of the restrainer is to check action on the unexposed grains, that is to prevent fog. It acts by increasing the barrier of negatively charged bromine ions which exists round the silver bromide crystals. This barrier to development (it will be recalled) exists in a complete state round unexposed crystals, and in a breached state in exposed crystals where a latent image is formed in the emulsion.

Without any restrainer the developer will be too active and will reduce the unexposed grains too readily. An excessive restrainer naturally is certain to check also the developing agent's effect on the exposed silver halide grains, and thus reduce desired developer activity. The solution must be accurately compounded so that the restrainer effectively minimizes fog during normal development, without unduly retarding the proper action of the developer which is sought. A correctly acting restrainer improves radiographic contrast by reducing or preventing fog. This is particularly important in the very low densities of the radiograph.

In Phenidone-hydroquinone combinations it is essential to include in addition to the potassium bromide restrainer an organic restrainer such as benzotriazole, which is widely used. The PQ combinations are less sensitive than MQ systems to the restraining action of bromide, and a large amount of bromide would be necessary to restrain the highly active PQ developers. Organic restrainers can act efficiently at much lower concentrations than potassium bromide requires. They are also able to minimize fog effectively with less retarding action on the development of exposed silver halide grains; organic restrainers are known also as *anti-foggants*.

THE PRESERVATIVE

Developing agents are easily oxidized and readily absorb oxygen from the air. If nothing is done to check this, it shortens the life of the developer. A chemical is therefore included which checks the rate of oxidation. This chemical is called the *preservative*. Sodium sulphite and potassium sulphite are both used as preservatives. The addition of a preservative to the developing solution does not entirely stop aerial oxidation, but it does reduce the rate at which it occurs and minimizes the more damaging effects.

As a result of being oxidized, either by air or as a natural consequence of normal developing action, developing agents produce certain oxidation products. Some of these can accelerate the process of further oxidation. The action of the sulphite preservative is to form sulphonates with the early oxidation products. These are comparatively inert, so that the accelerating action is stopped and the final oxidation products are not formed.

THE SOLVENT

The solvent used in making photographic solutions is almost always water, which has the advantages of being cheap and universally available. Unfortunately it is not universal in character as it comes out of the tap, for it then has dissolved in it various mineral salts. The nature and quantity of these depend on where the water supply originates and what treatment it is given.

However, in practice these dissolved substances are less of a photographic hazard than might be expected, and it is generally possible to use water from the tap with satisfaction. Distilled water of course is without dissolved salts, but the additional cost and effort of this process need not be contemplated when the tap water serves well, as is almost always the case.

The likely result of using water which is very hard (containing much dissolved mineral salt) is that the salts can react with photographic chemicals and produce precipitates. Such precipitates may form a chalky deposit or scum on the surface of films processed in the solutions. This will become obvious on drying and it is difficult to remove. Hard water can of course be softened before use by the addition of various agents which are available—for example the commercial product Calgon (sodium hexametaphosphate) in a concentration of ½oz. per gallon. In practice however it is not essential to do this. Water softening agents are included in the composition of modern developers, and special treatment of tap water is necessary only in extreme cases.

It need hardly be said that water used for preparing photographic solutions must be clean and free from obvious insoluble impurities such as grit and rust or any other unexpected additions. Water which stands for long periods in copper pipes can be contaminated by copper; only a very small amount of copper present in the water used to prepare solution leads to fog on films which are developed in them.

OTHER ADDITIONS

Developing solutions contain further ingredients in addition to the basic group. These additions are for particular purposes, such as water softeners, wetting agents and bactericidal substances. An important constituent is a hardener to harden the emulsions of films being processed: aldehydes are used as hardeners in developers. Some additions are provided in order to *buffer* the solution. A buffered solution is capable of accepting quantities of acid or alkali without much change in pH. Since pH values are so important in the activity of developing agents, adequate buffering helps to keep the activity stable; a later section (p. 139) explains the changes which occur in the developer with use and tend to alter its activity.

Buffering agents come in pairs. Examples are: sodium carbonate with sodium bicarbonate, and boric acid with sodium hydroxide.

DEVELOPING SOLUTIONS SUMMED-UP

To sum up developing solutions, their ingredients can be listed as follows.
(i) Developing agents to convert exposed silver bromide grains to metallic silver.
(ii) An accelerator, which is an alkali, to give the developer the desired activity.
(iii) A restrainer, for example potassium bromide and/or benzotriazole, to minimize fog by checking action on the unexposed silver bromide grains.

(iv) A preservative, which is usually sodium sulphite, to check oxidation and discolouration.

(v) A solvent, which is water.

(vi) Certain other additions, such as buffering agents and hardeners.

Alterations in these constituents have the following effects.

(i) Changes in the amount of developing agent and in the ratio of different agents to each other in the solution alter the time needed to reach a given contrast and density—that is, they alter the development time required.

(ii) Change in the amount of alkali alters the time needed to reach a given contrast and density; increasing the alkaline content shortens the development time and decreasing the alkaline content increases the development time required.

(iii) Changes in the pH are significant also in regard to the amount of swelling of the emulsion that takes place when the film is being developed. If the pH is relatively low in the alkaline region (say 9) the emulsion swells less from absorption of water: above pH 10 the swelling is increased, the gelatin of the emulsion absorbing several times its own weight in water. Thus swollen, it is very susceptible to mechanical damage and to high temperatures, which can liquefy it.

(iv) Changes in the amounts of hardeners which are present affect both the physical condition of the emulsion (by altering the extent to which it swells) and its sensitometric properties. If there is only very little hardener present, the emulsion swells more; more developer is absorbed; hence more is carried over with the film when it proceeds to the fixer in the next stage of processing; the softened emulsion may stick to the rollers of automatic processors, so that the emulsion is damaged and the machine is contaminated; the emulsion may leave the film base. If there is a high concentration of hardener present, the film cannot absorb the developer well enough to be developed in the time for which it is immersed; so the image lacks density and contrast; less developer is carried over in the emulsion because less has been absorbed; swelling is greatly reduced.

(v) Increasing the amount of restrainer reduces the fog level where fog exists but results in a longer development time being required to reach a given contrast.

(vi) Alterations in the amount of preservative affect the keeping properties of the solution.

(vi) Alterations in the amount of water naturally affect the dilution of the developer. The more concentrated the solution (up to a certain limit) the shorter the development time required.

Manufacturers' specifications on dilution should be followed: higher concentration than the recommended value may increase fog while greater dilution lessens the activity of the developer.

THE DEVELOPMENT TIME

Automatic processing is now in widespread use. If we are to define in relation to it the term *development time*, it can be done in part by saying that the development time is that period which the film spends in the developer section as it is conveyed through the processor. This interval will vary according to the full cycle-time of the processor, as the following figures show.

Cycle-time	Period of time in developer
7 minutes	130 seconds
3·5 minutes	68 seconds
110 seconds	30 seconds
90 seconds	26 seconds

Obviously as the cycle-time shortens, the period within the cycle which is available for the development of the image must shorten too. When the radiograph, processed and ready to be viewed, emerges at the end of the cycle it must be developed to the density and contrast which are wanted. So in any automatic processor the time available must equal the time required for correct development.

So we come to a further definition of *development time* as the period required for the image to develop to optimum density and contrast. The question now to be asked is: what are the factors which influence the development time?

In any developing solution, factors which alter the development time are as follows:

(i) the constitution of the solution;

(ii) the temperature of the solution:

(iii) the degree of exhaustion of the solution;

(iv) the agitation given to the solution and to the film which is being developed in it.

These matters are more fully considered in the following section of this chapter as conditions in the use of the developer which alter the development time and affect the quality of the radiographs which are obtained.

FACTORS IN THE USE OF A DEVELOPER

CONSTITUTION OF THE SOLUTION

It will be clear by now to the assiduous reader that the constitution of the developing solution must significantly affect the resultant image, especially in regard to its density and its contrast. These are important:

(i) the developing agents used and their relative proportions;

(ii) the degree of alkalinity;

(iii) the proportions, the natures and the conjoined functions of all the chemical agents which are present in the complete solution.

Modern radiographic developers are the results of sustained experience and research and they are very carefully compounded to meet the needs of the various processing systems which are used. These developers give high contrast, high speed and minimum fog and they have consistent activity when they are properly used.

In modern X-ray departments, almost all of the processing is done by the functioning of automatic processors and developers are available which are especially compounded for these systems. A very small proportion of the processing which is done is effected through a manual system. Manual processing too has developers which are compounded to meet the needs of such a method. In a later section of this chapter we consider the differences in the chemical requirements for automatic processors in contrast with manual systems.

TEMPERATURE OF THE SOLUTION

The temperature of a developing solution has marked effects on the activity of the agents used: a developer is more active as it becomes warmer. Taking the development time as the period needed for the image to develop to a point at which density, contrast and fog have optimum values, it can be said that lower temperatures imply longer development times and higher temperatures indicate shorter development times. At the one extreme, very low temperatures may make a developer almost inactive and at the other very high temperatures can fog the image and even physically damage the film, separating the gelatin from the base: physical damage is more likely if the emulsion is swollen and soft.

Different development agents are affected to different extents by changes in temperature: for example, hydroquinone loses activity to a greater extent than does Metol as the temperature of the solution falls. In practice a solution-temperature is chosen to give optimum speed for the developing agents which are present in any given combination and to achieve for them degrees of activity which are satisfactorily balanced.

In the table below we indicate the approximate times and temperatures which may be used in various processing systems. The reader can readily appreciate that the use of raised temperatures in automatic processors is one of the methods by which the development time is greatly shortened. This is an essential part in achieving the complete processing cycle within periods of time which are very much shorter than those which apply for manual processing systems. A developer-temperature around 31°C is now most widely used in automatic processors.

Processing system	*Developer temperature*	*Development time*
Manual processing	20°C	4 minutes
Automatic		
7 minute cycle	25°C	130 seconds
3½ minutes cycle	30°C	68 seconds
110 seconds cycle	31°C	30 seconds
90 second cycle	40°C	26 seconds

TIME-TEMPERATURE TECHNIQUE

The time-temperature technique of development is a practical method used in manual processing so that standardization may be achieved, or as nearly achieved as is possible without automatic systems. The technique is simple and consists of immersing the films for a certain length of time in a developer-solution which is at a certain temperature. In the table given above, the technique for manual processing is stated as 4 minutes immersion with the developer at the temperature 20°C. This has been the standard for many years, the assumption being made that the developer is an appropriately formulated X-ray developer which is properly made up and maintained. Indeed the manufacturers devise their developers for manual processing with the aim that in 4 minutes at 20°C the radiographic image should be developed to optimum density and contrast without a high fog level.

If the temperature of the developer in the tank alters from 20°C, an equivalent result may be given if the time of immersion is changed accordingly. For example, the temperature 18°C requires the time 5 minutes and the temperature 22°C needs the time 3 minutes if the results are to be the same. It should be noted, however, that if the range of variations in the developer-temperature is wide, there can be no expectation of achieving a standard result by adjusting the period of immersion for the film. The developer is compounded to perform at its best at a certain temperature and much variation from this may disturb the balance in the activity of the agents in solution and completely alter the result.

Those who undertake manual processing are often inclined to modify their practice so that it ceases to be strictly controlled as a time-temperature technique. The developer is at the required temperature and the film is put into the solution with the intention that it will remain there for 4 minutes. Nevertheless at intervals within the four minutes the film is taken out of the tank and is inspected under the safelights. If it 'comes up quickly' because it has been radiographically overexposed in the X-ray room, the 4 minutes development time is curtailed. If on the other hand the image seems to lack the expected density, then the film is developed for longer than the standard 4 minutes. The aim is to try to compensate in the darkroom for errors in the selection of radiographic exposures and so to avoid repeating radiographs.

It is not a sound practice and it cannot achieve standardized results which are consistently high in quality. For these, a strict time-temperature technique gives the best approach. A significant benefit from automatic processors is that the time-temperature method of development is inflexibly imposed when the machine is operating properly.

EXHAUSTION OF THE DEVELOPER

The activity of the developer must decrease with use since the composition of the solution alters as it is used. Functioning to produce a change in photographic materials, it undergoes chemical change itself in the process.

Let us consider this initially in relation to a tank of developer which is not part of an automatic processor and is being used to develop a number of films in a continuing series over a period of time.

The reactions involved are expressed below.

I Developer in use
Developing agents + silver bromide→
   silver + bromine ions + hydrogen ions + oxidized developing agents
II Developer standing
Developing agents + oxygen→
                oxidized developing agents + hydroxyl ions.

The following occurrences take place.
(a) Developer solution is taken out of the tank in the emulsion and on the

surfaces of the film. This physically removes some amount of all the ingredients in the bath.

(b) The developing agents are changed by oxidation both in the normal developing action in which they reduce silver bromide to metallic silver and through contact with the air. There is thus constant dimunition of the amount of active developing agent present in the tank. When all the developing agent is used up, the solution is completely exhausted.

(c) The oxidation products formed *may* retard the action of development. There is naturally a constant increase in the concentration of these products present in the tank. This effect, however, has little significance in reducing the activity of the bath in comparison with other factors mentioned under (b), (d), and (e).

(d) The bromine ions released with use as part of reaction I increase the bromide content of the solution. This exerts a restraining influence on developer activity.

(e) The alkaline content of the developer falls. Bromine and hydrogen ions are released in reaction I in the form of hydrobromic acid, and this is neutralized by the alkali present in the developer. This action uses up available alkali, and so the pH of the solution falls. There may be considerable reserve of alkali in the solution and it may be well buffered so that the pH is kept constant for some while, but in the end it is bound to fall. Since pH has marked effect on developer activity, the solution becomes less active.

(f) In the presence of reaction II, the sodium sulphite in the solution forms sulphonates and is used up doing so. There is thus dimunition in the amount of preservative present; if the sulphite becomes completely used up, the remaining developing agents will be left without a preservative and will rapidly succumb to oxidation. As a result of the reactions taking place, there is release of sodium hydroxide in the solution and this tends to a rise in pH, which will *augment* developer activity and may increase fog level.

Aerial oxidation and oxidation through normal development action thus have opposing effects on pH. However, when the solution is in use, the loss of alkalinity as described in (e) overwhelms the rise in pH that aerial oxidation causes. With this loss of alkalinity there are the other causes of reduced activity in the developer which have been shown. So used solutions are less energetic than fresh ones.

This means in practice that as the solution exhausts development times at a given temperature must be increased to reach a given contrast and density.

In an automatic processing system the development time used is short, is critical and cannot be prolonged to offset the effects of exhaustion since it must continue to take up the same time-interval within the processing cycle. So the activity of the developer-solution in the working tank of the machine must be kept constant. This is achieved by adding a solution which is called the replenisher.

The machine functions so that replenisher is added at a rate which is proportionate to the rate of exhaustion: when films are put into the processor, a pump injects replenisher and thus equilibrium is achieved. With the machine operating correctly, the films are developed to optimum density and contrast within the period of time that they travel through the developer-tank of the processor.

THE CONSTITUTION OF A REPLENISHER

Given an understanding of the processes which occur in the developer during use, it is easy to see in general outline the requirements of a replenishing solution which is to restore its activity.

(i) Since the developing agents are used up, the replenisher should contain them in somewhat higher concentration than did the original solution.

(ii) Since with use there is increased concentration of bromide which restrains the developer, bromide is not included in the replenisher. This does not really solve the problem of the formation of bromine ions, but at least does nothing to aggravate it.

(iii) Since the pH of the developer falls in use, the replenisher contains a high concentration of alkali (usually sodium hydroxide) to offset this.

(iv) Since the preservative in the developer is used up, some extra sulphite must be included in the replenisher. Its presence prevents aerial oxidation of the replenisher as its stands.

(v) There may be other additions to maintain adequate buffering of the solution.

A replenisher is designed to be used with a particular developer, and modern replenishers are formulated carefully and with scientific understanding. In a later section we consider the solutions used for developers and replenishers in automatic processing systems in comparison with those used with the manual technique.

REPLENISHING A MANUAL SYSTEM

As we have mentioned, there is still some processing which is undertaken with manual systems. For these there is no automatic addition of a certain amount of replenisher for every film processed and developer tanks must be replenished by hand.

There are, in fact, two tasks to be achieved when the replenisher is added: (i) to maintain the level of the solution in the tank, since it falls with use because a quantity is carried out as each film is passed by hand from the developer tank; (ii) to regenerate the solution chemically so that it remains active with use and the development time continues to be the standard 4 minutes at 20°C.

MAINTAINING THE SOLUTION LEVEL

In considering how much replenisher is required to restore the level of the solution in the tank, the question to be asked, of course, is: by how much does the solution fall? The short answer is: by varied amounts. When films are transferred from a developer tank to the next stage, they may be moved directly over or they may be allowed to drain developer from their surfaces back into the tank before they are carried over. Clearly the first practice carries a maximum amount of developer out of the tank and the solution-level falls quickly with use. A careful technique of draining for about 5 to 10 seconds results in marked reduction in the volume of solution which is carried out and slows the rate at which the level of the solution falls as the tank is used.

So factors which influence the fall in the solution-level are:
(i) the number of films processed:
(ii) the area of film processed;
(iii) the techniques of the individuals who undertake the processing. We use the word *individuals* with care, for each adapts an idiosyncratic approach.

REGENERATING THE SOLUTION

In order to maintain the activity of a tank of developer as it is used, the solution added to it should counteract the effects of exhaustion. In the ideal situation, the counteraction matches the rate at which exhaustion occurs and then the activity of the tank of developer is stabilized. The rate at which exhaustion occurs is clearly dependant upon the amount of chemical work which the developer must do. Factors which are important in determining the amount of chemical work to be done are:
(i) the number of films processed;
(ii) the area of film processed;
(iii) the radiographic subject and the film used.

The first two of the above are obvious in their significance but perhaps the last one needs some explanation. The task of the developing agent is to reduce silver halide to metallic silver and this must be done on *exposed* regions of the film. The reader should consider a film of a given size and then picture upon it different radiographic subjects: for example, a lateral view of the skull, two views of the ankle, two views of a foot, a view of the abdomen showing the gall bladder filled with contrast agent, a study of the stomach filled with barium sulphate. These radiographic subjects result in different patterns for the deposition of silver from the conversion of silver bromide and thus they may result in different amounts of chemical work for the developing agent to do. So the amount of work which is to be done by the developer per unit area of film put through it depends on the radiographic subject. It depends also on the size of film used for that subject and upon other factors such as the amounts of silver in the sensitive materials and the compositions of the emulsions used. In a general X-ray department, the proportion of silver developed varies over a considerable range with the different subjects examined. However, general departments are alike in handling more or less the same mixture of subjects and any one department over a period of time uses only one or two types of films. For any given busy department, the average quantity of silver halide developed per unit area of film will be more or less standardized. An average figure of 30 per cent of the total available silver (taking into account the size of film generally used for any particular examination) can thus be assumed. Special groups such as chest clinics, obstetric units and orthopaedic departments may have different averages for developed silver per unit area of film processed.

USING A REPLENISHER

To use a replenisher effectively in a manual system, it is necessary to correct simultaneously the physical condition of a lost volume of solution and the chemical condition of a lost degree of energy. The amount of replenisher added to restore the working level of the solution must bring sufficient regeneration to correct the diminished activity. In practice, the method most commonly used by anyone doing manual processing today is to pour into the tank of developer enough replenisher just to restore the solution to its proper working level. This is done as necessary on each working day and the amount added is that required to allow the solution to cover totally the films which are placed in it. The assumption is made that this amount is sufficient to correct the loss of chemical activity and the system seems to work effectively enough.

AGITATION OF FILMS AND SOLUTIONS

Agitation of the film and movement of the solution about the film during the period of development have two prominent effects: (i) within limits, the rate at which development takes place is increased so that shorter development times are required; (ii) uniformity of development is promoted.

In roller-type automatic processors, the film is in continuous movement after its entry until it is discharged at the end of the cycle. Further, the solution of the developer is actively circulated within the processor and so is itself in movement. Thus the developer has equal access to all parts of the film and this aids an even rate of development over the whole surface.

The certainty of a standardized degree of efficient agitation is a factor (only one among several) in ensuring that the short development times used in the processing cycle are fully effective.

Radiographs processed manually are suspended in stainless steel frames in a tank and usually given very little agitation. There is the disturbance of their entry to the tank and of their withdrawal, and that is usually as much agitation as they receive, apart from such movement of the solution as occurs with the entry and withdrawal of other films. The effect of agitation on even development is cause for regret that agitation is so much neglected when manual processing is done. Even a slight agitation given 4 to 5 times during 4 minutes immersion would do much to lessen the risk of development marks which a static condition allows when films are developed in a vertical plane.

These marks can commonly take two forms. They are (i) light streaks or 'streamers' beneath heavily exposed areas of the film, and (ii) dark streaks particularly beneath areas which have been lightly exposed. The light streaks occur in this way.

In a heavily exposed area there is considerable reduction of silver bromide to metallic silver, and this is accompanied by the release of bromine ions. There is thus a local bromide concentration which has a restraining effect on development. Agitation would sweep this bromide concentration away, but a static state allows it to sink down and restrain the developer in areas vertically below regions of high exposure. These areas therefore show light streaks.

The dark streaks occur in this way. In a static state developer from areas which are lightly exposed (this developer being largely unused) is allowed to drift downwards. Thus in regions vertically beneath these areas the developer is more active and dark streaks result. Agitation would sweep the unexhausted developer away.

Solutions which are not stirred properly also allow uneven development and the production of light and dark streaks. Stirring is important when solutions are being prepared for use in any system of processing. Even in an automatic one it must not be supposed that the method of use in the processor stirs the solution suitably. Inadequate stirring at the time of preparation can leave the solution in layers, with the active chemical agents insufficiently intermingled. As a result of this, films have been known to emerge from the developer with as little evidence upon them of visible images as they had when they entered the processor.

Chemical mixers with mechanical actions are available and are very useful pieces of equipment. They not only save the time and the effort of human beings: they make it certain that thorough mixing takes place even in the large volume of chemical solutions which must be mixed in some modern automatic processors.

DEVELOPERS IN PROCESSING SYSTEMS

CONSTITUTION OF DEVELOPERS

Progress in evolving machinery for automatic processing required progress also in another field: developers needed new formulations. Salient features in modern automatic processors are firstly the temperatures used, these being as we have seen higher than the standard 20°C of manual processing: and secondly the roller transport-systems which take the films through the processors. The higher temperatures increase swelling of the film and the abrasions of the rollers subject a swollen and softened film to physical stresses from which it needs to be protected. So the solution constituting the developer must contain agents to harden the gelatin of the emulsion during processing. These hardeners must act effectively in the alkaline solution of the developer.

The higher temperatures affect not only the physical condition of the emulsion but also the chemical condition of the developer: at higher temperatures it oxidizes more readily. So the new formulations have greater antioxidant properties than do those used for manual processing.

The high temperatures and the inclusion of the hardeners both result in an increased tendency of the developer to fog. So special attention must be given to anti-foggants and restrainers present in the developers used in automatic processors.

To sum up, the developers used in automatic processors contain the following.

(i) An organic hardening agent such as glutaraldehyde which acts in an alkaline solution.

(ii) A preservative such as sodium or potassium sulphite to combat oxidation.

(iii) Organic antifoggants such as benzotriazole and developer restrainers such as potassium bromide to minimize the growth of film-fog. The benzotriazole has a selective influence on unexposed silver halide grains. Potassium bromide inhibits the developer's action on both the exposed and the unexposed silver halide grains. Adjustment of the ratio of these two agents controls the growth of fog from the developer's activity.

(iv) Sodium carbonate or potassium carbonate to act as a source of alkali and also as a buffer. The alkali is important to the activity of the developer and the buffer controls the pH of the solution. This is usually between 9·6 and 10·6 in automatic processing. A relatively low alkaline pH reduces the swelling of the emulsions of the films developed.

(v) Sodium hydroxide or potassium hydroxide as a source of alkali and thus to be the accelerator or activator of the developer.

(vi) A sequestering agent to combat the formation of insoluble salts such as calcium carbonate which come from the use of hard water.

(vii) Hydroquinone in high concentration as a developing agent which acts most on the silver halide grains which have received the most exposure and has less effect on grains which have received little exposure. It thus functions to record those parts of the image which have the greater densities and it gives high contrast.

(viii) A developing agent which functions to record the lesser densities in the image by acting readily on the exposed silver halide grains even when they have received only slight exposure. Both Metol and Phenidone are suitable agents for this purpose, so one of them is included with the hydroquinone.

All developing agents are present in greater proportions in developers constituted for automatic processors than in those for use in a manual system.

In formulating a developer for an automatic processor, the manufacturer has certain considerations in view. These are:

(i) that in use the developer will be continuously replenished over periods of time of several months, solution being injected into the tank for each film that enters the processor;

(ii) that it is worthwhile to maintain the cleanliness of the processor by maintaining the mechanical strength of the film-emulsions;

(iii) that oxidation is more likely at higher temperatures and must be resisted;

(iv) that pH must be controlled through effective buffering.

These points can be contrasted with the conditions that apply for manual processing. Of such a system it can be said:

(i) that replenishment is not continuous but is intermittent and for a given tank of solution is not maintained over periods of months;

(ii) that maintaining cleanliness through the chemicalization is less critical since tanks are readily emptied and cleaned when being **recharged** perhaps weekly with fresh developer;

(iii) that since tanks of developer are emptied and recharged relatively frequently, the problems of oxidation and the changing pH do not have to be resolved with such long-term effectiveness as in the case of automatic processing. Oxidation is in any event occurring to a lesser extent at the lower temperatures which are used.

REPLENISHING DEVELOPERS

The replenishers which are used in automatic processing require special formulation since the conditions of their use are not the same as those which apply in a manual processing system. Once the developer tank of an automatic processor has been recharged with fresh chemicals, it will not be emptied for recharging and cleaning until perhaps two or three months have passed. During this time of use it is continuously replenished to maintain its chemical activity, for every film which enters the processor leads to an injection of replenisher into the tank of developer which is working within the machine. This can be contrasted with the system in a manual processor when tanks are recharged with fresh chemicals perhaps on a weekly basis and the replenisher is added as occasion arises to make good the fall in solution level: this might be done once a day.

In an automatic processor it is important that the additions of fresh replenisher to a seasoned developer-solution in the working tank do not have such effects on chemical activity as to alter the response of the film and produce changes in the radiographic image. The machine is initially charged with a solution which is compounded as follows.

Developer-replenisher plus *developer-starter* gives the *working developer*.

The developer-replenisher is more alkaline than the working developer is required to be and it contains no restraining bromides. It is therefore, through the alkalinity and the absence of bromides, a very active solution, liable to produce fogging.

The developer-starter is intended to reduce this high activity. To that end, it contains an acid such as acetic acid to lower pH and a bromide such as potassium bromide to act as restrainer. When the replenisher and the starter are combined to give the working developer, the resultant solution is an artificially seasoned developer. This is suitable for continuous replenishment with fresh developer-replenisher as the processor functions.

If the starter solution is omitted, the pH is too high. This results in too high a speed in the developer; increased oxidation; too much swelling of the emulsion; as a result of the swelling, greater likelihood of damage, absorption of more developer to be carried over to contaminate the fixer, diminished cleanliness of the processor.

In a manual system, the working developer with which the tank is initially charged is rich in restrainer. Replenisher is a more active solution without restrainers and it is added to the tank to maintain its activity as this declines with use.

The situation for the two forms of processing is displayed in the table below.

Type of processing	Initial charge in tank	Replenishing addition
Automatic	(i) Small amount of starter with acids and restrainers **plus** (ii) replenisher with high pH and no restrainers	Replenisher with high pH and no restrainer
Manual	Working developer rich in restrainer	Replenisher with high pH and no restrainer

Chapter 7
Film Processing: Fixing

When a film is taken from the developer, the exposed and developed crystals of the silver halide emulsion have become black metallic silver and a complete image has been formed. The unexposed silver halide is not developed. It is practically insoluble in water, and at this stage remains in the emulsion as a light-sensitive material. If left there, it will darken and spoil the image when any prolonged exposure to light takes place.

The fixing process is therefore required to fix or make permanent the image by removing the silver halide, leaving the metallic silver image unaltered against a translucent background. The silver halide is removed by being changed to a complex silver substance. The compound formed is soluble in water, and it therefore dissolves in the water content of the fixing solution and is further washed away in a later stage of the processing cycle.

Secondary purposes of the fixing bath may be to stop further action by the developer absorbed in the swollen gelatin of the film, and to harden the film. Some hardening, as already mentioned, is done by the manufacturer who makes the emulsion, but it is helpful if the film can be further hardened while it is being processed. Hardening is important both in protecting the film from damage and in controlling the extent to which it swells through absorbing moisture.

INTERMEDIATE RINSE

In manual processing it is customary to use between development and fixing an intermediate stage known as a *rinse*. This is discussed in detail in Chapter 8, and for the moment it will be left alone.

CONSTITUTION OF THE FIXING SOLUTION

THE FIXING AGENT

The fixing agent is the constituent which converts the silver halide. To be suitable for the job the fixing agent is required to:
(i) react with silver halide to form a soluble compound;

(ii) leave the gelatin undamaged;
(iii) have no appreciable effect on the silver image;

SODIUM THIOSULPHATE

The most commonly used fixing agent is sodium thiosulphate, known to succeeding generations of photographers as 'hypo'. In an earlier nomenclature it was given the chemical name hyposulphite of soda, but today this is considered incorrect. Although the formal name is now sodium thiosulphate, the old abbreviation is firmly fixed, one might say, in common usage. It may be wrong to the pedants, but every photographer knows exactly what substance you mean when you say 'hypo'.

The chemical action of the hypo with silver bromide is to form a somewhat polysyllabic compound. The reaction can be expressed simply as follows.

Silver bromide + sodium thiosulphate→

sodium salt of monoargento-diothiosulphuric acid + sodium bromide
These compounds which form are soluble and are removed in water. The chemicals provided for use in modern X-ray departments are in liquid form. The old practice of mixing a fine white powder of anhydrous sodium thiosulphate to be dissolved in water is no longer with us and we now combine solutions of liquid concentrates with given volumes of water. Combining solutions with active stirring is quicker and simpler and it evades the nuisance of fine powders floating about in the air. The problem of an unpleasant smell which produces an acrid taste at the back of the mouth is still commonly encountered today but certain manufacturers seem to have almost eliminated it.

AMMONIUM THIOSULPHATE

Ammonium thiosulphate is another fixing agent in widespread use for proprietary products supplied as liquid concentrates.

The reaction between ammonium thiosulphate and silver bromide can be expressed thus:

Silver bromide + ammonium thiosulphate→

ammonium salt of monoargento-dithiosulphuric acid
+ ammonium bromide

It is thus similar to the action of sodium thiosulphate in that the result is an argentothiosulphate and a bromide which are soluble in water. These ammonium silver complexes are highly soluble in water and can be washed out of the film very quickly.

The ammonium complexes which form are less stable than the sodium complexes produced when hypo is the fixing agent. This is significant in practice because if the films are not completely washed, subsequent staining and deterioration in the image will be quicker in onset than if a hypo fixing bath is followed by inefficient washing.

Ammonium thiosulphate solutions fix more rapidly than their sodium thiosulphate counterparts in equivalent concentrations and rapid fixing solutions are therefore based on ammonium thiosulphate.

In addition to the fixing agents, other constituents are present in X-ray fixers. These are considered below.

THE ACID, THE STABILIZER, THE BUFFER

Development must not be allowed to continue in the presence of fixing agents. The function of an intermediate bath between the developer and fixer is to stop the action of the developer before the film reaches the fixing stage. Developer carried into the fixing bath in or on the film and continuing its action can have certain possible effects.

(i) Development continuing in the presence of the fixing agent can cause *dichroic fog*. This is an unmistakable stain which appears greenish-blue when examined by reflected light, and pinkish when viewed by transmitted light; hence its name which means showing two colours. The stain is really a deposit of silver finely divided, and it is produced by the action of the developer reducing silver salts which the fixer has put into solution. It can thus occur both when the fixing bath (which is usually acid) is contaminated by developer (which is alkaline), and when the developing bath is contaminated by the fixer. So it is sound practice never to let these two meet.

(ii) Developer transferred to the fixing bath can produce another type of stain—that of the brown final oxidation products of oxidized developer. This becomes particularly obvious under the influence of electrolysis which may be applied to the bath for the purpose of silver recovery. (Electrolytic silver recovery is discussed in detail later in this chapter.)

(iii) Prolongation of development after the film leaves the developer can produce streaks on the radiograph.

In order to preserve the film from these ills, it is usual to include in the fixing solution a suitable acid. Since the developer needs an alkaline environment before it can act, acidification of the fixing bath halts the further action of any developer which may be left in the film; some developer is *bound* to be carried into the fixing bath. The acidity of the fixer is important also in its effect on the efficiency of hardening agents as discussed in the next section.

Strong acids spoil hypo and precipitate sulphur with an accelerating deterioration of the bath. So a weak acid is used, and acetic acid is frequently chosen. There is still some tendency by the thiosulphate solution to decompose and precipitate sulphur, even although the acid is not strong. To prevent this, it is usual to include in the solution a preservative or stabilizer. This can be a sulphite, a bisulphite, or a metabisulphite; with acetic acid as the acidifier the preservative is often sodium sulphite.

An alternative method of providing for acidification and stabilization is to use one compound to do the work of two. Such a compound would be an acid sulphite such as sodium metabisulphite or potassium metabisulphite; these are commonly used.

There is another function to be considered—that is buffering the solution. The bath is acidified to a pH of about 4·0 to 5·0, but in use this figure tends to rise owing to the carry-over of some alkaline developer in the films. It is therefore general practice to buffer acid fixing baths so that the pH will be maintained. Pairs of agents used for this purpose are sodium acetate and acetic acid; and sodium sulphite and sodium bisulphite.

To sum up: (i) the fixing solution must include (a) an acid, (b) a stabilizer, and (c) a buffer. Some of the compounds used are able to serve in more than one capacity. (ii) A typical combination is: acid—acetic acid, stabilizer—sodium sulphite, buffer—acetic acid and sodium acetate. (iii) Sodium metabisulphite and potassium metabisulphite each can be used for the double function of providing both an acid and a stabilizer, and they have some buffering action as well.

THE HARDENER

The emulsion layer of a film absorbs moisture and swells during processing. As Fig. 7.1 shows, it can become several times thicker than it was in the dry state. This swelling is most marked during the water-rinse and washing stages because where solutions have a high salt concentration (as in the developer and fixer) only a limited amount of swelling takes place. For the same reason, swelling is greater in soft water than in hard.

Hardening of the emulsion during fixing, as the graph shows, results in its being less swollen at the end of the wet processing cycle. Efficient hardening has certain beneficial effects.

(i) The temperature at which the gelatin softens is raised. This means that much higher temperatures can safely be used for processing films.

(ii) The gelatin absorbs less water, and therefore can be dried more quickly.

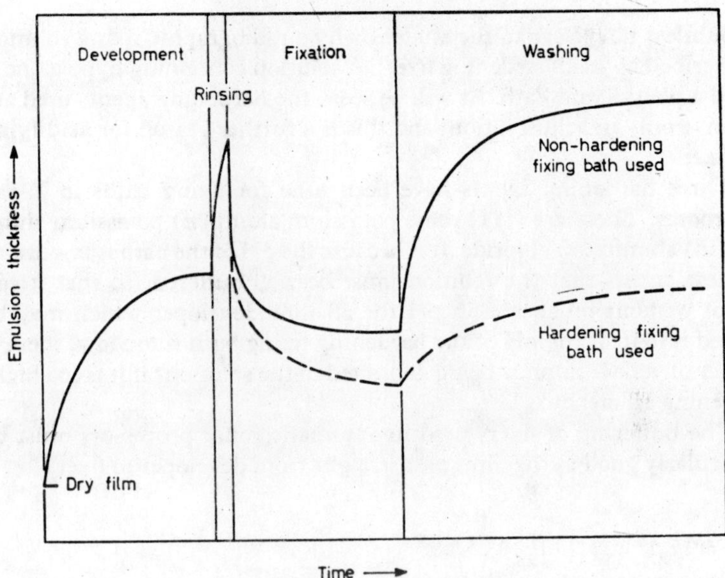

Fig. 7.1. Changes in emulsion thickness during processing. *By courtesy of Ilford Ltd.*

(iii) The film is much less susceptible to physical damage such as scratches, abrasions, and other marks on the surface.

(iv) The radiographs can be put safely through rapid driers at high temperatures.

All these points are of practical importance in the functioning of modern automatic processors with a complete cycle time of a few minutes: the most usual cycle time now is 1·5 to 2·0 minutes. The hardening of the film ensures that it will be washed and dried in the times available (since the hardened emulsion absorbs less solution) and that the cleanliness of the processor will not suffer from the film's adhesion to the rollers, a trouble which is particularly likely to occur if a soft emulsion is put through the drier.

X-ray films are hardened by manufacturers by means of hardening agents incorporated in the emulsion, but it is necessary to do some further hardening during processing if the desired results are to be obtained. Hardening *can* be a separate stage of the processing cycle, and it can be done during development as is done in automatic processing by roller processors. It is conveniently, commonly and in radiographic darkrooms universally done during the stage of fixing.

Hardening agents are incorporated as constituents in fixing baths; it is doubtless now clear to the student why a radiographic fixing solution is described as 'acid hardening fixer'. A solution containing hypo alone is called a plain fixing bath. As will be seen, the hardening agents used are effective only in acid solution, and this is a further reason for acidifying the fixer.

Three hardening agents have been used for fixing baths in X-ray darkrooms. These are (i) chrome potassium alum, (ii) potassium alum, and (iii) aluminium chloride. It is because the pH of the bath is important to these agents that the solution must be well buffered, so that it can accept without much rise in pH the alkaline developer which may be carried into it. If the pH of the hardening fixing bath is too low, there is danger of yellow sulphur being deposited in the solution; if it is too high, hardening efficiency is lost.

The buffering of fixers used in automatic roller processors must be particularly good as the films pass straight from developer to fixer.

CHROME ALUM AS HARDENER

Chrome alum was commonly used as a hardener at one time and a fresh solution of it is a very efficient hardening agent, said to be more efficient than a solution of potassium alum. Chrome alum as a hardener has a great disadvantage; it does not keep its efficiency for more than a few days. Once the solution has been made up, this loss of hardening action will occur whether it is being used or is simply standing in a tank and the hardening action will fall to zero in a few days; it is a fact that very prolonged keeping will restore the hardening action, but perhaps this is not very useful in view of what happens first!

Chrome alum is therefore suitable for a hardening fixing solution which is to be used soon after preparation and not used for long.

Chrome alum is critical in its demands concerning the pH at which it works effectively and the range is 3·5 to 4·7. Above 4·7 there is little hardening action, and chrome alum hardens most efficiently at the lower pH; but where it forms part of a hardening fixing bath there is the risk of sulphurization at that level of acidity.

POTASSIUM ALUM AS HARDENER

Potassium alum retains its hardening properties well with time, almost indefinitely, and has its greatest efficiency at a higher pH—from 4·5 to 4·9. At raised pH, hardening continues up to the region of 5·5 but it does not survive a pH above 6.

In acid hardening fixing baths there is danger at pH values beyond 5·5 that a white 'bloom' (a precipitate of aluminium hydroxide with potassium alum hardener) may appear on the film.

ALUMINIUM CHLORIDE AS HARDENER

Aluminium chloride can be used in a concentrated hardener solution. It is normally associated with the rapid ammonium thiosulphate fixers and allows hardening to be completed in the very short time that the film remains in such a bath. The optimum pH for its hardening action is 4·1 to 4·4.

In the composition of any acid hardening fixing bath sufficient hardener is allowed for the bath to keep its hardening properties as long as it is in use, and for it to harden films efficiently during the length of time allowed for their immersion.

THE SOLVENT

The solvent and diluent for fixing solutions is always water, and the reader is referred to page 133 where water as a solvent for photographic chemicals is discussed.

OTHER ADDITIONS

Boric acid is introduced into the solution to function as an anti-sludging agent. The sludge in question is the white precipitate which appears in fixing baths when the pH rises too high, particularly with potassium alum and aluminium chloride hardeners. Boric acid delays the precipitation of this sludge.

FIXERS USED IN AUTOMATIC PROCESSORS

The formulation of fixing solutions which are to be used in automatic processors must be undertaken carefully with regard to the special problems which may arise. The fixing agent used is ammonium thiosulphate because this is suitable for the concentrated solutions which the manufacturers provide to prepare the chemical charges of the machines.

Any intermediate rinse between the developer and the fixer is omitted and the film is mechanically taken straight from the developer tank into the fixer tank. The purposes of the rinse as it is used in manual processing are to halt developer-action and to diminish the amount of active developer which the film carries over into the fixer. In an automatic processor the omission of the rinsing stage helps to shorten the cycle-time and the film carries very little developer out of the tank because the squeegee action of the transporting rollers removes solution from the surfaces of the film. The absence of a rinse raises two significant points, as follows.

(i) The rapid change in pH between the two solutions (developer and fixer) causes the gelatin of the film to swell, nullifying the effect of the hardener contained in the developer. If the film is to be successfully dried in the shortened periods implicit in automatic processing, it must be re-hardened in the fixing solution.

(ii) The pH of the fixer will rise owing to the carry-over of developer absorbed in the emulsion and this rise may be sufficient to cause the hardener to be thrown out of the solution. The fixer must therefore be buffered particularly well in order to prevent an undue rise in pH from occurring. High buffer capacity is an essential characteristic of the fixers used in automatic processing.

Any fixing solution in use accumulates silver thiosulphate complexes; these (a) retard fixing action and (b) inhibit the rapid removal of fixer by the wash-water. In the case of manual processing a gradually slowing fixing rate probably does not matter very much up to a certain limit. In automatic processing, fixing must be completed and adequate washing must be given within specific and very short periods of time. For these reasons there are certain recommended levels above which the silver concentration in the fixing tank should not be allowed to rise. The levels are: 5–7 grammes of silver per litre in machines with cycles less than 3 minutes;

9–10 grammes of silver per litre in machines with cycles of 3 minutes.

Fixing solutions for automatic processors have the following constituents:

(1) ammonium thiosulphate as the fixing agent;

(ii) a salt such as aluminium chloride to harden the film while it is in the fixer;

(iii) acetic acid to keep the pH in the acid range and to buffer the solution well so that it stays at 4 to 5 pH;

(iv) sodium sulphite as a preservative for the fixing agent.

Fixers for automatic processors are supplied as liquid concentrates which are diluted with water to give solutions of correct working strength in accordance with the manufacturers' instructions.

FACTORS AFFECTING THE USE OF THE FIXER

The first stage in fixing a film material is diffusion of the fixing agent into the gelatin of the emulsion. This is followed by a chemical action involving fixing agent and silver bromide and oxygen from the air to form soluble complexes and soluble halides in accordance with the relationships given on page 150. These substances go into solution, and in the last stages of fixing are diffused to some extent out of the emulsion.

The process is accompanied by an observable effect—the disappearance of visible traces of the unexposed and undeveloped silver halide on which the fixer is acting. The milky-yellow regions of the image as it comes out of the developer vanish in the fixing bath, and the deposits of black metallic silver are seen, not against an opaque yellow ground, but on a clear transparent base.

When this observable effect is complete the film is said to be *cleared*, and the time which is taken by this is called suitably enough the *clearing-time*. The time taken for the whole process in its three stages is known as the *fixing-time*. In any processing system it is important that the film not only is fixed within the time that it stays in the fixing bath but also is effectively hardened by the action of the hardeners present in the solution.

In a manual system of processing it is possible of course to give films long immersion in a fixing bath. They might be left for an hour or more or even forgetfully abandoned overnight.

Sodium thiosulphate given time exercises a weak solvent action on the silver image itself, particularly in an acid solution; ammonium thiosulphate can do this too, somewhat more quickly. The result can be a film which emerges from the fixing bath as a pale shadow of what it was when it went in.

Several factors affect the rate of clearing and the fixing rate. These are listed below.

(i) The type of fixing agent used.

(ii) The concentration of the fixing agent.

(iii) The temperature of the solution.

(iv) The presence of aluminium salts such as potassium alum or aluminium chloride used as hardeners.

(v) The film material—screen-type or direct-exposure film.

(vi) Agitation of the film during fixing.

(vii) Exhaustion of the fixing bath.

THE FIXING AGENT USED

We need be concerned here only with the two fixing agents which have been previously discussed—sodium thiosulphate and ammonium thiosulphate. As mentioned in the previous discussion, ammonium thiosulphate is more rapid in action than sodium thiosulphate when they are compared in equivalent concentrations.

THE CONCENTRATION OF THE FIXING AGENT

For wet films it is true to say that higher concentrations of fixing agent result in shorter clearing times.

THE TEMPERATURE OF THE SOLUTION

Temperature affects the clearing-time, which decreases as the temperature of the solution is raised. Generally at higher temperatures diffusion processes take place more quickly and the gelatin is more readily permeable. It is, however, unnecessary to control the temperature of fixing baths in radiographic darkrooms as strictly as that of developing solutions. There should not be too marked a difference between the two, and obviously if the fixer is at too high a temperature the gelatin will swell too much, may soften unduly, and can give rise to many difficulties.

THE PRESENCE OF HARDENERS

Potassium alum and aluminium chloride lengthen the clearing-time of solutions in which they are present. Where speed in fixing is a sole consideration it might be logical to leave them out but if they are left out the film takes longer to dry: its lack of hardness makes it absorb more water. So in automatic processing a hardener is included in the fixing solution to shorten the drying time, despite its lengthening of the clearing time. The amount is adjusted to ensure that fixing takes place in the time allotted to it. If there is too much hardener the fixing may be so slow that it does not occur at all in the film's progress through the tank.

The physical hardness of an emulsion does not have much effect on the fixing rate. An unhardened emulsion offers less hindrance to diffusion, but at the same time it is more swollen and diffusion paths are consequently longer.

THE TYPE OF FILM MATERIAL

Various features of a photographic emulsion alter the rate at which the material clears. These are: (i) the silver halide used: silver bromide fixes more quickly than silver iodide; (ii) the grain size: small grains not unexpectedly dissolve in less time than larger grains; (iii) the thickness of the emulsion layer: since most of the fixing time is taken up by diffusion of soluble salts out of the emulsion layer and not by chemical action, and since diffusion can take place more rapidly in thin layers, thinly coated materials clear more quickly.

AGITATION OF THE FILM

Since the fixing process mostly depends on diffusion, agitating the film increases the rate at which it clears. Agitation prevents the collection of a layer of exhausted fixer near the film surface; fresh fixer can then swirl against the film and will significantly decrease the time required for clearing. In automatic processors, the circulation of the fixer and the mechanical movement of the film through the tank are both important to accomplish complete fixing in the very short times that each film stays in the fixer. According to the cycle time of the processor, the fixing period varies from 15 to 131 seconds. Radiographs manually processed receive little agitation in the fixer. Lack of agitation in the early stages is regrettable. If the film is agitated in the first few seconds of its arrival in the fixer bath, any developer carried with it is soon neutralized.

EXHAUSTION OF THE FIXING BATH

Practical experience again soon teaches us that a used fixing bath takes longer to clear films than a fresh one does. Indeed this longer time is taken as an indication of the state of exhaustion of the bath. With use the following changes occur in the composition of the solution and slow its action in a manual system of processing.

(i) There is increasing dilution of the bath as water from the rinse is carried in and fixer is carried out with the passage of films. There is thus reduction in the concentration of hypo; another cause of reduced concentration is that the fixing agent is used up. From either cause this decreased concentration materially affects the clearing rate.

(ii) There is steady accumulation of soluble silver complexes—the argentothiosulphates resulting from the reactions on page 150. When these compounds are in solution silver ions are liberated, and the presence of these ions retards the chemical action.

(iii) There is steady accumulation of soluble halides in accordance with the previously mentioned reactions. In fixing solutions used for processing radiographs, these halides will be bromides and iodides. Both slow down the fixing action, particularly the soluble iodide even although it may be present in a very small amount.

REGENERATION OF FIXING SOLUTIONS

REPLENISHMENT IN AUTOMATIC PROCESSORS

From what has been said in the preceding paragraphs, it is clear that as a fixing solution is used the time taken for the film to be completely fixed becomes longer. If the fixing solution is in no way regenerated, the duration of its useful life depends upon the following factors:

(i) the number of films passing through the solution;

(ii) the amounts of silver halides and the silver bromide/iodide ratios within the emulsions of the film materials which are processed;

(iii) the area of silver halide on each film which is left for removal in the fixing bath.

In regard to this last point, it will be recalled from the previous chapter that different radiographic subjects result in different amounts of silver halide being made developable: the rest must be removed by the fixing solution. It can be said of any radiograph that where it is not developed it must be fixed and it has been estimated that in the average run of radiographs through a busy general X-ray department about two-thirds of the total area of silver halide which is processed is not developable and must be removed in the fixing solution. In a system of automatic processing the fixing must be accomplished unvaryingly within the time allotted for the film to pass through that section of the processor. So the fixer must be regenerated as it is used. To meet this requirement, the machines function to inject into the working tanks certain amounts of a fixer replenisher as films are processed. The squeegee action of the rollers which transport the films removes solution from their surfaces: so very little is taken out of the fixing tank as each film leaves it. In order to make room in the tank for the injected replenisher, certain amounts of the fixing solution are bled off.

The fixer replenisher is constituted similarly to the fixer and contains the following:

(i) a fixing agent to replace what is used;

(ii) acetic acid to provide hydrogen ions and buffer the solution so that it stays in the 4 to 5 pH range;

(iii) a hardener to offset the loss of hardening powers;

(iv) sodium sulphite to preserve the fixing agent.

The soluble silver complexes and the soluble halides which are mentioned in the previous section on the exhaustion of the fixer should not accumulate since as the fixer is used some of the solution is bled off and unused replenisher is injected.

When the processor is freshly charged with new fixer in its working tank and it begins to be used, the replenisher should then be automatically added at such a rate that after a small initial rise in pH the pH is then reasonably constant and the amount of silver present in the fixer does not much change.

The replenishers are supplied as liquid concentrates. These are then mixed with added water in accordance with the manufacturer's instructions and given volumes of working-strength replenisher are thus obtained.

REPLENISHMENT IN MANUAL PROCESSING SYSTEMS

As we have previously explained, a fixing bath becomes progressively much weaker in its action as it works if no system of regeneration is used to halt such decline. The effects of using a fixing bath which is nearly exhausted are as follows.

(i) Long clearing time and eventually inadequate fixing. There is a tendency for the film to retain unfixed silver halide and unstable silver complexes which may not be eliminated by washing. The end result may be a stained radiograph.

(ii) The film may be inadequately hardened.

(iii) The radiograph may have developer stains.

(iv) The radiograph may be marked with deposited scum.

The duration of useful life for a fixing bath depends upon the following factors:

(i) the number of films passing through the solution;

(ii) the silver halide-content of the emulsions which are processed;

(iii) the area of silver halide which is left on each radiograph for removal in the fixing bath;

(iv) the operator's technique. Dilution of the bath by the transfer of rinse-water into it and of fixer out of it with the passage of films will vary. An operator who drains the film carefully over the rinse and over the fixing bath in turn, so that the drainings return to their source, will minimize but not prevent this dilution.

To keep a fixing bath in useful action within a system of manual processing there are clearly two things to be done: (i) to maintain the level of the solution as it falls with the passage of films out of the tank; (ii) to sustain its chemical activity to an acceptable standard such that the clearing times are not over-long and films can be adequately fixed.

The level of the solution is simply maintained by adding fresh fixer as it falls. This helps also to sustain the chemical activity since the added solution contains: (i) fixing agent to replace what is being used; (ii) acid to counteract the changing pH which is rising because alkaline developer is carried over into the fixer; (iii) hardener to offset the loss of hardening power; (iv) sulphite to maintain the quantity of preservative which is present.

Despite this regeneration, the used solution continues to accumulate soluble silver complexes and soluble halides which result from the chemical actions indicated at the beginning of this chapter. These accumulations retard the fixing action and extend the clearing time. In a manual processing system, the increase in clearing time has been taken to indicate when a fixing solution is exhausted. It has been said that the fixer should be discarded when it takes twice as long to clear the film as it did when it was fresh. Other methods for estimating exhaustion are: (i) to consider the solution exhausted after it has been in use for a given amount of time (say, a fresh charge of fixer is prepared for use and the previous one discarded from the tank every Monday morning); (ii) to assess the silver-content by means of silver-estimating papers and discard the solution when the quantity of silver in it has reached a certain pre-selected amount.

An advisable system for maintaining and using fixer tanks in manual processing is a two-bath technique. This means simply that two separate fixer tanks are established and when the film is taken out of the developer it is put into the first fixer tank for its initial fixing. When it has cleared it is passed into the second tank where the fixing process is completed. Such a technique causes the first fixer tank to exhaust more rapidly than the second but allows its use to a point of greater exhaustion than could be tolerated if it were a single tank which must do all the fixing that was to be done for each film. When it is time to discard the fixer in the first tank, the second is put into the position of being the first tank in use and it receives the films as they come from the developer. Newly charged with fresh fixing solution, the previous first tank assumes the role of being the second.

SILVER RECOVERY

In a photographic context the term *silver recovery* means the reclamation of silver after it has been used for its intended photographic purposes. There are two main sources of such silver as is recoverable: these are (i) exhausted processing solutions; (ii) discarded film materials and photographic papers.

The photographic industry as a whole uses about one-quarter to one-third of all the silver put to industrial use and it is said that about two-thirds of the quantity used by the photographic industry is potentially to be recovered. A diagnostic X-ray department using films is of course part of the industrial consumption of silver and silver is to be recovered from our used fixing solutions and from exposed and processed radiographs which are being discarded. In used fixers, silver is present in the silver complexes which result from the chemical action of the fixing agents. In processed radiographs, the silver is the black metallic deposits that form the photographic densities of exposed and developed films and constitute the images on them.

It has been said of the fixer solutions which are used to process medical X-ray films that the amounts of silver recoverable potentially if not in practice are 3,000 to 6,000 grams for every 1,000 square metres of film processed; and that every kilogram of discarded radiographs (exposed and processed films) could yield from 6·4 grams to 25·5 grams according to the type of film used. What are the reasons for seeking to recover any portion of these amounts?

REASONS FOR SILVER RECOVERY

The reasons for silver recovery come under two main headings according to whether they relate to the economy or to the environment. The reasons are as follows:

(i) silver is a natural resource which is becoming scarcer and so its conservation is important;

(ii) silver commands a high price and so its recovery is profitable;

(iii) recovering this valuable commodity helps to save costs;

(iv) recovery from fixer solutions can result in more efficient use of the chemicals, greater permanency in the images which are fixed, a diminution in the costs of chemicals and in some special processes the recycling of fixers for further use;

(v) fixer solutions which are discharged down the drains with their content of silver in no way removed are wasteful in the views of economists and in the judgement of ecologists are polluting to the environment. So it is better not to send large amounts of silver down drains.

SILVER RECOVERY IN X-RAY DEPARTMENTS

The above considerations certainly answer the question: why should silver recovery be practised in an X-ray department? The next question to follow is: can the silver be recovered to the full potential extent? The answer to that one is: probably no.

Important factors which influence the amounts of silver actually recovered from used fixers in X-ray departments include (i) the efficiency of the recovery system and the recovering apparatus which are used; (ii) the types of films which are processed; (iii) the radiographic subjects, since these influence the area of the film which is developable and the area which, remaining to be fixed, will consequently put silver complexes into the fixer; (iv) the amounts of silver carried out of the fixer tank on the surfaces of the processed films to be lost irrecoverably in a state of dispersion in the washing water.

In automatic systems of processing only minimal amounts of fixer solution are carried over by the films as they pass from the fixer tank into the washing section of the processor. This is mainly because the squeegee action of the rollers which transport them removes much of the solution. So in a properly functioning automatic processor the loss of silver through this carry-over could be said to be contained.

In manual processing the amount of solution which is carried over by each film varies with the practice of whoever is moving it from the fixer into the wash tank. If the film is barely drained and is moved quickly into the wash-water, it will take with it an appreciable amount of the fixer solution. If the film is held carefully over the fixer tank and the solution from its surfaces is allowed to drain back into the tank, then clearly the amount to be carried into the washing water is very much less.

In a system of manual processing a two-bath technique for the fixing section has already been described. When this is used, the silver content of the second bath is kept to a minimum since most of the chemical action for the fixing of each radiograph is carried out in the first tank. Furthermore, since the fixing is completed and the action of the hardeners is fully accomplished in the second tank, the first tank can be allowed to reach a state of being more heavily loaded with silver complexes than would be acceptable if it were the only fixer in use. Silver recovery can be more effectively carried out from used fixers when the silver content is higher.

Within X-ray departments, the recovery of silver is undertaken in practice from used fixer solutions but is not attempted from scrap films. To recover the silver from these it is usual to sell them to a firm that purchases such material and refines the silver in it. This procedure implies the availability of large amounts of scrap film, for the refiners are not likely to judge it economic to deal with quantities below a certain minimum: small amounts would not be worth the cost of collection. From time to time departments do have large collections of scrap films which are being discarded: for example, the removal of out-of-date radiographs from old records. It is then to be recommended that the radiographs should go for the recovery of the silver which they bear. To do otherwise is reprehensibly wasteful.

RECOVERING SILVER FROM FIXER SOLUTIONS

There are several methods of recovering silver from used fixer solutions. We enumerate these as follows:
(i) electrolytic methods, based upon the fact that if two electrodes are put into a fixer solution which carries silver in it and a direct current is

passed from one electrode to the other then nearly pure silver plates on the cathode;

(ii) metallic replacement, based upon the fact that when a metal such as copper or iron or zinc is put into a solution which has a silver salt in it an exchange takes place in which the base metal dissolves to replace the silver and the silver is deposited out of solution;

(iii) chemical methods (called sludging), based upon interactions occurring when certain chemicals are added to a silver-loaded fixer and silver is precipitated in a finely divided state;

(iv) galvanic methods, based upon a process which immerses in the fixer solution two dissimilar metals in contact with each other, with the result that silver from the solution plates out on the immersed metal sheet.

We need concern ourselves here only with the methods that radiographers may encounter in X-ray departments. We limit our discussions to the techniques of electrolysis and of metal replacement, the other two categories receiving here no further consideration.

Electrolytic silver recovery sounds a simple process indeed, for it entails putting two electrodes into a silver-salt solution and establishing a voltage between them. Silver then plates out upon the cathode.

The process is a straightforward one when the solution for electrolysis contains a simple silver salt in which the silver is present in the form of positively charged silver ions. The silver ions are naturally attracted to the cathode, their charge is there neutralized, and silver is deposited. It requires only a small potential difference to be maintained between the electrodes, and the greater the electrolytic current flowing the more rapidly is silver deposited.

The first problem in electrolysis of a used fixing bath is that the silver which loads it is not a docile positive ion. It will be remembered that we are dealing here with complex argentothiosulphates in solution. The ions involved are negatively charged, and will migrate not towards the cathode but away from it (Fig. 7.2).

These complex ions do make some concessions in so far as they undergo dissociation, and give rise to a very small proportion of positive silver ions. These few positive ions move to the cathode, and silver is deposited. As these few silver ions are reduced, there is further dissociation to a limited extent to make up their number, and thus a slow continuous deposition of silver can theoretically take place.

It can be seen, however, that the reluctance of the complex argentothiosulphate ions to approach the negative electrode results in a deficiency of them in the region of the cathode, and a deficiency also of the positive silver ions which they produce on dissociation. The cathode therefore will quickly be at a loss for silver ions. Since it is a determined

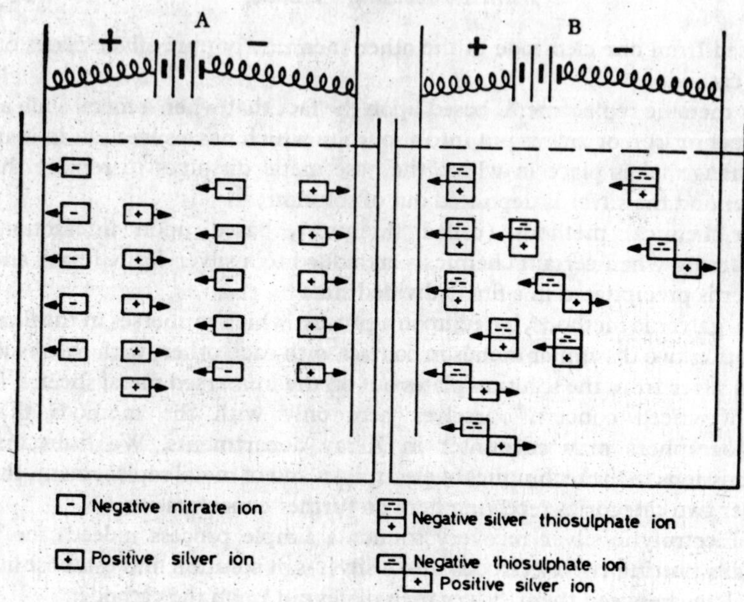

Fig. 7.2. A: electrolysis of a simple silver salt solution (silver nitrate). B: electrolysis of a used fixer.

In the used fixer the complex silver thiosulphate ions are negative and are attracted to the anode. They can dissociate to give a small proportion of positive silver ions.

acceptor of positive ions, in the absence of silver the cathode attempts to plate out some of the thiosulphate ions of the fixing salt itself. This has a disastrous result, for the thiosulphate ions break up. One of the products formed is silver sulphide, and this has the power to react with unexposed silver halide. Films put into a fixing bath where silver sulphide has formed become the victims of sulphide fog, and the fixing solution is soon unusable.

These disasters are avoided in a solution which is violently agitated all the time that silver recovery is in progress. Agitation forces the argentothiosulphate ions to go where they are wanted—towards the cathode—and this reduces the risk of sulphiding which is promoted by lack of silver ions near the negative electrode.

In a silver recovery system where the fixer is static and is not agitated, sulphiding can be avoided if the voltage across the electrodes is kept sufficiently below the critical level at which sulphiding begins. It is not possible to give a fixed figure for this since the value is dependent upon variables which include the type of fixer and the work it is doing.

The two electrodes in a silver recovery unit are usually a carbon anode (or anodes) and a stainless steel cathode upon which the silver plates as the unit operates. Every so often the cathode is removed and the recovered silver is stripped by chipping or breaking it away from the steel cathode. A control system allows the unit to be operated from the alternating mains at the correct voltage and current values.

The area of the cathode and the value of the current are importantly related in an entity which is called the current density: this is milliamperes per unit area of cathode. For any particular recovery unit, the optimum current density for its operation is indicated by the manufacturer. If the current density at which a unit is operating is higher than it should be, silver sulphide forms. An indication that this event is imminent appears in the colour and texture of the silver that plates on the cathode for it becomes brown-tinged and loose instead of the firm creamy-white deposit that it should be. If a silver recovery unit operates at a current density which is below the recommended value, than the process is wasteful: silver is not being recovered at a high enough rate. So the unit is not recovering silver to maximum efficiency and potentially recoverable silver is being needlessly lost.

The situation may be reviewed as follows.

(i) If there is no agitation of the fixer solution and the silver recovery unit operates in a static tank of fixer, then it must be of the type which functions at a low current density. Such a unit usually has a cathode which is in the form of a stainless steel plate, large in area to keep the current density low.

(ii) If there is brisk agitation of the fixer, then units operating at high current-density may be used. These give a faster rate of recovery and are more efficient. It is usual to make the cathode in the form of a screw (like a many-bladed ship's propellor or the screw-formed cutting part of an ordinary domestic mincing machine used in our kitchens). The agitation is achieved by rotating this screw-cathode while the unit operates and also in certain units by recirculating the fixer.

(iii) Sulphiding of the fixer occurs when there is an insufficiency of silver available at the cathode. This lack of silver at the cathode can arise from two causes: (a) the fixer has not been used sufficiently for its content of silver to be high enough to provide the silver ions for plating out silver on the cathode; (b) the fixer solution which is immediately adjacent to the cathode has had the silver ions plated out from it and, because the solution is not agitated, a new supply of silver-laden fixer is not forced into contact with the cathode.

(iv) Sulphiding is more likely to occur when the following conditions operate:

(a) the silver-content of the bath is very low, either because the fixer has not yet done enough work or because the current-density is too high for the amount of agitation being given;

(b) the fixer has become insufficiently acid with use, for the more alkaline the fixer is then the more probably will sulphiding occur and a pH value in the 4 to 5 range appears to be optimum for electrolytic silver recovery;

(c) the sulphite concentration in the bath is low (it falls with use of the bath and when it is high there is less tendency for the sulphiding reaction to occur);

(d) the fixer is based on sodium thiosulphate (as opposed to ammonium thiosulphate fixers, which can tolerate a higher current-density without sulphiding).

(v) The indications of sulphiding are muddy (not granular), black silver on the cathode, a dark, cloudy fixer solution and a smell of bad eggs.

PRACTICAL ELECTROLYTIC SILVER RECOVERY IN AUTOMATIC PROCESSING

An automatic processor which is operating properly has a system of replenishment whereby certain amounts of fresh fixer solution are injected into the working tank as the films enter the machine. In order to make room in the tank for these injections, equivalent amounts must be bled off and discarded. Before the solution goes down the drain, silver that is available in it should be recovered and can be recovered by passing the solution from the outflow point of the processor to an electrolytic unit for the recovery of the silver.

Such units which are intended to operate on the overflow from automatic processors function at high current-densities with screw-type cathodes which rotate to agitate the fixer while silver recovery is in progress. From the electrolytic unit the emerging desilvered fixer is usually discarded down the drain. In some special systems the desilvered fixer is recirculated in the automatic processor and used again.

Self-contained and automatically operating electrolytic units may be used to recover silver from the outflowing fixer of automatic processors. A unit of this type basically comprises two separate tanks. The first of these receives the fixer from the automatic processor and it is called a receiving tank, a balance tank or a holding tank. No electrolytic plating out of the silver occurs in it and its function is to hold the discharged fixer until the level in the balance tank has reached a certain measure: a device in the tank can sense when the critical level has been attained.

In reaction to this device, the fixer in the holding tank is allowed to go at a pre-determined rate into the second tank: this is the plating one where the electrolysis actually occurs. When the fixer goes into the plating tank, the electrolytic unit is automatically switched on and functions as it should to recover silver. The electrolytic unit is automatically switched off when the recovery of silver from the volume of fixer in the plating tank has reduced the concentration of silver in the fixer solution to about 0·5 g per litre. When the level of the solution in the balance tank falls to a certain point, the unit is switched off until more fixer from the processor raises it to the level which again initiates a metered flow into the plating tank.

Fig. 7.3 shows a flow diagram for such an automatic recovery unit

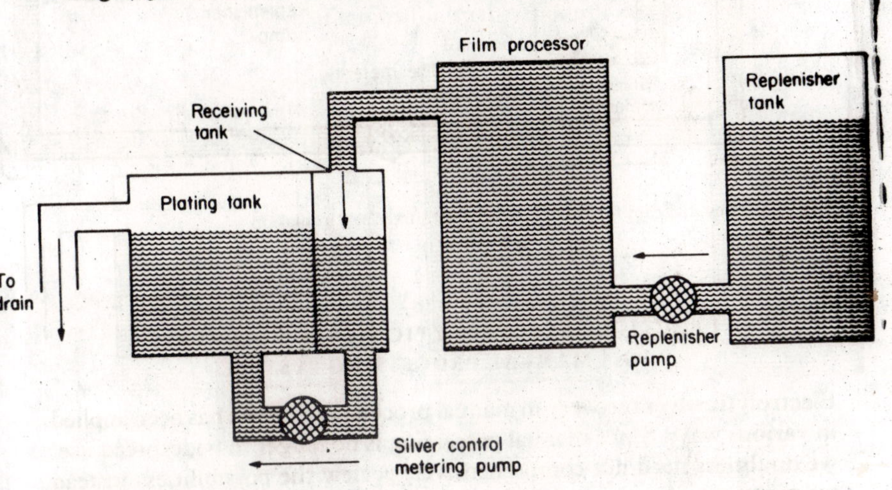

Fig. 7.3. Flow diagram for silver recovery

with metered control of the fixer and Fig. 7.4 shows the flow diagram for such a unit which incorporates a re-cycling system for the fixer.

The advantages of a metered unit which functions automatically are as follows:

(i) the recovery is at a rate which is optimum for the silver-content of the fixer;

(ii) because of this optimum recovery rate, sulphiding should not occur and at the other extreme there should be minimum waste of silver which is not recovered;

(iii) the automatic operation adapts the unit to fluctuating work-loads;

(iv) in the plating tank high current-density is used;

(v) the unit requires for its efficient operation very little attention from the staff of the X-ray department and this is a worthy advantage for those who are very busy.

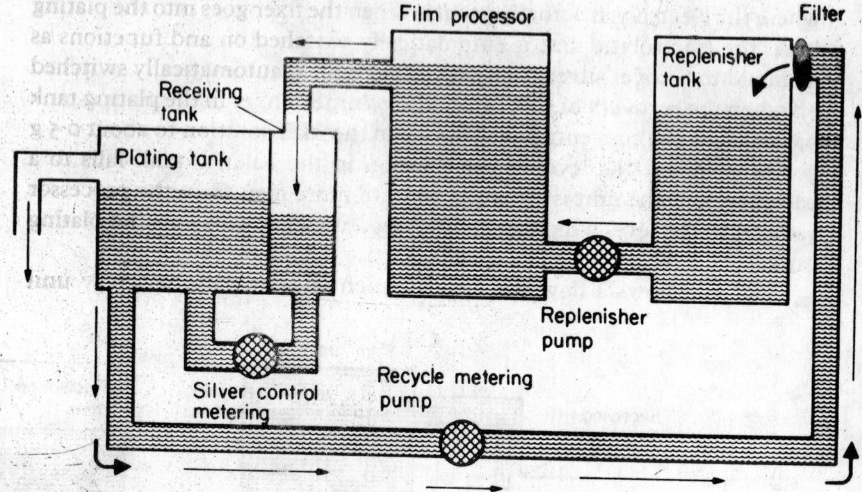

Fig. 7.4. Flow diagram for silver recovery with fixer re-circulation.

PRACTICAL ELECTROLYTIC SILVER RECOVERY IN A MANUAL PROCESSING SYSTEM

Electrolytic silver recovery in manual processing systems has been applied in various ways. Since manual processing is no longer in widespread use, we doubtless need not comprehensively review the possibilities: instead we mention only two systems.

(i) An electrolytic silver recovery unit can be operated in a tank which is being used to fix films simultaneously with electrolysis of the solution. In this case, the fixer receives no positive agitation and so the unit must function at a low current-density. The cathode is a stainless steel plate with a large area and it is placed to one side of the tank.

It is important to remember that the unit must not be switched on in a tank which has just been recharged with fresh fixer solution. There is then no silver present to be recovered and silver sulphide will form to wreck the fixer. Only when the fixer has been in use for a while and has a certain content of silver (say, above 5 g per litre) should the recovery unit be switched to operate.

The rate of recovery is slower than the rates which are achievable with high current-density units. To be efficient the recovery of silver should take place at the same rate as silver is released into the working fixer. When the department is closed and no films are being processed, either the recovery unit must be switched off or its current must be reduced to a very low value.

(ii) Another method is to save the discarded fixer when the tank is being given a fresh charge. A silver refiner could provide a service to collect it, purchasing the silver recovered from the used solution. Alternatively, the fixer to be discarded could be put through an automatic silver recovery unit if the department has one which is serving other processors. In that case, it is important to be sure that the recovery unit can handle the volume of fixer which is being put into it.

SILVER RECOVERY BY METAL REPLACEMENT

The method of recovering silver by the replacement of metals rests upon the fact that if base metals such as copper, iron and zinc are put into a solution which contains silver salts, the base metals dissolve and the silver is deposited out of solution in exchange. This reaction can be used to recover silver from fixing solutions which it is not proposed to use again: so it can be employed to treat fixing solutions which issue as the outflow from automatic processors.

It is usual to apply this method by means of a self-contained vessel or silver recovery cartridge. Such a cartridge consists of:

(i) a holding tank to contain the fixer whilst silver is being recovered from it;

(ii) a charge of base metal in which the reaction is formed and the exchange takes place.

The holding tank is a moulded plastic body with an air-tight cover. The important points are that (i) it should be made of an acid-resistant material; (ii) it should be air-tight to prevent the escape of an unpleasant smell of fixer; (iii) it should be leak-proof; (iv) the passage of the fixer through it should be such that the fixer solution to be desilvered rises from the bottom of the tank to leave at the top: such a system allows the fixer full and free access to the charge of base metal and desilvered fixer can be led from a pipe at the top of the cartridge to be discarded down the drain.

The charge of base metal can be embodied in steel wool. This is a cheap material available in various forms: for example, as disc pads of suitable size. These can be arranged like a pile of pancakes, just lightly touching the sides of the cartridge holding-tank and supported on a base clear of the floor of the tank. In the exchange process, the steel wool pads are converted to silver wool pads. The pH of the fixer which holds the silver is important in the action which takes place. Steel wool dissolves in the acid at a pH below 4, while if the pH is above 6·5 the replacement is slow and the process is wasteful.

A new practice is to embody the charge of base metal as an iron-impregnated synthetic foam. The foam has great stability, does not deteriorate in the fixer and is resistant to corrosion. It retains its shape and does not become a messy sludge. The impregnation of iron provides a considerable total surface area of iron to take part in the exchange: it is said that this results in the cartridge's having a working life (that is, the period of time before the charge is fully loaded with silver) and a recovery capacity which are double those of a similarly sized cartridge charged with steel wool.

A metal exchange cartridge can be connected between an automatic processor and the drain if there is no intention to use the fixer again. There should be an external bypass for safety's sake so that if the discharge from the recovery unit becomes blocked accidently the processor is safe from the effects of the obstruction. If two such units are put in series, silver will be recovered to a greater extent. When this is done, the first unit (nearest to the processor) will exhaust earlier than the second since it is dealing with fixer that contains more silver. An economical method of running the two units in series is to move the second one up to first place when the first is exhausted and insert a cartridge with a fresh charge of base metal to become a new second unit. Sometimes a metal exchange unit is installed in series with an electrolytic system: the arrangement is for the metal exchange cartridge to act as the tailing unit for the other.

The effluent desilvered fixer from metal exchange cartridges is discharged down a drain since the fixer is of no further photographic use. The drain chosen should preferably be separate from the one which carries away the outflows of developer and of wash-water from the processor: if the three outflows (desilvered fixer, developer and wash-water) share a slow-flowing drain, the precipitation of an iron complex may block the drain. If it really is not possible to assign a separate drain to the outflow from metal exchange cartridges, care should be taken to site the entrance to the drain so that the effluence goes into it at a point where the rate of flow is usually high.

MONITORING SILVER RECOVERY SYSTEMS

The method chosen by an X-ray department to recover silver from its fixer solutions may be an electrolytic one or may be by metal replacement or indeed may be a combination of the two. Whatever it is, the ability to check on the efficiency of the process is important. The tests are simply made by means of the silver-estimating papers which are commercially available.

The papers are made up as little booklets containing a number of strips of chemically impregnated paper. When a paper strip is dipped into the solution which is being tested, the paper becomes stained: the depth of tone in the stain is related to the quantity of silver in the solution. A comparator chart is provided and from this the tone of stain can be compared with a set of standards which equate the colour to the amount of silver present, giving an assessment in grams per litre of the tested solution.

The essential test to make is to check the amount of silver present in the solution which is flowing out of the silver recovery unit. A unit which is operating efficiently should discharge an effluent which has a content of silver that is less than 1 g per litre. This test should be made at the beginning of every working week as one item in a programme of weekly monitoring of an automatic processor with which the recovery unit is associated. The checking should be done whether the silver recovery system is or is not regularly serviced.

If appreciable silver is found to be present in the outflow of waste fixer, then the facts should be reported to the appropriate people who are responsible for the servicing of the unit. This routine monitoring by the staff of the X-ray department is valuable in maintaining the efficiency of the silver recovery system which is used.

The functioning of the silver recovery unit can be assessed as a percentage of silver removed if the silver-content of the fixer is tested at two places: (i) at the inlet point of the recovery unit, which gives the silver-content of the fixer as it leaves the automatic processor and enters the recovery unit: (ii) at the outflow of the recovery unit, which gives the silver-content of the presumably desilvered fixer as it goes to the drain. The two values can be compared and the percentage of silver which has been removed can be calculated.

If the operating conditions are near the unattainable ideal situation, well over 90 per cent of silver may be removed in the time that the fixer is in the recovery unit. In practice in some circumstances all is going well if about 90 per cent of the silver is removed.

When a silver recovery system has been installed, tests can be made to establish the theoretical yield of silver from it. For such testing, a number of samples are taken of the fixer which leaves the automatic processor which is associated with the recovery installation: the samples should be accumulated over a period of three months. From the accumulated samples a volume is removed and its silver-content is checked by means of silver-estimating papers to give a value expressed in grams per litre. This value is then related to the number of litres of working strength fixer which have been used in the processor over the three-month period of the sampling. The resultant figure indicates the number of grams of silver theoretically to be recovered in the three-month period.

If the fixer which flows out of a silver recovery unit is to be discarded and is not to be re-cycled, it is good practice to take from it as much of the silver which it holds as can possibly be removed. To this end, the silver recovery unit may be associated with another secondary or 'tailing' unit into which it passes its outflow of fixer. A metal replacement unit may often function as the tailing unit of an electrolytic one: it is to be noted that once a fixing solution has been through a metal replacement recovery unit there is no possibility of using the solution again for a photographic purpose. So from the tailing unit the fixer is discarded down the drain.

COMPARISONS BETWEEN SYSTEMS OF SILVER RECOVERY

For an X-ray department which sets up a system to recover silver from used fixer solutions the methods to be considered are (i) electrolytic recovery and (ii) recovery by metal replacement. The two methods have their relative advantages and disadvantages as below.

ELECTROLYTIC METHOD

In favour of the electrolytic systems the following points can be made.
(i) The process yields silver which has a high degree of purity and this makes it economically acceptable to the refiner. For the hospital authorities as a whole who are concerned with silver recovery on large scales, the cost of running electrolytic systems is economic for the quantities of silver which are recovered. So both for the refiners and for the hospitals which recover the silver, the economics are favourable.
(ii) It increases the life of some fixer baths and it allows re-use of the fixer.
(iii) Less silver is lost when an electrolytic recovery system is combined with a process of continuous recirculation.

Against the electrolytic systems, the following points must be considered.
(i) The equipment required is costly (but could be rented).
(ii) These systems require some time and attention. The functioning unit must be controlled and checked for its maintained efficiency; the silver must be stripped from the cathode; the equipment must be cleaned;

the stripped silver may be dried and must be treated with strict security precautions as a precious metal.

RECOVERY BY METAL REPLACEMENT

In favour of the recovery of silver by metal replacement, the following points can be mentioned.

(i) The equipment is not costly and its installation is simple, with no electrical supply involved.

(ii) When it is used properly, the efficiency at first is as high as 98 per cent.

(iii) The method adapts easily either to automatic processing or to a manual system.

(iv) The process requires relatively less attention. When the charge of base metal becomes exhausted by being fully loaded with silver, the usual practice is for the servicing company to remove the entire self-contained recovery unit and replace it with a new one.

Against the metal replacement method, we find the following points.

(i) The fixer cannot be used again in a photographic process

(ii) The high initial efficiency falls sharply in the late stages of use when the charge of metal is nearly exhausted.

(iii) Assay and refining of the silver are relatively more difficult.

(iv) Some iron is contained in the effluent and there may be problems in regard to the drains which carry it away.

Chapter 8
Rinsing, Washing, Drying

THE INTERMEDIATE RINSE OR STOPBATH

The rinse is the stage in the processing cycle which may be between development and fixing. Its object is to prevent film materials from carrying active developer with them into the fixer. It has already been seen that the presence of developing agents in the fixing bath can result (i) in dichroic fog; (ii) in staining from the brown final oxidation products of oxidized developer; (iii) in increased alkalinity of the fixing bath as the developer solution contaminates it. When necessary, the correct use of the intermediate rinse minimizes or prevents these troubles.

In automatic processing units the rinse is omitted. Its omission saves time in the processing cycle, and its inclusion has proved unnecessary. Risk of staining is reduced by agitation of the film during its period of travel through the wet parts of the processing cycle, and the quantity of developer carried by the film into the fixing bath can be brought to a minimum by the squeegee action of rollers; furthermore the fixing solution is well buffered.

In manual processing there are two possibilities for this intermediate stage.

(i) To *slow* the action of the developer and to remove it from the surfaces of the film by simply diluting it with water. This is done by a *plain rinse bath*.

(ii) To *stop* the action of the developer by neutralizing it in the emulsion layer and also to remove it from the surfaces of the film. This is achieved by putting the film in an acid solution known as an *acid stopbath*.

In X-ray departments where a manual system of processing is used, the rinse is of plain water. Fixing baths are always acid so that the action of the developer is stopped at that stage, and the previous acid bath is unnecessary. It may be appreciated that a plain rinse *must* be followed by the use of acid fixing solution.

PLAIN RINSE

The plain rinse can be (i) a static bath, or (ii) a bath of water continually renewed because it is in the form of a spray (a spray rinse) or because there is running water continually entering and leaving the bath (a running rinse).

The static bath is extremely simple—it is just a tank full of water—but it must be warily regarded as a potential source of damage by being kept in use too long. As films pass through it, the liquid contents become loaded with developer, and what began as plain water becomes an alkaline solution. It will cease to be effective in slowing the action of the developer. The most important thing to remember about a static rinse is that it must be renewed frequently. This is sometimes called a dip-rinse.

A spray-rinse is an advantageous system since the water is always fresh, being provided as a number of jets directed on the film, and it is economical since the water flows only when films are passing through the rinse. It is, however, liable to certain inefficiencies. Errors can arise through low water pressure, careless use of the rinse, poor positioning of the jets, and lack of maintenance of the sprays.

The running rinse is a system whereby there is a flow of water through the tank, the water entering at low level and leaving at the top. It is a commendable and efficient system; the principal disadvantage is lack of economy in the use of water.

WASHING

The washing stage in the processing cycle follows fixing. When the film comes out of the fixing bath, it carries in its emulsion layer (i) the argentothiosulphates which have been formed in the chemical action of the fixer; (ii) residual sodium thiosulphate, or alternative fixing agent; (iii) remaining salts which are the other constituents of the bath. If no effort is made to remove these, more than one form of disaster awaits the film.

The results are (a) the colourless argentothiosulphates decompose after a while to form silver sulphide, which produces a yellow-brown stain; (b) the residual fixing agent decomposes, and substances are produced which attack the silver image and form silver sulphide, resulting similarly in a yellow-brown stain and loss of the image; (c) all the residual salts crystallize on the film surface and make the radiograph difficult or impossible to view. Since all these substances are water soluble, they can be removed by water, the process being one of diffusion.

The object of washing thus is to remove from the emulsion substances which it has acquired during fixing. They will deteriorate the image if they are allowed to remain. It can be done by subjecting the film to a flow of water, or by putting it into a series of baths of clean water, the water being changed for each bath.

Student radiographers may recall with horror their meeting with an exponential relationship in the absorption of X-ray beams, but one thing about it is easily remembered: that exponential absorption results in the radiation never being totally absorbed. Some fraction tantalizingly remains. Diffusion of residual salts into the washing water results in their exponential removal; this is never complete and some fraction always remains. The aim of washing is to reduce the residual salts not to zero but to a level so low that they can do no harm.

The question then arises as to what this level is. All the substances to be removed wash out at more or less the same rate, and it is usual to express the level of what remains in terms of one salt only; the thiosulphate fixing agent. Tests can be done to determine the amount of hypo remaining in an emulsion, and the results are expressed in micrograms of the agent per square inch of film. The lowest level measurable by usual tests is 5 microgm/sq. in. (about 0·8 micrograms per square centimetre). The level above this which in fact is safe depends upon several considerations, which include conditions of storage; perhaps the most important is the length of time for which it is expected to keep the films. A distinction has been made between what is termed normal commercial storage (which would be a few years only), and what is termed archival storage (which is an unspecified period considered to be permanent or 'for ever'). In the latter case, for many photographic records the thiosulphate content may be required to be so small as to be undetectable. For radiographs it has been suggested that a maximum level for permanent records is 40 microgms/sq. in. or about 5 micrograms per square centimetre. (This is 20 microgms/sq. in. or about 2·5 micrograms per square centimetre for each emulsion.) In practice it is probably unnecessary to achieve so slight a content, since most hospitals have not the filing space to keep their films permanently, and are doing well if they can keep them 10 years.

THE WASHING RATE

The term washing rate is a convenient expression for the rate of removal of thiosulphate in the water bath, and it is affected by various factors which will be reviewed in due course. Before we do this, the diffusion process itself is now considered more closely.

At the time when the film is put into the water there is high thiosulphate concentration in the emulsion, and (we hope) none in the water; there is thus a big difference between salt concentrations of the two. In these circumstances, the thiosulphate diffuses out of the emulsion into the water, and eventually the relative concentrations are evened, the level becoming the same in the emulsion and in the water. If matters are left like this, further diffusion of thiosulphate from the emulsion is unlikely to happen.

If the film is now put into a fresh bath of water instead of being left in the previous one, there is again difference in concentrations of thiosulphate between the emulsion and the water. The process of diffusion begins again and continues until equilibrium is reached. Passing the film through several changes of water thus results in the removal of certain fractions of the thiosulphate content, until eventually what remains is so slight as to be disregarded or as to be unmeasurable. For each change of water the washing rate begins at a maximum and falls to nothing when the state of equilibrium is reached.

It can be appreciated that a sufficient number of changes of water is more important to adequate washing than the volume used; a certain volume used as a static bath gives a very much less efficient result than a smaller volume used to provide several changes. Water is most economically and efficiently used when it is employed to give as many changes as possible of as small a volume as possible, and when time is allowed for each change of wash to reach the point of equilibrium just described. It may be difficult to achieve this in practice and keep the processing cycle within a realistic time-limit.

FACTORS AFFECTING THE WASHING RATE

THIOSULPHATE CONCENTRATIONS IN EMULSION AND WASH-BATH

The importance of the difference in the concentration of thiosulphate in the emulsion and in the wash-bath has been explained already. The concentration difference can be maintained at a maximum if a constant supply of completely fresh water impinges on the emulsion, as by the use of a spray, the water running at once to an outlet. This gives very rapid washing, and saves time but not water. Both in automatic processors and in manual systems, washing is by a continuous flow of water: in automatic processors the water is actively agitated.

THE TEMPERATURE OF THE WASH-BATH

The washing rate increases if the temperature of the water is raised, but there is an obvious limit here. If the water is warmer than 77°F (25°C), the gelatin may be removed from the film base, particularly if it has not been adequately hardened at an earlier stage. At temperatures below 60° F (16°C) the washing rate is very slow.

THE NATURE OF THE FIXING BATH

The hardening agents used in the fixing bath affect the rate at which thiosulphate is removed in the wash. It was found that where potassium alum is the hardening agent and the pH of the fixing bath is at a level to give efficient hardening, the washing rate is slow. Increase in the pH of the fixer improves the washing rate, so that washing can be done in a shorter time. It will be remembered, however, that increased pH results in loss of hardening action. It follows that with potassium alum and aluminium chloride hardeners, the needs for efficient hardening action in the fixer and for the rapid removal of thiosulphate in the following wash can be in conflict.

Chrome alum hardener in the fixing bath seems to have no effect on the subsequent washing rate. Since chrome alum has the disadvantage of losing its hardening power in a few days (as discussed in the previous chapter), the fixer may soon be a non-hardening one.

A neutral or alkaline fixer promotes rapid washing, but, as well as its failure to harden, its inability to halt quickly the action of the developer encourages the formation of stains. The situation can be summarized by saying that the use of acid hardening fixer solutions is incompatible with a rapid washing rate, but that for the sake of other advantages which accrue from the use of these fixers some sacrifice in regard to the washing rate is necessarily accepted.

AGITATION

If agitation is applied, fresh water is brought continually against the films and the washing rate is improved. In radiographic darkrooms where manual processing is done, some agitation is provided by the flow of water through the tank in which washing takes place. In automatic processors, the water is positively agitated.

SOME PRACTICAL POINTS

In radiographic darkrooms with manual processing, the method used for washing is to immerse the films in a large tank, or in a series of tanks, through which water is kept flowing. This method is not particularly economical of water, but it is adapted to the washing of a large amount of material, and it makes minimum demand on the attention of the operator, an important consideration since the psychologists tell us that we cannot do two things at once.

In such tanks, the water in practice often enters at the bottom and leaves near the top. This is not the ideal arrangement since the hypo content tends to sink to the bottom of the bath; it is better for the outlet to be at the bottom, the tank draining by a syphonic arrangement. When films are put into the tank, the point to be remembered is that the films should enter near where the water leaves, and should leave near where the water enters. The reason here is that this allows films to have their last washing with water which comes fresh to the tank, and has not been heavily loaded with hypo by films newly arrived from the fixing bath. An arrangement of the inlet and outlet for achieving this is siting the inlet at the bottom of one side of the tank, and the outlet at the top of an opposite side, the flow of water being in the direction counter to the travel of films through the tank.

If only one tank is used, it must be recognized that if a batch of films is placed in the tank and is adequately washed, placing another batch of films alongside the first introduces more hypo which is diffused into the bath. This can contaminate the first group of films. The risk is minimized by careful observation of the correct progression for films through the tank. It is better still if two separate tanks are available through which films are progressed; equally well the tanks can be used completely to wash one batch at a time, each tank being employed alternately to take the films as they first come from the fixing bath.

In automatic processors washing takes place in dissimilar conditions. We can begin with the difference that the progression of the films, one after the other through the processor, ensures that the washing section contains only one or at most two films at any given time. There is rapid circulation of the water and active agitation of the water in a small tank. The water may be changed at a rate which is as high as 40 times an hour. This can be contrasted with the rate considered acceptable in a manual system, which is the complete change of a large volume of water 4 times in an hour, the tank being a big one holding several films.

Another dissimilarity for the two systems is in the temperatures of the water used. Manual systems use the mains supply of water as it comes out of the tap (cold water supply) and no attempt is made to heat it. In many automatic processors, also obtaining their supply from the mains, the temperature of the water used for washing is raised within the processor, perhaps to 30°C (86°F).

The film's ability to withstand higher temperatures is altered by the hardness of the emulsion. If it has been well hardened, the emulsion will not swell and soften as it does when it is unhardened: hardened, it can then safely be washed in warmer water; but not higher than 35°C (95°F) for this causes too much swelling of the emulsion.

We may next consider these questions: how much washing must be done and how long does it take? The amount of work to be done in washing any film depends obviously (i) on how much residual thiosulphate is there to be removed; and (ii) on what level of remaining thiosulphate is considered acceptable for the film to be kept. The amount of thiosulphate to be removed depends upon the fixing conditions; upon the presence or absence of a squeegee action by rollers which clear surface fluid from the films; upon the type of film; upon the type of radiograph; and upon the hardness of the emulsion. The acceptable level for remaining thiosulphate depends as we have seen upon what period of time is set for the keeping of the radiograph, the acceptable level of remaining salts being lower for very long keeping periods.

The answer to the question as to how long the washing takes clearly depends (i) on how much washing is to be done; (ii) on the methods by which it is undertaken. In automatic processors the time allowed for the washing of each film may be as short as 18 seconds or as long as 65 seconds. In manual processing systems, films usually stay in the washing tank 20 to 30 minutes, although if the water in the tank is being changed at an appropriate rate washing may be adequately done in 10 minutes. Even 10 minutes is much longer than the longest washing times allowed in automatic processors. Important to the short washing-times used in automatic processors is the squeegee action of the transporting rollers which takes from the films' surfaces water that is loaded with thiosulphate: this would otherwise need to be removed in the washing section of the processing cycle.

DRYING

So far all the stages of the processing cycle have had at least one common factor—they all have made it necessary for the film to become wet. In fact it becomes very wet indeed, and by the end of the washing stage an emulsion contains several times its own weight in water if it has been through a manual system of processing. In an automatic processor the situation is different because (i) emulsions are harder and absorb less water: (ii) the squeegee action of the transporting rollers removes much fluid. It is clearly necessary to dry films before they can be used conveniently and the object of this last part of the processing cycle is to remove most of the water in the gelatin. The final product must be an undamaged emulsion free from dust particles, crystalline deposits, stains and marks. It is described as being a dry film, but the term is a relative one; it is very much *drier* than it was. A fully dehydrated emulsion is brittle and will crack, so this extreme state is to be avoided. At the end of the drying process, the film looks and feels dry, but it should contain about 10–15 per cent of its own weight of water.

FACTORS AFFECTING DRYING TIMES

The length of time required to make a film look and feel dry is related to the quantity of water to be evaporated. In automatic processing units drying is rapid, and the most important factor in achieving this is physical removal of excess water, usually by means of the squeegee action of rollers.

An unhardened emulsion (as shown in Chapter 7) swells more in washing than a hardened one, and it therefore holds more water when the film comes out of the wash-bath. Unhardened emulsions thus take longer to dry than hardened ones do. Where rapid drying is to be done, the correct hardening of the emulsions is significant from two aspects; (i) because less water will be present in the emulsion to remove, and (ii) because a hardened film is better able to withstand the raised temperatures which may be used. Rapid drying devices which transport films by rollers require strict adherence to the manufacturer's recommendations on hardening since emulsions which are too soft in the heat stick to the rollers.

The most usual method of drying photographic materials is by air: there are three features which are important. These are (i) the temperature of the air; (ii) the humidity of the air; (iii) the flow of air past the emulsion.

Raising the temperature of the air increases the rate at which moisture evaporates from the gelatin and thus shortens drying time. The temperature selected for the operation of any given drying system is governed (i) by the length of time that this part of the processing cycle is intended to occupy and (ii) by the amount of drying to be done. In automatic processors the following circumstances apply:

(i) the period of time allowed for drying is very short, ranging from about 25 seconds to 135 seconds, according to whether the cycle time is 90 seconds or up to 7 minutes;

(ii) there is relatively little drying to be done because the rollers have removed the surface wetness and the well-hardened emulsions absorb relatively little water;

(iii) movement of the film and high-speed circulation of the air accelerate the drying process and as a result a given temperature can achieve more in a given time;

(iv) very high temperatures have proved to be unnecessary, as a consequence of the little drying to be done and the accelerated process, and the range used is approximately 40°C to 50° C (about 105°F to 120°F).

In manual processing the following circumstances apply:

(i) the period of time allowed for drying does not need to be controlled within critical limits and can be allowed to be long, in fact 'as long as it takes' for the film to appear dry;

(ii) in contrast to the situation in an automatic processor, there is much more water absorbed in the emulsions and there is copious fluid on the surfaces of the films when they are taken from the washing tank and put to be dried;

(iii) the temperatures used vary over a range according to the drying method used and may be from about 40°C (approximately 105°F) to about 50°C (approximately 120°F);

(iv) drying is done by means of hot-air drying cupboards or by means of rapid-drier machines which work at higher temperatures than the cupboards do and dry only one film at a time.

The position in regard to the temperatures to be used for drying films could be summarized by saying that the air temperature should be just that which is high enough to accomplish drying in the time which can be allotted to it.

The humidity of the air is significant in this way. The difference in percentages of water in the gelatin and in the air surrounding it determines the rate at which water is removed from the emulsion. The lower the humidity of the air, the more rapid is the loss of moisture from the emulsion to it.

Flow of air past the emulsion is very important, more important than temperature. Adequate flow of air, even if it is relatively cool, can dry films much more quickly than hot air which is static. The air in a drying cabinet is moved by a fan, and saturated air in the immediate neighbourhood of the film surfaces is swept away, and is replaced by fresh air of lower humidity. This accelerates the drying process.

Chapter 9
Processing Equipment

In this chapter will be given some closer account of the practical methods which are used to obtain development and permanence of the latent radiographic image, discussed so far mainly from the viewpoint of chemical and physical theory. In particular some of the equipment designed for this work will be described and its salient features explained.

It is not impossible to process a radiograph using equipment as unambitious as three large dishes and a sink with a running hot and cold water supply. The practical procedure would be to fill one dish with a working developer solution, the second with cold water (for a rinse bath) and the third with an acid, hardening fixing solution; the sink would be used initially for a warm water jacket (to bring the developer in its dish to a working temperature) and then to provide a means to wash the processed radiograph.

Such a processing system unquestionably could be made to yield the desired product, being a radiographic image which is visible and permanent; but no doubt the reader has already recognized a complete unsuitability to the circumstances of a contemporary radiodiagnostic department. The inappropriate features which must strike us surely with a series of dull thuds are:

1 only one film may be processed at a time (and it takes rather a long time at that);

2 processing cannot really be standardized and for success depends significantly on the manual dexterity of the operator;

3 adequate temperature control of the developer is virtually impossible to maintain;

4 solutions exposed in shallow dishes, having a large surface area, quickly oxidize;

5 before and during processing, a radiographic emulsion fares better if it is not subject to handling (damage occurs especially readily when an emulsion is wet and softened).

In order to avoid these difficulties, the routine processing of radiographs is undertaken with equipment of which the basic components are a number of deep tanks. The advantages of these relate conversely to the drawbacks and hazards of the processing dishes.

1　Temperature control is easier when the volume of solution is large and the surface exposure relatively small.

2　Oxidation is decreased in a tall tank, because the surface area is reduced. Often a lid can be used and this will further lessen the exposure to air. The solution therefore keeps better.

3　Several films may be processed simultaneously.

4　There is no direct handling of vulnerable emulsions.

5　Processing can be more nearly standardized. Both plane surfaces of the film are equally exposed to the action of a solution, unless a tank is improperly crowded. Agitation may be performed mechanically or manually at defined intervals.

The principles of tank processing are embodied in several forms of equipment, which may be categorized broadly in two groups:

1　a number of tanks built within a larger one, making a self-contained— or almost self-contained—processor which is operated manually;

2　a number of tanks assembled together, likewise to provide a single processing unit, but in this case associated with mechanical means to move films from one tank to another and thus providing an automatic method of processing.

In view of the widespread, almost ubiquitous use of automatic processors within the United Kingdom, these are the equipments to receive most of our attention now. However, a brief consideration of a manually operated system may offer helpful introduction to basic principles, which must be realized with greater sophistication in automatic machines.

MATERIALS FOR PROCESSING EQUIPMENT

A considerable amount of study has been given to the correct selection of substances suitable for the manufacture of items of processing equipment. The following factors are relevant to the problem.

1　The material should have no effect on the photographic properties of the solution concerned. For example galvanized iron might be fairly suitable for a washing tank, but when it is used for developing or fixing solutions the zinc in it is liable to react with sodium bisulphite and give rise to chemical fog, as a result of the formation of sodium hydrosulphite.

2　The material should be capable of resisting the most corrosive fluid with which it is likely to be in contact. Again galvanized iron can be taken as an example: it is readily attacked by fixing solutions and carry-over from the fixing bath could be a danger to washing tanks made of this substance.

3   The period of time during which a material is likely to be exposed to chemical action and the probable dilution of the solutions concerned. These considerations might make some substances suitable for a washing tank or a plumbing system but not for storage of chemicals or for use as developing or fixing tanks.

4   The cost of the material. Tantalum for instance appears to be inert to all photographic solutions but is too expensive for any but small items of equipment.

5   The mechanical adaptability of the material for constructional purposes. Glass for example is highly resistant to chemical actions but is too fragile in many situations, especially of course if the equipment is large.

In selecting a material for photographic use the first criterion is obviously its chemical suitability. If this is satisfactory then the other factors mentioned can be considered. Costs and mechanical adaptability *are* important but become irreleva. t if the substance concerned has chemical characteristics which are inappropriate.

Consideration has to be given not only to the material of which any article is constructed but also to those substances which may be used with it to make joints or watertight connections. For instance any solder containing tin will cause fog, as also will cheap rubber if sulphur and metallic sulphides are present as impurities.

It is to be remembered, too, that any coated material, for example steel lined with rubber, is only as good as the thickness and durability of the coating substance. If the coating is worn, scratched or cracked, or if it contains blemishes or pores, the exposure of the base metal which is likely to result can contaminate solutions or cause corrosion. Coating materials should be neither brittle nor thin. To prevent the formation of pinhole defects they should be used in at least three applications.

The association of different materials has a further danger if the article concerned is manufactured from one metal plated by another. If the plating wears off or becomes damaged the effect of two metals in solution is to form an electrolytic cell: the resultant process of electrolysis leads to the destruction of one of the metals. Whenever possible metal equipment should be made from a single metal or alloy and electro-welded from the outside. If two dissimilar metals must be used electrolysis between them can be decreased if they are separated from each other by a layer of some insulating material.

Among metals, stainless steel is very suitable both chemically and mechanically for all types of processing apparatus. The best steel for the purpose, because it is most resistant, is of the kind described as having an 18/8 analysis (18 per cent chromium, 8 per cent nickel) and containing 2–4 per cent molybdenum: it should have a carbon content no higher than 0·2 per cent and preferably less than 0·08 per cent. The ability of these steels to resist corrosion is found largely in their highly polished surfaces. If they become dirty or scratched, chemicals are likely to affect them.

Modern processes have made available a wide range of synthetic thermoplastic materials which are easy to manufacture and resistant to most photographic solutions. They are less expensive than steel and are widely employed in X-ray processing equipment.

The plumbing associated with a processing area no doubt is a matter which student radiographers may well feel to lie beyond their scope and control. However, it is to be observed that the previous discussion of materials appropriate or inappropriate for the manufacture of processing equipment is relevant equally to agents for the disposal of discarded processing solutions.

Provided they are well diluted, exhausted developers and fixers can be passed without special treatment into the normal drainage system. Brass or copper pipings, however, should not be used, owing to their readiness to corrode. Whenever possible a material should be chosen which is resistant even to full strength processing solutions. The following substances are applicable: for large drains—earthenware pipes with joints set in acid-proof cement; for smaller connections—18/8 molybdenum stainless steel, steam-quality screwed iron piping, or synthetic substances such as polythene or polyvinyl chloride (P.V.C.). Iron or plastic pipes are the usual ones recommended for drainage from a processing area.

All outlets should have detachable strainers of stainless steel. The fitting of plugs to give easy access to pipes which turn through an angle is often a useful measure. Some water in association with processing products tends to form a gelatinous deposit which can obstruct a drain over a period of time. The possibility of reaching likely sites of obstruction easily should be available.

Pipes for the water *supply* are in a less hazardous position than drainage systems. Brass or copper piping is very satisfactory. Rigid P.V.C. can also be used, though it may be brittle. Lead is relatively expensive and owing to its soft nature must be well supported.

It should be observed that developer is not immune to the presence of copper; indeed one part in 1,000,000 of this metal is capable of contaminating a solution. It is good practice when preparing such solutions first to run off the static contents of any supply pipes before using the water. Condensation on copper pipes above a developing tank may result in droplets falling into the solution and this has been known to fog films during development.

PROCESSORS FOR MANUAL OPERATION

Manually operated processing units are available in a number of models and sizes; and although minor differences in their specifications may be noticed these processors share similar basic features of design.

GENERAL CONSTRUCTION

Fig. 9.1 illustrates the typical features of a manually operated processor. Essentially, the processor consists of a large master tank which includes certain smaller tanks and divisions. From left to right in the drawing, these are as follows:

(a) a lidded tank for the developer;

(b) a tank or compartment, usually having a separately tapped cold water supply, which provides a means to rinse films between developing and fixing solutions;

(c) a tank for the fixer;

(d) a large compartment, with its own cold water inlet-valve, in which developed and fixed films are washed.

It can be seen that (a), (b) and (c) make a processing section of the whole unit and (d) a washing section which can be filled and emptied of water independently of the other part of the master tank.

When it is operational, the processing section of the master tank also is filled from the mains with water but this is controlled in temperature and constitutes a water jacket for the two tanks which contain the processing chemicals. The purpose of the water jacket is to maintain these solutions—significantly the developer—at a correct working temperature continuously over as long a period of time as may be required.

CONTROLS

In Fig. 9.1, certain controls are indicated on the front of the processor. The first of these from the left is a thermometer regulator (see page 192), operating in conjunction with a thermostat and an immersion heater in the water jacket. The functions of this equipment are:

1   to raise the temperature of the water jacket to a preselected degree;

2   to maintain this temperature whilst the unit is operational.

The next three controls are inlet valves for the rinse, the water jacket

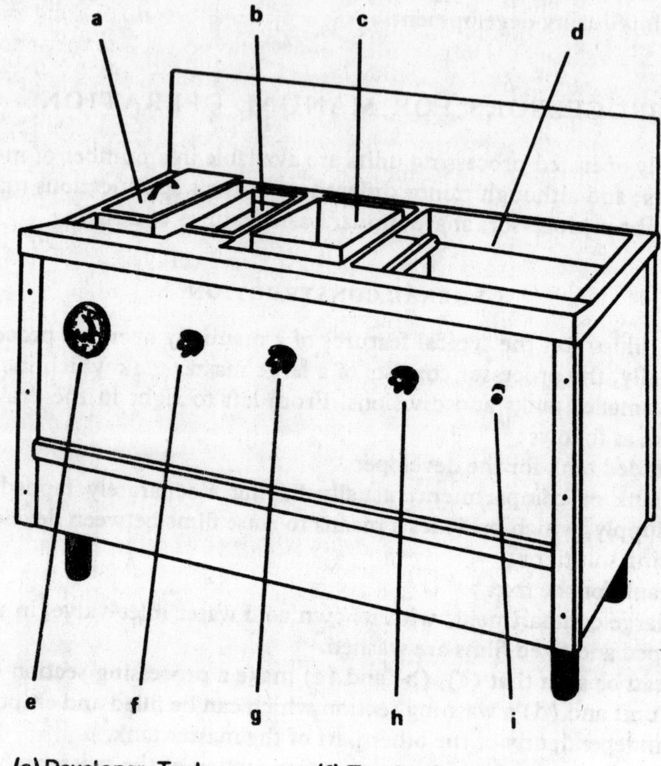

(a) Developer Tank   (f) Tap for Spray Rinse

(b) Rinse Tank   (g) Tap for Water Jacket

(c) Fixer Tank   (h) Tap for Running Wash

(d) Running Wash   (i) Push Button ON/OFF Switch

(e) Thermostat

Fig. 9.1. A typical manually operated processor.
By courtesy of Wardray Products (Clerkenwell) Ltd.

itself and the wash. Finally, there is an ON/OFF switch for the electrical supply, which is taken in the usual manner by means of a three-core cable, a 3-pin plug and an earthed outlet socket on the darkroom wall.

It is necessary to be able to empty the various parts of the processor for cleaning and other purposes, such as a change of chemistry. In the case of the processor sketched in Fig. 9.1, the developer and fixer tanks are emptied into the water jacket by means of a supplied siphon; this has some advantage, as the solutions are thereby diluted before they enter the hospital's general drainage system. The water jacket, the rinse and the washing section all drain by means of a single gate valve, usually accessibly situated below the processor at the front. However, variants of this arrangement are found: for example, sometimes the wash section has its own outlet valve. Students should examine any manual processor encountered in their hospitals and note any difference of detail—in whatever respect—from the unit we have described.

MATERIALS

Typically, a manual processor of the nature depicted in Fig. 9.1 is constructed on a strong steel, or chemically resistant iron, framework. The internal and external faces of the master tank are made from panels of PVC. The space between the inner and outer walls is usually filled with a substance such as expanded polystyrene, which reduces heat loss from the water jacket and helps to stabilize temperature; resin-bonded plywood also has been used.

The edges and corners of the master tank are capped with stainless steel, for greater strength and durability. The solution tanks and any lid provided are also likely to be moulded PVC or similar plastic material; stainless steel would be equally suitable but is more expensive.

TANK CAPACITIES

The individual capacities of solution tanks in a processor vary from model to model and naturally influence both the dimensions of the total unit and the through-put of films which the processor may adequately handle. Typical specifications are given below.

Capacity Films hour	*Developer Tank*	*Fixer Tank*	*Dimensions of Processor*
20	1 × 14 litres (3 gall.)	1 × 14 litres (3 gall.)	570 mm long × 650 mm deep (22½ in. × 25½ in.)
30–40	1 × 25 litres (5 gall.)	1 × 23 litres (5 gall.) or 2 × 14 litres (3 gall.)	1220 mm long × 690 mm deep (48 in. × 27 in.)
50–60	1 × 45·5 litres (10 gall.) or 2 × 23 litres (5 gall.)	1 × 45·5 litres (10 gall.) or 2 × 23 litres (5 gall.)	1420 mm long × 690 mm deep (56 in. × 27 in.)

A series of much smaller tanks, in a table-top category, can be obtained, which are suitable only for the processing of dental radiographs.

TEMPERATURE CONTROL

In a manually operated processor, the developer is the only significant solution of which the working temperature must be closely controlled. As we have said, this control is given by maintaining the temperature of the water jacket at an appropriate level.

Within the United Kingdom at least, this operation implies the use of equipment which will raise the temperature of the ambient (cold) water supply. In tropical regions of the world the reverse may be true and the task of the equipment must be to cool the ambient water supply. More readers of this book are likely to be involved with the first situation than with the second, so we will consider at this point how the water jacket in a manual processor of the type shown in Fig. 9.1 is heated.

Depending on the size of the volume of water to be warmed, the electrical power of the immersion heater concerned may vary from 600 watts up to 2 kilowatts. The heated element is usually placed at the base of the water jacket, like the element in an electric kettle, from which in principle it is no different.

However, users of kettles as a rule are expected to switch off the electrical current when the water is hot enough for its purpose; and generally this occurs when the water boils. The case of the processor is very different. The heater must switch off automatically when the water in the master tank has reached a temperature which the operator must pre-select; and similarly it must switch on again as soon as—and as often as—the temperature of the water falls significantly below the required level. This piece of expertise comes from an instrument called a thermometer regulator.

A THERMOMETER REGULATOR

A thermometer regulator allows the heating system of the processor's water jacket to be in continuous operation, even during unattended periods, such as the weekend, when processing is not expected to be undertaken. This is necessary because a heated water jacket is not a rapid method of altering the temperature of processing solutions. Some hours are required for the stabilization of temperatures within the contents of each tank. If the jacket's immersion heater were switched on and off by the operator only as each day required, there would occur both an extravagant use of electrical power and a crucial failure to bring the

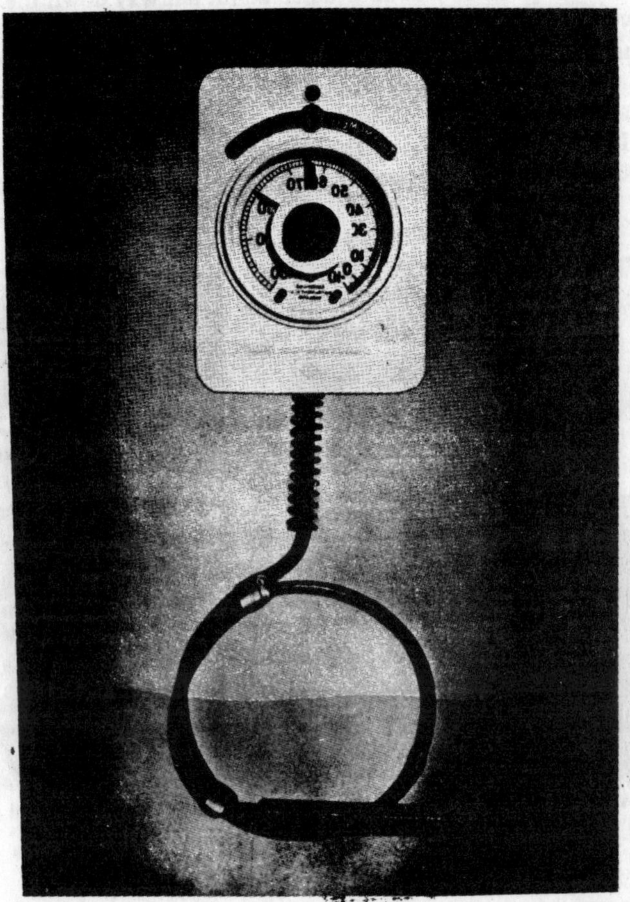

Fig. 9.2. A thermometer regulator. *By courtesy of Ilford Ltd.*

developer quickly enough to its correct working temperature when it was needed.

Fig. 9.2 illustrates a thermometer regulator. Its main features are:

1 a large dial with calibrations between zero and 100 deg. F (37 deg. C), or a range approximating to this;

2 two pointers on this dial, a coloured one (usually blue or red) which can be manually adjusted with a key to lie opposite the chosen value of temperature, and a black one which records the temperature actually obtaining in the water jacket;

3 a lead covered capillary tube terminating in an expanded portion or

bulb which in practice will be situated about halfway down the depth of water concerned, in order to record its mean temperature. This bulb is the sensitive element in the thermometer: its principle is the expansion and contraction of a volume of gas, a more accurate indicator than the response of a column of mercury.

In Fig. 9.3, which illustrates the practical arrangement in a typical processing unit, the thermometer and the regulator can be seen in circuit.

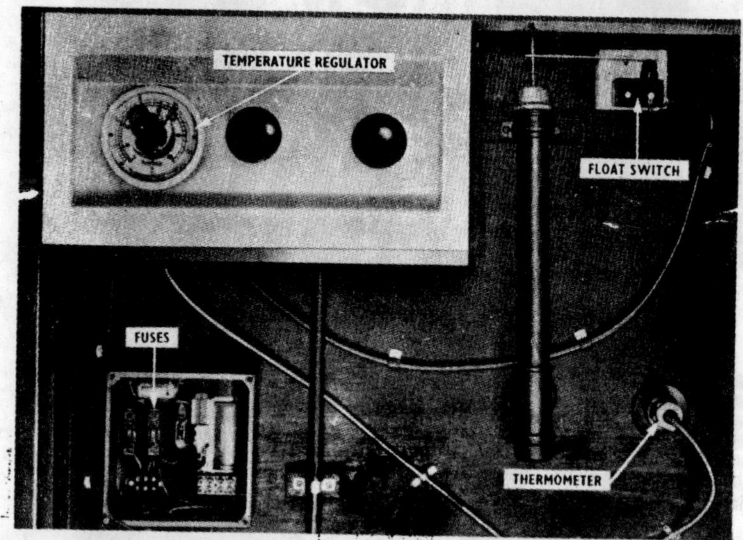

Fig. 9.3. A thermometer regulator in operation in a manual processor. The front panel of the processor has been removed. *By courtesy of Kodak Ltd.*

The thermometer bulb is connected by means of its capillary tube to the regulator and the heater also, through a connection box with fuses. As the temperature of the water jacket rises, the black pointer on the regulator dial will move round the scale until its position coincides with that of the previously set coloured pointer. When this occurs, a microswitch in the regulator operates a control switch in the heating circuit and the current supply is terminated. When the temperature falls sufficiently, the two pointers are again separated on the dial and a similar sequence of events results in the restoration of the heating current. The processes alternate continuously.

A thermometer regulator of this kind is simultaneously a measuring and a regulating instrument.

A FLOAT SWITCH

Electrical heating equipment which is to remain in operation during hours when premises may be empty and the equipment unsupervized must be made safe against the possibility of its becoming the source of a fire. In the case of an unprotected water jacket of a film processer, a fire-raising sequence of events could begin with the occurrence of a leak from the tank. This might either reduce the water-level in the tank to below the site of the thermometer bulb, or empty the tank. In either circumstance the regulator is no longer in charge of the situation and cannot terminate the current supply: dangerous over-heating of the electrical element may then occur, as in effect it is attempting to heat not a contained volume of water but the ambient air of the room. An appropriate safety device to meet such a situation is the float switch—and associated float chamber—which are seen in the processor depicted in Fig. 9.3.

The float chamber is a long, narrow cylinder which contains a float: it is attached to the front of the water jacket and is in communication with it. The level of the water in each of the two compartments is necessarily the same; if this level falls in the main tank, it is bound to do so equally in the chamber containing the float and the float itself will fall correspondingly. On the float is mounted a light rod, positioned horizontally so that, as the float moves downwards with the falling water-level, the distal end of the rod operates the contacts of a small electrical switch. This switch is so connected that it will open-circuit the heating element as the float descends through a critical level and re-establish the circuit when the water jacket is filled again to above this level.

A float switch of the type described is a very simple device but it requires regular maintenance. In areas where the water is hard, an accumulation of salt on the sides of the float chamber or on the float itself may prevent free movement of the float. If it becomes completely or effectively immobile, of course it will fail to operate the circuit-breaking switch. At least once a year, a competent electrician should check the electrical equipment of the processor and this inspection should include a survey of the float switch.

METHODS OF COOLING SOLUTIONS

We have considered so far only equipment which raises the temperature of solutions from their standing value to the level required for correct processing procedure. In climates where the ambient temperature normally exceeds 24°C (75°F) it becomes necessary to cool solutions before they may be employed in accordance with standardized techniques for the manual processing of radiographs.

The working temperatures of processing solutions can be reduced either if the ambient temperature of the darkroom is held sufficiently low or by the use of a refrigerator unit which will cool the water jacket, in a manner comparable with its heating in more temperate climates. If seasonal variations are such that cooling is required during some months of the year and heating at others, the supply circuit should have a switch of the throw-over type, in order to avoid the possible accident of attempting to conduct both processes simultaneously. In some circumstances sufficient reduction of the darkroom's ambient temperature can be obtained if a system of air-conditioning is in use. In this case no modification of the processing equipment is necessary.

However, in many cases cooling of the water jacket becomes essential and usually this is effected by a separate refrigerating unit which—unlike the heating element described in the previous section—is not an integral part of the processing unit itself. If room temperatures are *not* appreciably above 90°F (32°C), a small refrigerator may simply be attached by a bracket to one end of the processor: from it, stainless steel pipes carrying the coolant pass into the water jacket, one going to the front of the processing tanks and the other to their rear. An adjustable thermostat provides control of the water jacket's temperature. In the use of a cooling pipe running through the water jacket we have a close analogy with the principle of heating by means of immersion devices, such as those earlier described.

PROCESSING HANGERS

Films are suspended for processing in metal frames known as hangers. These are designed:

(a) to support the film and allow it to be manipulated without handling of the emulsion;

(b) to permit a number of films to be processed simultaneously and to keep them separate from each other during the procedure.

There are two general varieties of hanger: these are the channel type and the tension type.

CHANNEL HANGERS

In this design of hanger the frame is a double structure on either side of the film and forms a groove which holds each of its edges. At the top of the frame a hinged lip can be raised to allow the film to be inserted and this is then closed. A hanger of this type is illustrated in Fig. 9.4.

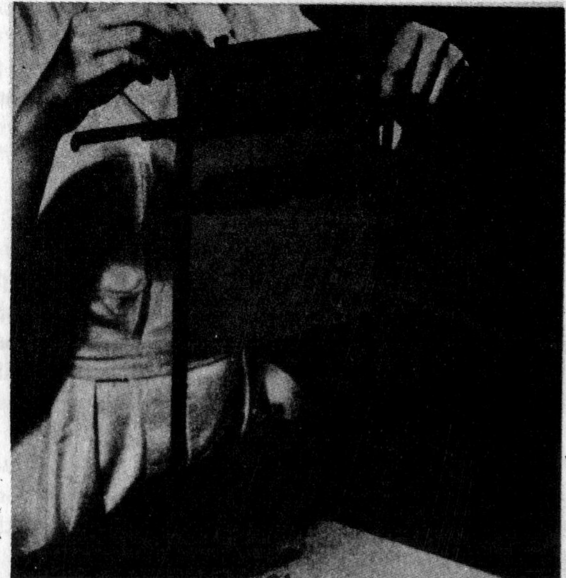

Fig. 9.4. A processing hanger of the channel type. *By courtesy of Ilford Ltd.*

The good features of the channel hanger are:
1   it is quick to load;
2   the film is securely held and in normal conditions is unlikely to suffer accidental release during processing.

Less convenient features are as follows.
1   Since the sides of the frame overlap the edges of the film this area is protected during drying and radiographs dried in these hangers remain wet at the edges long after the rest of their surface is ready. In practice this makes it necessary to remove films from channel hangers and suspend them by another means for drying.
2   Channel hangers are difficult to clean. If inadequate attention is given to them, chemical deposits and other residues are prone to accumulate in the grooves. If a film is not removed from its hanger for drying, the heat may raise the temperature of the metal sufficiently to melt the emulsion in contact with it. This mishap not only damages the immediate radiograph but has the capacity to inflict similar harm on its successors, since the sticky emulsion remaining in the hanger may adhere to another film when the hanger is again heated in the drier.
3   While the film cannot readily become detached, it is not a close fit in the channels. The play available creates some tendency for the larger sizes

of film to bow away from the vertical plane under the pressure of attempted immersion in a deep solution. This may bring one surface of a film into contact with its neighbour or—if the hanger is worn and the top of the frame either broken or missing—may in fact pull the film from the hanger. Any hanger, whatever its pattern, which is in a state of even slight disrepair, should be discarded until it can be serviced or replaced.

TENSION HANGERS

Tension hangers have a steel-rod framework which normally does not touch either plane surface of the film. Each of four small clips perforates one corner of the radiograph and maintains it within the hanger; the lower two clips are attached directly to the frame and the upper two by means of a spring bar, the purpose of which is to hold the film under slight tension and keep it flat. A typical tension hanger is illustrated in Fig. 9.5.

In loading this hanger it should be inverted and the film attached first to the two lower clips. The upper clips in turn can then be brought to meet the parallel edge because of the mobility given them by the spring

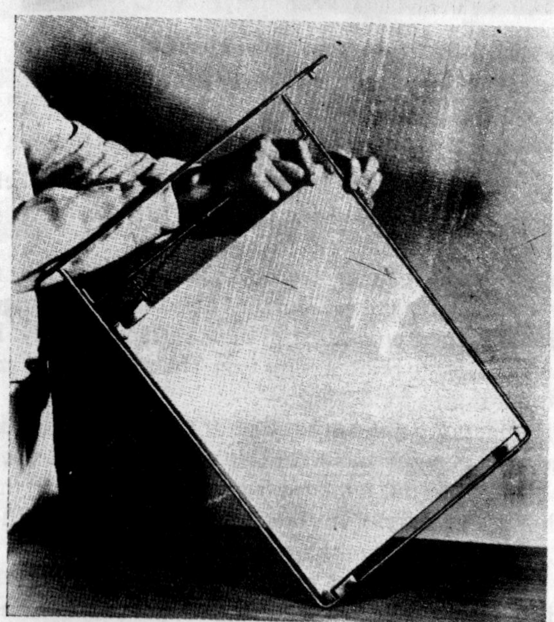

Fig. 9.5. A processing hanger of the tension type. *By courtesy of Kodak Ltd.*

bow. If the film is not flat in the hanger it is usually because it is incorrectly placed in the lower clips and adjustment to these should be made if required.

Tension hangers have the convenience that they can be used to suspend films in a drier and are easier to keep clean than those of the channel type. However, they require rather more care in loading and sometimes during processing a film will pull free from one of the clips; both these features are accentuated if the film used has the rounded corners now presented by manufacturers.

HANGER BARS AND CLIPS

Hanger bars are virtually essential accessories to the use of the channel type of hanger, since they are designed mainly to support the film during drying. Their appearance is illustrated in Fig. 9.6 and is largely self-

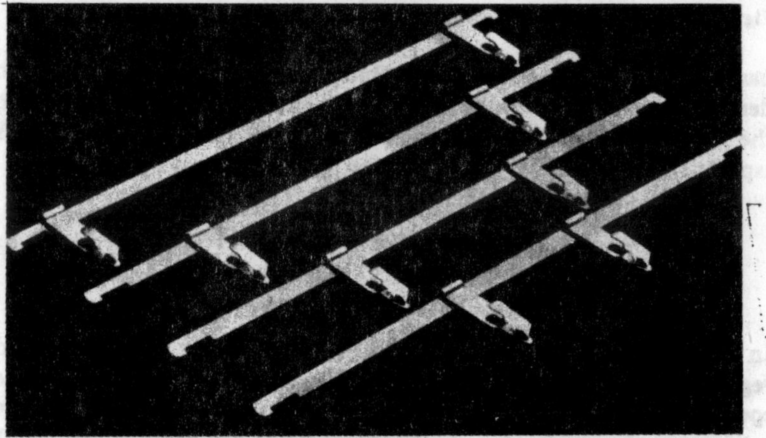

Fig. 9.6. Hanger bars. *By courtesy of Kodak Ltd.*

explanatory. The position of the clips along the bar is adjustable so that each is appropriate for any size of radiograph. A film can be attached to a bar either before being put into a channel hanger or after removal from it before entry into the drying cabinet. Some care must be exercised in positioning the clips to avoid bowing of the film.

DENTAL HANGERS

A special type of hanger is used for the processing of dental radiographs. This is illustrated in Fig. 9.7 and is self-explanatory in appearance. The

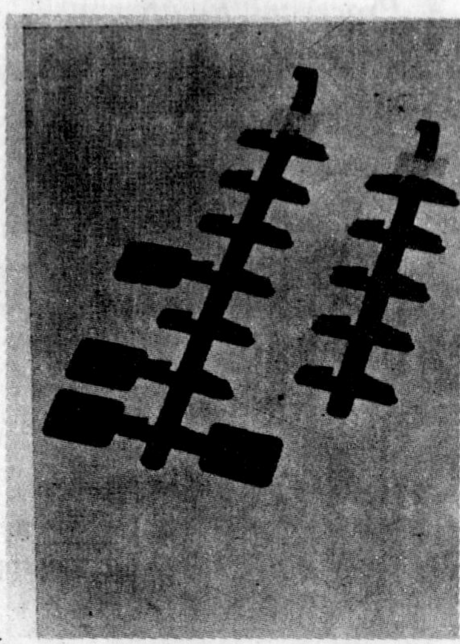

Fig. 9.7. Processing hangers for dental radiographs. *By courtesy of Kodak Ltd.*

hanger usually includes an ivorine tablet for record purposes. In attaching dental radiographs to these hangers the technician should avoid impaling the film at the point where its surface is embossed to identify the tube aspect. This can lead only to doubt and confusion.

CARE OF PROCESSING EQUIPMENT

MANUAL PROCESSORS

In a processing area cleanliness is next to godliness. A little attention regularly given to a processor is worth far more than a large-scale attack sporadically conducted. The technician who has for the darkroom's equipment the pride of a ship's engineer for his engines and can be discovered habitually going round with a cloth in his hand is of inestimable value in the production of good radiographs.

Modern materials are easy to maintain in smart condition simply by being regularly and often wiped over with a clean damp cloth; the operative words are 'regular' and 'often'. In the case of many plastic materials, stains usually penetrate beyond the surface. If they are not removed within a few hours of formation their subsequent removal may be very difficult indeed. Warm water and a little soap solution are effective in the first instance.

The steel capping on some processing units may be polished after washing by the use of impregnated wadding, such as 'Dura-Glit'. Deposits on the surface may be removed with fine pumice, and troublesome rust deposits usually respond to a 5–10 per cent warm solution of citric acid followed by simple washing. Abrasives and wire wool never should be employed for this purpose.

When chemicals are changed the opportunity should be taken to scrub tanks thoroughly with clean warm water and a long-handled brush. Very hot water is detrimental in action to hard rubber and will distort tanks of this kind. At no time should it be used indiscriminately on tanks of plastic material. Narrow tanks require a double-sided brush and one designed for the purpose is easily obtainable.

A hard scale sometimes forms on the sides of developing tanks and can be difficult to remove by scrubbing, particularly if it is of long standing. A 10 per cent solution of acetic acid put into the tank for a while may help to loosen the deposit and it can then be dislodged with a scrubbing brush. After this treatment, thorough rinsing of the tank with clean water is essential.

The presence of bacteria in the processing water is a potential hazard to radiographs. As a result of their action sulphites may be converted to sulphides which affect photographic emulsions and produce chemical fog. Because of this risk it may be thought advisable to sterilize processing tanks from time to time. This can be done by filling them with a bacteriostatic solution. For this purpose a suitable substance is dichlorophen, obtainable as the proprietary preparation 'Embatex'. Four ounces (115 ml) of 'Embatex' to 10 gallons (45·5 litres) of water is an appropriate strength. Alternatively a domestic bleaching preparation such as 'Parazone' or 'Domestos' may be used in a dilution of 1 + 5. Such a solution should not be left for any length of time in stainless steel tanks, as a reaction between the metal and the bleach will occur. After sterilization, tanks should be thoroughly washed before further use.

The tendency of static volumes of water to accumulate slime is well known to us all. The water jackets of processing units are prone to gather bacterial growth because such micro-organisms flourish in conditions of warmth and where light intensity is low. Their presence not only is unpleasant to sight, touch and sometimes to our sense of smell, but is likely to promote corrosion of the unit's structure and can effectively insulate processing tanks: this will retard the transfer of heat from the water jacket to the developing solution.

The growth of algae can be prevented in a water jacket by the introduction of chemical agents. The water jacket of a manual processor typically may hold about 20 gallons (90 litres) of water. One ounce (28·5 g) of sodium pentachlorophenate added to this makes an appropriate bactericidal solution. 'Embatex' in the proportion of 1 oz. (28·5 g.) to 10 gallons (45·5 litres) may be used equally well, or 'Kirbychlor' tablets (sodium dichloro-s-triazinetrione).

CARE OF HANGERS

Processing hangers are made of stainless steel of a specified quality such as was described in a previous section. They repay regular attention. A hanger which is dirty or damaged, or one which is not the correct size for the film but employed because of shortage, almost certainly will originate a number of artefacts during processing. Indeed it is not an unknown occurrence for a film even to be torn if it is forced past the edge of a neighbouring film which is partly adrift from its hanger in a processing tank.

As well as being periodically inspected for serviceable condition, hangers should be cleaned on a regular rota. Abrasives must not be employed for this purpose. Dry scrubbing with a stiff brush, if undertaken at frequent intervals, is simple and effective. It should be combined with a regular wash in clean hot water to dissolve any obstinate chemical residues.

Hangers which have been allowed to become very dirty may need more powerful treatment. A suitable cleanser for this purpose is 5 oz. (64 ml) of glacial acetic acid with the addition of water to make 80 oz. (1000 ml) of fluid altogether. Glacial acetic acid can be obtained from the pharmacy. Hangers should be steeped in this solution for an hour and then scrubbed in three changes of hot water.

PROCESSING PROCEDURE

To process a radiograph by means of manually operated equipment requires much more time than would be taken by any automatic processor now available; but when such processing is correctly performed, in properly controlled conditions, there is no doubt that images of lasting high quality may be expected to result.

An operator may readily acquire the necessary knowledge and adroitness to process quite large numbers of radiographs—perhaps several hundred in a working day, given a processor of sufficient capacity—but attention to detail is always necessary and a certain care is continuously demanded. The following is a description of the procedure to be followed. (It is understood that the darkroom is in safelight.)

1   The film is unloaded from its cassette (see p. 121).

2   The film is identified by means of a suitable marker, if this has not already been done before the entry of the cassette to the darkroom.

3   The film is placed in a processing hanger of an appropriate size (see pp. 197–198).

Throughout these three manoeuvres—as at any time when a film is handled—the operator should exercise care to avoid finger-marking the emulsion.

4   The lid is removed from the developing tank and the loaded hanger is suspended in the solution, subject to a satisfactory check that the solution's level is adequately high to cover the film completely.

5   The time is then noted from a darkroom clock, which should have a large, clear dial and a central sweep seconds hand; or an interval timer is set appropriately for the period of development (usually 4 minutes)

In the working situation it is rare for there to be only one film in need of processing at a time and the operator often must fill the tank to capacity with a succession of loaded hangers. It is important not to overcrowd a processing tank—although in a busy department there is an obvious temptation to do so—as films may be marked by accidental contact with each other; or they may become partly dislodged from their hangers, to their own and others' detriment. A 23-litre tank cannot safely contain more than six hangers at once, without a risk of their jostling each other at some time.

6   If possible, some agitation of the solution should be made by slightly raising and lowering each hanger in turn, whilst keeping the film below the surface of the solution. Ideally this should be repeated once during the development period.

7   The lid of the developing tank should now be replaced. Its primary purpose is to protect the solution from the occurrence of aerial oxidation, as much as possible; and from contamination by dust and similar matter. However, it also enables the darkroom to revert to white light at intervals during processing operations, if so wished.

8   When the appropriate development time has elapsed, the hanger is removed from the solution and transferred to the rinse tank where it is subjected usually to a continuous stream—but sometimes to a fine spray— of water for a period of 5 to 10 seconds. A busy operator who is concerned with several films at once is prone to hurry this stage of the process, unless well trained and self-disciplined: films are sometimes whisked from the developer, without time being allowed for an adequate drainage of solution from the emulsion surfaces; and they may be dipped once through the rinse and be immediately taken from it. When there are a number of hangers in the developer tank, they should be lifted one at a time in the same careful sequence as they were introduced. If the rinse is

of the preferred running type—as opposed to a spray—hangers should 'queue' in it: this will ensure that all have several seconds immersion, since each waits in the tank for the departure of its forerunner.

9   After rinsing, hanger and film are put in the fixer for an interval of which the duration is much less critical than in the case of the developer but should be at least twice the clearing time (see p. 15).

10   For the last 'wet' stage of processing, the operator transfers the radiograph in its hanger to the washing section of the processor, again taking care to allow some drainage of solution to occur when the hanger is elevated above the fixer. The film is now fully impervious to white light: no safelighting is needed for this part of the processing cycle, which may occupy about 15–20 minutes.

11   Following this, the film is dried by means of one of the available equipments, such as those described on p. 269.

AUTOMATIC PROCESSORS

The use of automatic equipment to process radiographs is now very widespread. In the United Kingdom it is considered that manually operated processors are appropriate only if the daily throughput is fifty films or less: consequently nearly every radiodiagnostic department possesses an automatic processor and usually possesses several, since the recommended provision approximates to one processor for two radio-diagnostic rooms.

A variety of automatic processors are marketed by a number of leading manufacturers. Here, we may consider them only in broad terms which relate to their features in common. All automatic processors possess:

1   a system which mechanically transports films through the processor;

2   systems which provide for (a) the replenishment of chemical solutions (developer and fixer) and (b) their recirculation;

3   systems for the temperature control of processing solutions (these include the washing water in certain examples);

4   a system concerned with the circulation of water (mainly for film-washing purposes);

5   a system for drying films.

PROCESSING CYCLES AND PRODUCTION CAPACITY

The term *processing cycle* refers to the processing time, the period during which one film passes through the processor. This period begins with the insertion to the equipment of an unprocessed film and is completed when a dry—but now processed—emulsion is delivered again to the hand; for reasons which are clear, the processing time is sometimes described as the dry-to-dry cycle.

Different machines offer different dry-to-dry cycles and some have a built-in speed regulator which enables one of several available cycles to be selected. This facility makes the processor suitable for application to the needs of different developers and to the needs of various types of emulsion (for example, a single-sided fluorographic film in distinction to a double-sided direct exposure film), which may have different optimum development times. In one example, for instance, the speed regulator can alter the interval during which the film is in the developer from 19 seconds to 40 seconds, in six steps having a difference of a few seconds between each step. (Overall processing cycle: variable between 90 and 200 seconds.)

The processing cycles most commonly employed at present have durations between 90 and 115 seconds. These machines have been described sometimes as *rapid cycle* processors. Other processors may offer much longer processing times, such as $3\frac{1}{2}$ minutes (*half-cycle*) and 7 minutes (*full cycle*) but these are now obtained only to special order, as a rule.

In the case of a machine with a built-in speed regulator, alterable at the turn of a control knob, this is not intended to be employed merely between one film and the next, as a means of attempting to compensate for incorrect radiographic exposure (a manoeuvre unlikely to succeed anyway): what is obtained is flexibility, so that a processor may be used satisfactorily in various circumstances but should achieve standardized results from the relevant emulsions and chemistry in every instance.

Up to a point and in the case of the rapid cycle equipments, the actual length of the dry-to-dry period is not of supreme importance to many radiodiagnostic departments: in the generality of users who will notice differences of 5 to 10 seconds? What may be of considerably greater significance is the production capacity of the processor, which is usually stated as the number of films which it is able to accept in one hour. If it is to have any real meaning, this number must be qualified: it is important to know the size of films to which it relates.

A processor which may have a certain production capacity when only small films are processed, has a lower capacity when large films are considered. Usually a manufacturer publishes a specification in terms of 35 cm × 43 cm sheet film (the largest used) or of sheets of mixed sizes. Sometimes both expressions are included. For example, one manufacturer has made the following statement about the output of a processor: 385 sheets of film per hour, average of intermixed sizes (250 sheets of 35 cm × 43 cm size film per hour).

The data above refer to a large processor: typically the capacity of a 'small' machine might run at about one-third of these values; whilst a processor of intermediate capacity might be able to accept 175 × 35 cm × 43 cm films per hour.

Even these facts about the capacity of a processor may not be all that the purchaser of the equipment wishes to know. In the practical situation, an hour may be a less realistic period to consider than the busiest few minutes in that hour. We may ask ourselves how effectively our chosen processor will dispose of a number of films, arrived almost simultaneously at its 'in-tray'. This load might contain, for example, the contents of 4 or 5 cassettes from a fluoroscopic room and perhaps the same quantity from a cranial examination in an adjacent room. The important question is: how soon after the insertion of one film, may another be introduced?

A significant specification here is the film feed time or feeding speed. Typical rates for a 'large', a 'medium' and a 'small' processor are as follows: 158 cm per minute; 100 cm per minute; and 50 cm per minute. In practice, many machines have an ability to accept the next sheet of film a mere 15 to 25 seconds after the introduction of a forerunner, having dimensions 35 cm × 43 cm and fed lengthwise. This interval is so short as only rarely to occasion any hiatus in the darkroom's activity.

FILM TRANSPORT SYSTEMS

A film introduced to an automatic processor is moved by means of a system of rollers in one or other of two ways: (a) vertically through a series of deep tanks or sections of the processor; (b) horizontally through a number of shallow trays. Vertical transport is the commoner method.

VERTICAL ROLLER TRANSPORT

Fig. 9.8 is a schematic general diagram in side elevation of an automatic processor, showing the principles of the vertical roller system. It can be seen that the processing unit is divided into three sections, one each for developing, fixing and washing. These are an integral part of the unit but virtually they are tanks; they may be made of stainless steel or of a moulded plastic. The rollers are arranged in a rack in each processing tank and this can be lifted out for cleaning. Materials used for the construction of the rollers vary: hard plastics and different categories of rubber are commonly employed. It may be that in one processor not all the rack rollers are of the same substance, depending upon their particularity of function. For instance, rollers which convey a film from the washing section of the processor should have a squeegee action and

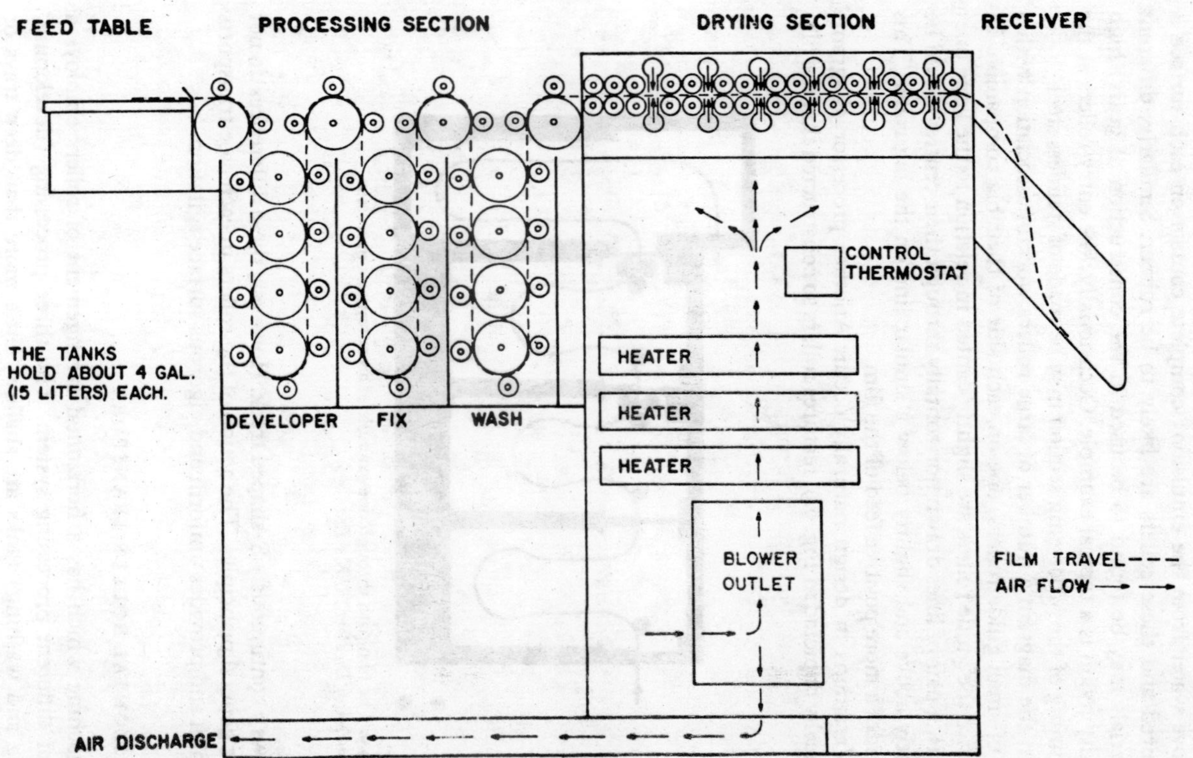

Fig. 9.8. Sectional diagram of an automatic processor employing rollers and deep tanks. *By courtesy of the Pako Corporation.*

remove water from the emulsion; complete contact on each surface is required and these rollers are likely to be rubber. Similarly, different materials may be found to be used in the construction of gears: high density nylon is a typical example. Occasionally, the entry rollers at the beginning of the processing section may be made of stainless steel.

In the diagram a number of large rollers work in association with a pair of small guide rollers, one on each side of their big companion. In practice the guide rollers are slightly canted in relation to the large one; that is, a pair of lines drawn horizontally through their centres would lie slightly above and slightly below a similar line on the big roller. This provides a more positive feed of the film.

Variations in design naturally occur. Another processor, diagrammatically depicted in Fig. 9.9, features rollers so constructed that the film

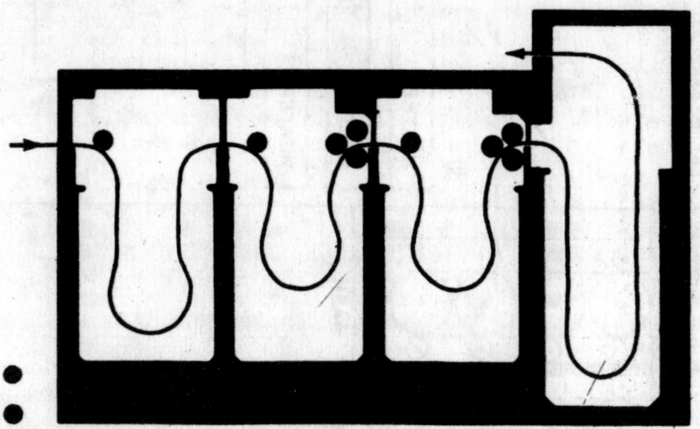

Fig. 9.9. The film path through one example of an automatic processor. *By courtesy of Du Pont (U.K.) Ltd.*

follows a continuously S-shaped track. However, these differences do not affect general principles. The action of the rollers in each case transports the film and provides uniform and vigorous surface agitation.

HORIZONTAL ROLLER TRANSPORT

A machine which has a horizontal arrangement of rollers employs a rather different processing system. The three processing (developing, fixing and washing) tanks are shallow, little more than deep trays or dishes, each with a capacity of about 3 litres. (The deep tanks associated with a vertical roller system may contain 10–15 litres of solution.) Rollers arranged horizontally in parallel pairs—one roller above the film and its fellow beneath—move each sheet in a linear path across the tanks in succession. Fig. 9.10 illustrates this path.

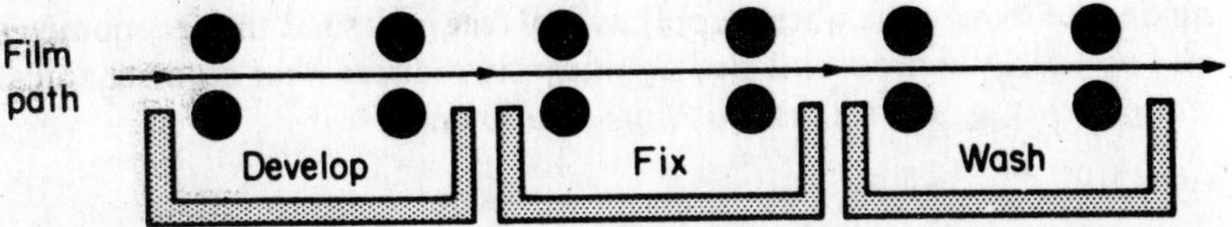

Fig. 9.10. Diagram to illustrate the film path through a processor employing shallow tanks.

The films are not immersed in the respective solutions. Instead, injection systems draw developer, fixer and water from each appropriate tank and feed the solution to applicators. Each applicator has one head positioned over the film plane and another head positioned beneath the film plane: the function of these heads is to distribute the solution evenly over the surfaces of the emulsion whilst the film is in transit through the tank concerned. Afterwards, surplus fluid is collected by intermediate receivers—situated on either side of the lower distributing head—and from there is returned to the processing tank.

THE MOTOR DRIVE

Whatever may be the characteristics of the rollers, automatic processors require to be driven. The energy to move the rollers comes, through a main drive shaft, from a direct current motor, which is often variable in speed. The drive-speed determines the length of the processing cycle and may be controlled through a printed circuit regulator. Adjustments are carried out by means of an external indexed knob. In a typical example, seven different settings of this control change the cycle time between 90 and 200 seconds, in 20 second intervals. The index is often arbitrarily chosen and reference should be made to the manufacturer's data sheet for details of the cycles.

It is usual for the processor's drive to be activated and de-activated automatically by the passage of a film, so that the processor is not motoring during idle periods. An electronic sensor energizes the drive—as well as other electrical components, such as recirculation pumps and the dryer heater—as soon as a film is introduced. When the processed film leaves the dryer and if the sensor detects no other in its train, the processor is automatically switched to a standby condition, in which no power is supplied to the drive. This effects an electrical economy of about 50–60 per cent.

Obviously, there should be an interval between the presentation of a 'last' film to the processor and the moment of the 'switch-off' Three minutes is a typical interval but in some equipments the time is adjustable over a range between zero and about eight minutes. A processor's standby mode usually taps the water supply as well (see p. 225). It thus economizes on two energy sources and also significantly reduces wear on mechanical components, gears, rollers, bushings and so on.

REPLENISHMENT OF SOLUTION

Regular additions of fresh solutions are essential to the automatic processing of radiographs. All automatic machines, even those operating on a 7–8 minute cycle, depend on accelerated chemical reactions, compared with manual processing. The required rapidity of these reactions cannot be obtained from partially exhausted solutions: adequate solution activity needs to be assured at all times and is achieved by arrangements which inject fresh solution to each processing tank, from each of two large reservoirs containing respectively developer and fixer.

Such a system provides for a fall in solution level, as well as for diminished chemical activity, and this, too, is an important need. However, in the case of roller-operated processors, the squeegee action of the rollers in removing surface fluid from the film, significantly reduces the carry-over of solutions, relative to what may happen—and in practice does happen—when a film is manually processed. During automatic processing very little volume of solution is lost and—as additional fluid is introduced—a regular outflow of used developer and fixer occurs. It is inherent in this sequence of events that both developing and fixing solutions in theory may continue in use indefinitely, without its being necessary at any time completely to empty and replace the contents of either tank. In practice of course tanks should be regularly drained and cleaned.

The power needed to transfer the developer and fixer from their respective reservoirs to the appropriate processing tank is provided by an electric pump (the replenisher pump). There is one pump for each solution, although both may be powered from a single motor. The operation of these pumps occurs automatically but it is necessary for the delivered quantity of solution to relate to the area of emulsion being processed, if circumstances of either over-replenishment or under-replenishment are not sometimes to occur.

In practice, radiographers do not usually think of an overall area of film put through a processor and are more likely to compute workloads in more familiar terms of the numbers of films and their sizes; but of course the two forms of expression have similar significance.

A replenishment system in an automatic processor consequently must include a means to monitor film-throughput; and the monitoring or sensing system in turn must trigger the developer and fixer replenisher pumps.

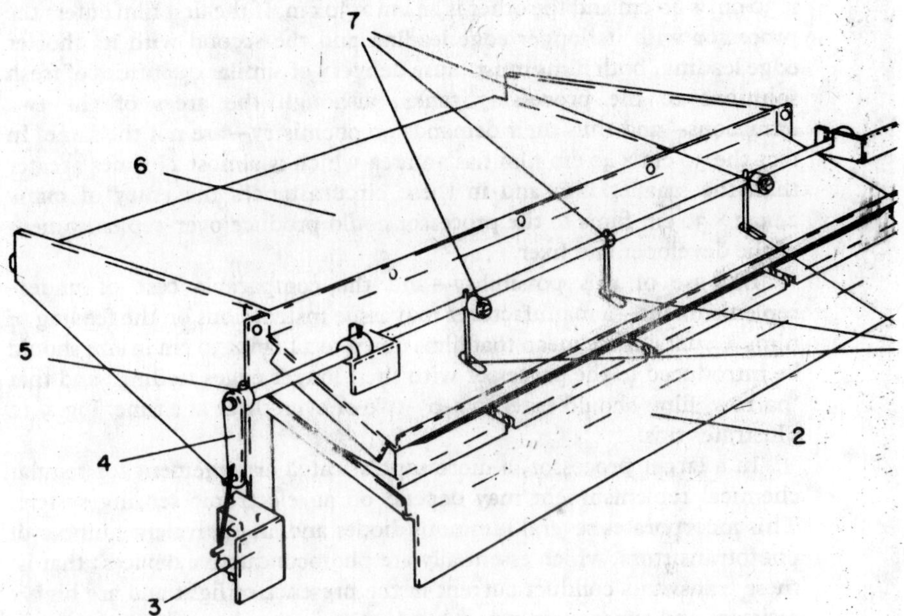

Fig. 9.11. A detector assembly for control of replenishment:

1 Detector fingers.
2 Developer drip guard.
3 Microswitch.
4 Control level.
5 Clamping screw.
6 Feed tray.
7 Retaining screws.
By courtesy of 3M United Kingdom Ltd.

The means by which a processor may monitor film-throughput varies between different models. A simple device consists of a row of detector fingers (see Fig. 9.11) which 'feel' the film as it enters the processor from the feed-tray. As these fingers rise they activate the replenisher pumps through a microswitch. So long as a film is beneath the detector fingers, the switch is energized and the pumps are operative: in this way the delivered quantity of solution is proportional to the length—and thus to the surface area—of the film being processed.

It is perhaps already evident to the reader that this monitoring system might fail to result in correct chemical replenishment, unless all films were fed to the processor in a recognized procedure. For example, let us consider two frequently used sizes of film which share a dimension: one is 30 cm × 40 cm and the other is 24 cm × 30 cm. If the first film enters the processor with its longer edge leading and the second with its shorter edge leading, both films must cause delivery of similar quantities of fresh solutions to the processing tanks, although the areas of the two emulsions—and thus their demands on chemistry—are not the same. In fact the 30 cm × 40 cm film has an area which is almost $1\frac{1}{2}$ times greater than the smaller film and in these circumstances the entry of many 24 cm × 30 cm films to the processor could produce over-replenishment of the developer and fixer.

Because of this possibility—and the comparable case of under-replenishment—a manufacturer may issue instructions on the feeding of films. Usually these mean that films down to 24 cm × 30 cm in size should be introduced to the processor with their longer edges leading; and that 'narrow' films should enter two-by-two or even three at a time. Fig. 9.12 illustrates this.

In a larger processor, a more sophisticated arrangement for regular chemical replenishment may depend on an electronic sensing system. This incorporates several luminous diodes and an equivalent number of phototransistors, which essentially are photoconductive devices; that is, these transistors conduct current in the presence of light and are highly resistant and consequently non-conductive in the absence of light.

The processor's feed-tray normally reflects infrared light from the luminous diodes towards the phototransistors, which are suitably positioned in relation to the feed-tray to receive a maximum amount of this reflected light. In these circumstances the phototransistors are conductive: they transfer a voltage to a special amplifier which reverses the input signal and holds de-energized a pilot relay, associated with control of the replenisher pumps.

Introducing a 'green' (that is, unprocessed) film to the feed-tray interrupts the reflection of infrared light to the diodes. The phototransistors become non-conductive, the amplifier then being deprived of its significant voltage: the pilot relay is thus energized and the consequence is a triggering of the replenisher pumps.

The electronic sensor which is described in essentials above controls the replenisher pumps, through a time pulse switch, in such a way that pre-set quantities of developer and fixer are delivered to the processing

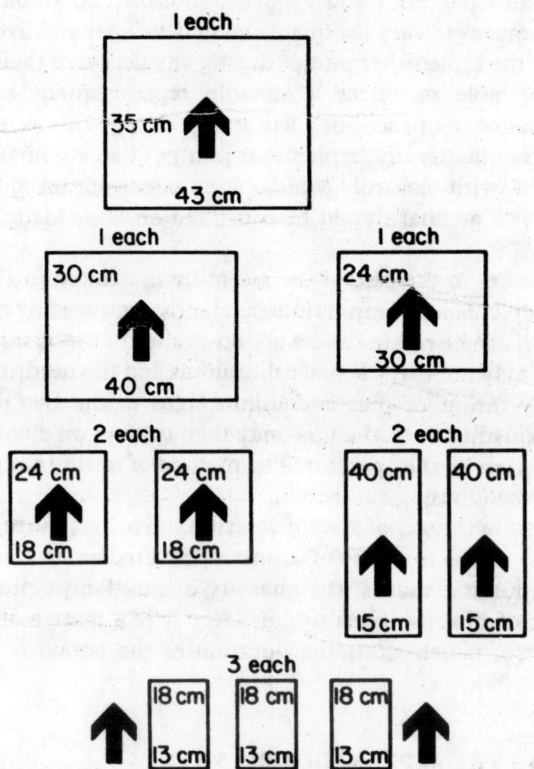

Fig. 9.12.

tanks, in discrete pulses which succeed each other every 95 cm of film put through the processor. The width of the film is taken to be a medium of the variety which might be processed and is estimated as 35 cm.

REPLENISHMENT RATE

It is important for the reader to recognize that the systems just described for the automatic replenishment of a processor's chemistry, whilst they relate the delivered quantities of solution to the area of emulsion processed, are not sufficient in themselves as a means to control replenishment. The added solution quantity which is requisite to maintain chemical activity (and thus constitutes optimum replenishment) includes other factors than the numbers and sizes of the films processed: for instance, the type of emulsion and the nature of the radiographic subject are both relevant to determinations of a correct replenishment technique (see Chapters 6 and 7). Because of this, an automatic system should offer means to vary the quantities of developer and fixer which are delivered by the replenisher pumps during any period of their operation; we must be able to select a suitable replenishment rate for the circumstances of the processor's use and to change this as our case may require. Consequently, the replenisher pumps of an automatic processor are provided with controls which alter the solution flow and the manufacturer's manual should be consulted on their identification and use.

For instance, in the case of the assembly illustrated in Fig. 9.11, the flow of the replenisher pumps is independently regulated by means of two knobs, which can be rotated and work on a range of 0–300 ml per minute. Such knobs may not carry actual calibrations and the needful indications are made by means of plus and minus signs in the two directions of rotation. Adjustments of the flow may then depend on a trial-and-error experimentation by the operator. The method of testing a replenishment rate is described in the next section.

In the case of the sensor system described on p. 212, the replenishment rate depends on the quantity of solution delivered on each occasion that the pumps pulsate: that is, the quantity of solution pumped when the throughput of film has been 95 cm. Here it is a matter of adjusting a timing control which alters the duration of the period of the pumps' activity.

MEASURING THE REPLENISHMENT RATE

Measurement of the replenishment rate is a simple test to make with most automatic processors. Reference to the relevant operator's manual is necessary for identification in the equipment of the two replenisher supply lines, one of which delivers developer and another of which performs the same service for the fixer. To prevent confusion between them they are often different in colour, red being a common indicator of the developer and blue of the fixer; sometimes they are actually labelled DEV and FIX, or D and F.

In a typical instance, these pipe lines each terminate in a swan neck or hook which normally is hung over the rim of the processing tank concerned, so that solution flowing from the pipe enters the tank. To make the test it is necessary to unhook the swan neck from the tank and hold it over a calibrated beaker (see Fig. 9.13), so that the quantity of solution delivered may be collected and measured.

When this experiment is to be made, the operator should notice the levels of the developer and fixer in the replenisher tanks, as they can

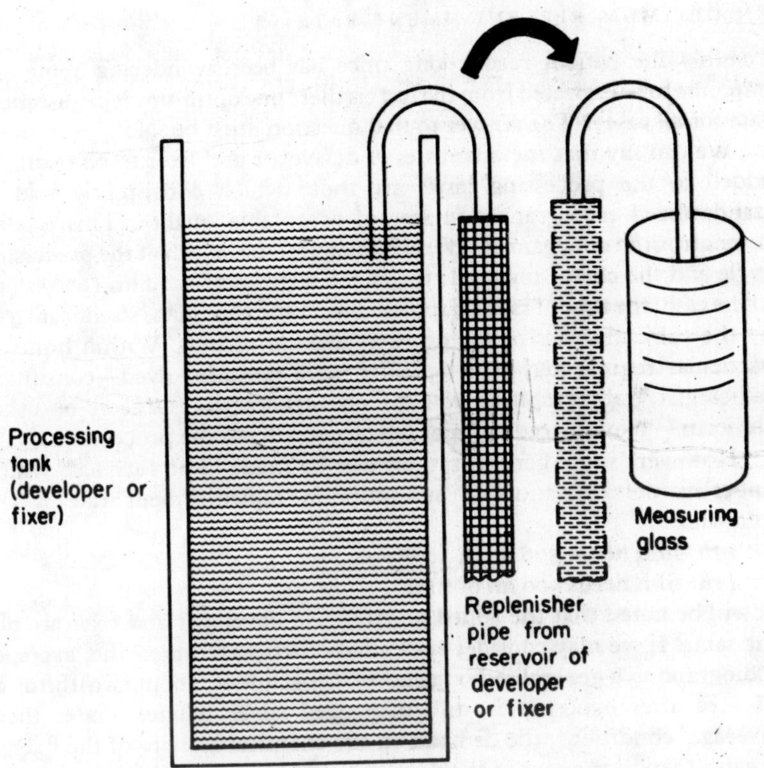

Fig. 9.13. Measuring replenishment rate.

influence the results obtained. Ideally, these reservoirs should be about half full. A nearly empty tank tends to reduce the quantity of solution delivered, whilst a full tank may have an opposite effect, because of changing pressure in the system. To standardize the test it is best to perform it always at similar solution levels.

To complete the test, the instructions of the manufacturer should be followed on the procedure for correct assessment of the replenishment rate. For example, in the case of replenishment by film length during traverse of the film (see p. 212), it is common to establish the replenishment rate in terms of feeding one 35 cm × 35 cm film to the processor and measuring the quantity of solution which then enters the measuring glass. A more accurate result can be obtained if the operator in fact introduces a sequence of three 35 cm × 35 cm films and divides the yielded quantity of solution by three to obtain the replenishment rate.

AN OPTIMUM REPLENISHMENT RATE

Possibly the patient reader long since has been wondering about the outcome to be expected from the test; is there one optimum replenishment rate for all cases? The answer to that question must be 'No'.

We can say that the quantities of developer and fixer to be regularly added to the processing tanks are those which consistently lead to standardized radiographic images of acceptable quality. This quality comes from an amalgam of several influences: the length of the processing cycle and the chemistry used; the characteristics of the film (emulsion) in the case; the type of radiographic subject; and—perhaps significantly— by the subjectiveness of the decision-making process. Within limits, a particular regime may be adopted because those involved—consultant radiologist, radiographer, perhaps an orthopaedic surgeon or other clinician—'like' the radiographs which come from the processor.

However, some generalizations can be made. The rationale which underlies determination of an optimum replenishment rate is the following:

1   1 m^2 film needs 500 ml of developer;
2   1 m^2 film needs 900 ml of fixer.

It will be noted that the added quantities of developer and fixer are not the same. If we may consider such a hypothetical entity as the 'average' radiograph in a general radiodiagnostic department, about two-thirds of its area after exposure is still unchanged silver halide. Under these 'average' conditions, the demand on the chemical activity of the fixer is greater than in the case of the developer and consequently—in a general department at least—its replenishment rate should be higher.

Optimum replenishment rates may be more difficult to determine for specialised radiodiagnostic departments. For example, when a high proportion of the work consists of chest examinations, these radiographs generally exhibit low average density and will require less developer replenishment and more fixer replenishment than 'normal'. The converse is valid when a large proportion of the films processed show higher than average density; for instance, the processor might be serving a suite of gastrointestinal rooms.

From the expression stated above for the general determination of optimum replenishment, the correct replenishment rate may be calculated in the following way.

replenishment rate =

$$\frac{\text{film length (m)} \times \text{film width (m)} \times \text{replenisher volume (ml)}}{\text{m}^2}$$

To attach some values to this formula, we may consider the case of the 35 cm × 35 cm film to which reference was made on p. 215 and which was introduced to a processor for a test of the replenishment rate. In this instance the required quantities of developer and fixer is as follows.

Developer

$$\text{Replenishment rate} = \frac{0.35 \times 0.35 \times 500}{1}$$
$$= 61.25 \text{ ml}$$

Fixer

$$\text{Replenishment rate} = \frac{0.35 \times 0.35 \times 900}{1}$$
$$= 110.25 \text{ ml}$$

Thus, we should adjust the flow controls of the replenisher pumps until these are the solution quantities seen to be delivered to the measuring glass.

In the case of replenishment initiation by the diode scanning system which was described on p. 212, the film length to be considered was 0.95 m and the film width 0.35 m. When the same formula for replenishment is applied to this area of film the resultant replenishment rates are:

    developer—166 ml
    fixer   —300 ml.

The operator should adjust the appropriate controls until these are the quantities of solution pumped on each occasion.

REPLENISHMENT RATES ON MACHINES WITH LOW THROUGHPUT

Something has been said of the way in which the determination of optimum replenishment rates can be influenced by the type of radiographic studies made, the subjective image-evaluations which often occur and other factors. Apart from these considerations, the processor which does very little work—from this cause alone—may pose a special problem. Typically, this might be a rapid cycle processor serving an operating theatre suite and handling the occasional run of a few films, in irregular periods during any week, or even month.

Let us consider first what may happen to the developer in these circumstances. The effects which reduce the activity of a working developer solution are discussed elsewhere in this book (see Chapter 6). In the present context, the important feature is aerial oxidation. When the daily throughput of films is very low, aerial oxidation may become excessive and there may also be an excessive loss of volume from evaporation of the solution, particularly in a warm ambience. The few films subsequently processed do not result in the injection of a sufficient quantity of fresh developer to annul these effects. A gradual depletion occurs and radiographic quality is not maintained. In these circumstances, if the developer replenishment rate is set at an abnormally high level it may be possible to compensate for the changes and preserve a consistent standard of processing.

So far as the fixer is concerned, the most significant occurrence is a loss of water from the solution by evaporation. This results in:

1   an increased ('over'-) concentration of the working solution;
2   a relatively rapid reduction in its volume.

Again, some increase in the replenishment rate is the required remedial action, which may both restore the optimum fixer concentration and maintain the solution's level in the processing tank.

REPLENISHER TANKS

External reservoirs of developer and fixer are necessary to the operation of automatic processors. From these come the fresh working solutions with which the processing tanks must be regularly supplied. The capacities of associated replenisher tanks vary with the needs of different 'sizes' of processor. A particularly high capacity may be necessary when the replenisher tanks are a reservoir for more than one processor in a radiodiagnostic department. Typically, a processor with a throughput of 300 films (mixed sizes) per hour would be supported by replenisher tanks having each a capacity of about 100 litres.

An important aspect of the use of these replenisher tanks is not to allow either of them at any time to become empty. When this happens and the tank is subsequently refilled, air locks in a replenisher line may occur. An air bubble can block the flow of a solution just as effectively as may a kink or a solid obstruction in a pipe line and often is not easily located and dispersed. Under-replenishment and a succeeding chemical exhaustion are the consequences of such a mishap.

THE RECIRCULATION OF SOLUTIONS

Automatic processors of the deep tank variety usually provide for positive recirculation of the developer and fixer solutions (and sometimes of the wash water as well). The impulsion is obtained from individual, high-output, magnetic-drive pumps. Typically, the solution might be drawn from a side opening in the processing tank and returned through an inlet

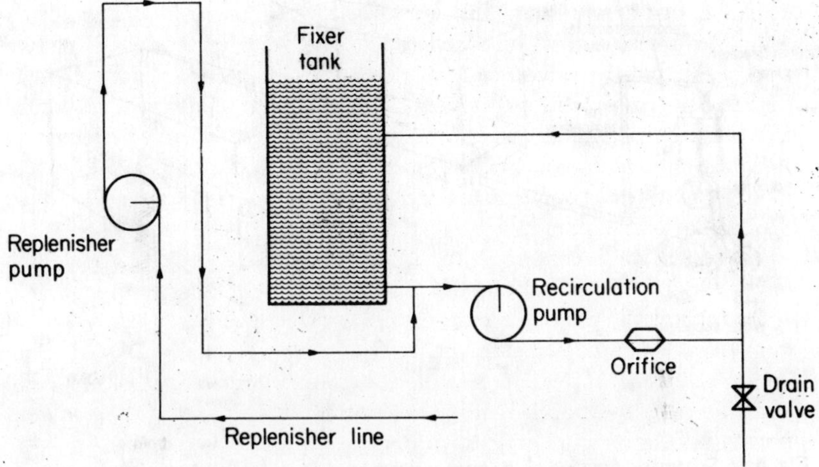

Fig. 9.14. Fixer recirculation in an automatic processor. (Schematic.)

in the bottom of the tank; or vice versa, like the arrangement for recirculation of the fixer which is sketched in Fig. 9.14.

The purposes of the recirculation systems for developer and fixer are:

1   to afford better thermal control, particularly of the developer;
2   to obtain more even flow and distribution of the solutions;
3   to maintain solution activity;
4   to allow solutions to be filtered before re-entry into the processing tanks and thus to ensure the removal of any accumulated particles;
5   to increase agitation of the solution.

Generally, recirculation rates are of an order to move a solution through a processing tank about six times in a minute.

TEMPERATURE CONTROL

Automatic processors require accurate methods of temperature control, particularly, of course, for the developer. However, because of the accelerated processing cycles, the temperatures of the fixer and—to some extent—of the washing water are much more significant than in the case of a manually operated machine; these solutions, too, generally have supervision of their working temperatures.

In many cases, the circuit of one solution through the processor can be deployed to allow the temperature of this one to influence the temperature of another solution. Fig. 9.15 shows such an example: warm water, destined for the washing tank, follows a route beneath the fixer tank and thus maintains this solution at its processing temperature.

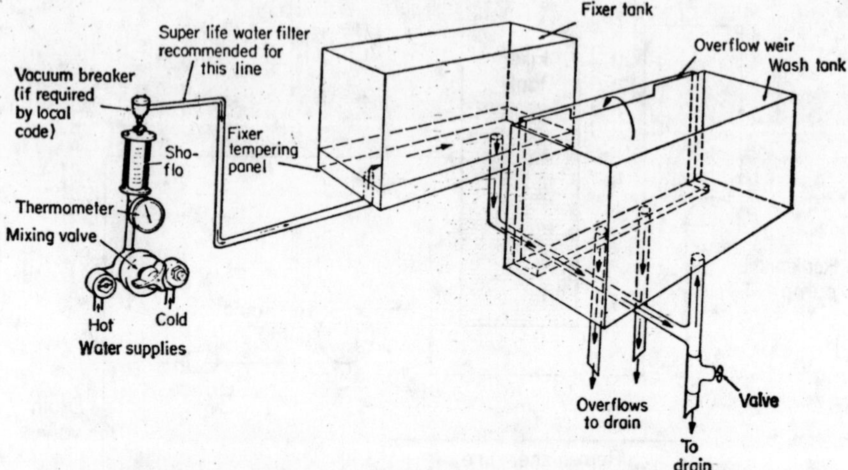

Fig. 9.15. Schematic drawing of the wash water system of an automatic processor. *By courtesy of the Pako Corporation.*

Sometimes, the very proximity of the developer tank to the fixer tank, together with the characteristics of the thin wall between them, ensures sufficient conduction of heat from the developer to the fixer that the same purpose is achieved.

Not all processors are the same in their utilization of available tools for altering the temperature of a solution. Below are described three such devices which are variously found in employment in different models of processor.

IMMERSION HEATER WITH THERMOSTAT

A heating element placed at the base of the processing tank is a suitable means of raising the developer to its required working temperature: this is 25°C–35°C, depending on the developer and the duration of the processing cycle. (Rapid cycles need higher working temperatures.)

It is necessary to include thermostatic control of these heating elements by instruments which are similar to the thermometer regulator, described on p. 192, and will maintain the developer at a preselected temperature, once this value has been reached.

HEAT EXCHANGERS

A heat exchanger is a device which can be used either to raise the temperature of a solution or to make it cooler. One is shown schematically

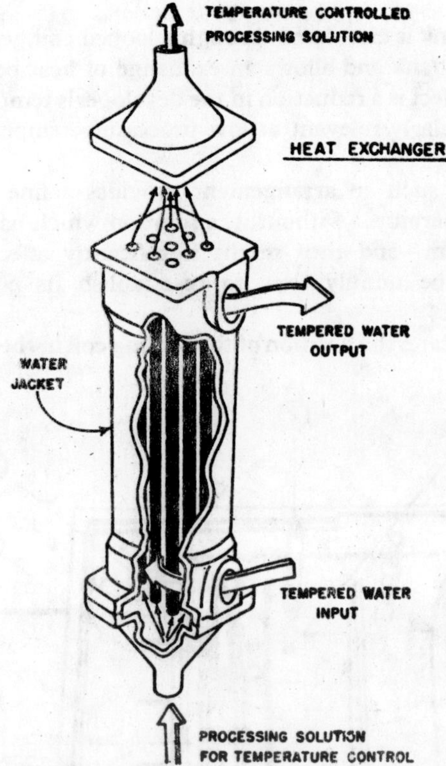

Fig. 9.16. A heat exchanger.
By courtesy of X-ray Sales Division, Eastman Kodak Co., Rochester, New York.

in Fig. 9.16 and essentially consists of a number of narrow tubes contained within another of much greater calibre.

The processing solution (as a rule, the developer) passes through the narrow tubes. During this progress, its temperature will be influenced by the temperature of the relatively larger volume of solution (water) in the outer tube or jacket and it will either lose heat if the jacket is cooler or gain heat if the jacket is hotter than is the processing solution itself. Warmed water in the jacket may conveniently be obtained from the wash tank of the processor by a suitable circuitry. Alternatively, warmed water at a preselected temperature may be obtained directly from a mixing valve, such as that described on p. 223.

Application of a similar principle of heat exchange is found in a cooling coil for the developer in some other processors. In this instance cold water from the mains may be fed to the washing tank and from the bottom of this tank is circulated through a looped coil, which is situated in the developer tank and allows an exchange of heat between the two solutions. The effect is a reduction in the developer's temperature, which might be particularly relevant at low processing temperatures ($25°C$–$27°C$).

In any case, such an arrangement provides a fine control of the developer's temperature: without it, a solution which had become even slightly too warm—and thus might significantly affect radiographic quality—would be unduly slow to re-establish its correct working temperature.

Fig. 9.17 indicates the position of the cooling coil in the developer tank

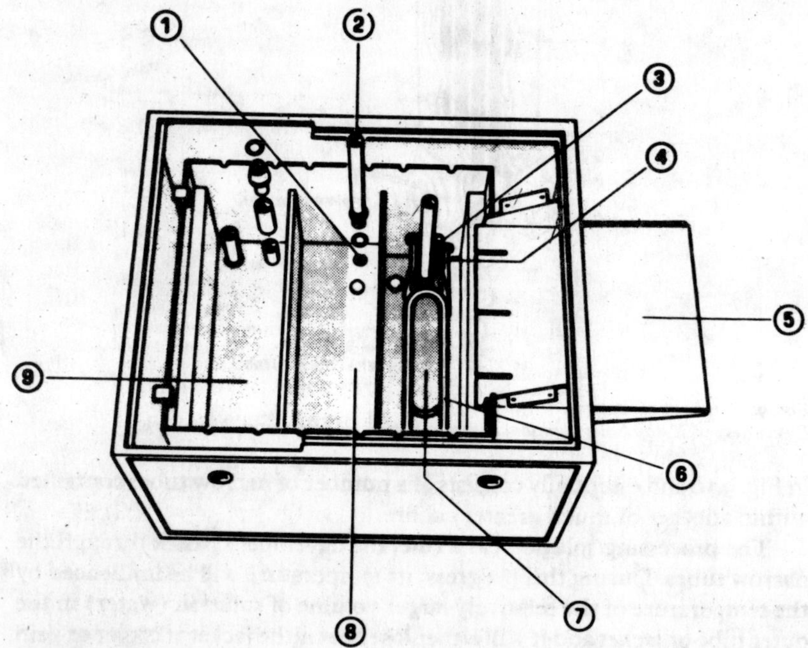

Fig. 9.17. The processing tanks of an automatic processor.

1 Tank drain.
2 Standpipe.
3 Developer heater.
4 Thermometer probe.
5 Feedtray.
6 Cooling coil for developer.
7 Developer tank.
8 Fixer tank.
9 Washing tank.

By courtesy of 3M United Kingdom Ltd.

and shows also the heating element and the probe of the thermometer regulator. In some cases it is possible for this cooling coil to be short circuited when the processor is operating in circumstances which do not require such chilling of the developer: for example, when the developer's working temperature is relatively high (34°C–35°C) and greater than the temperature of its immediate environment.

In an alternative system, employing the same principle, incoming mains cold water is fed to the developer coil before it is taken to the wash tank. This effects a stronger cooling of the developer and enables the processor to tolerate room temperatures in excess of the processing temperature and also to switch fairly quickly from a short processing cycle (90 seconds) to a longer one (3 minutes or more), should it be required to do so.

WATER MIXER

A water mixing valve is illustrated diagrammatically in Fig. 9.18. It operates by combining hot and cold water from the tap supply to produce

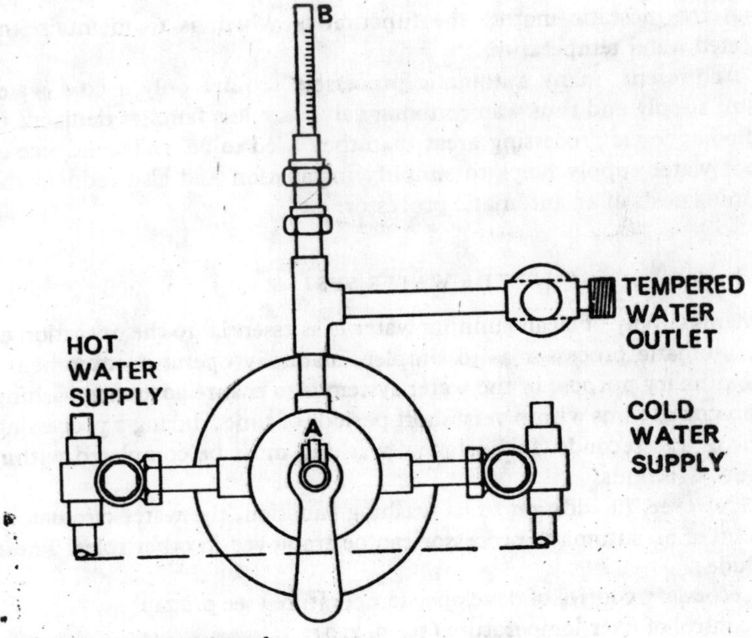

Fig. 9.18. A water mixing valve.
A   Manually adjusted handle for selection of the tempered water.
B   Column thermometer in outlet pipe.
By courtesy of Kodak Ltd.

a mixture at some desired temperature. Possible applications of such a tempered water supply occur in automatic processors, for washing purposes and for heating chemical solutions.

A water mixer is a compact and relatively inexpensive means of controlling water temperature. It is properly described as a thermostatically controlled, manually adjusted, mixing valve. Reference to Fig. 9.18 demonstrates its main features, of which a short account is given below.

1   Separate inlet ports for the hot and the cold mains supply.

2   An outlet port for the tempered water.

3   A handle for selection of the desired temperature, which is manually adjusted by the user. Such a valve might be capable of supplying water at any chosen value between 15°C and 38°C, irrespective of fluctuations in the temperature or pressure of the supply. In some valves, the handle may be removable after adjustment to avoid fortuitous tampering with this control.

4   A thermometer, of which the bulb is inserted in the outlet pipe. The one in the diagram is of a column type but a dial thermometer is equally suitable.

5   A thermostatic motor, the function of which is to maintain the selected water temperature.

At present, many automatic processors require only a cold water mains supply and thus water mixing valves are less familiar denizens of radiodiagnostic processing areas than they used to be. Independence of a hot water supply helps to simplify installation and also reduces the running costs of an automatic processor.

THE WATER SYSTEM

A mains supply of clean running water is as essential to the operation of an automatic processor as to simpler, manually operated equipments. The primary purpose of the water system is to ensure adequate washing of processed films within very short periods of time: during a processing cycle of 120 seconds, for instance, washing must be completed within about 20 seconds.

However, in addition to its washing function, the water circulatory system of an automatic processor can be employed in other roles. These include:

1   secondary control of developer temperature (see p. 221);

2   control of fixer temperature (see p. 220);

3   maintenance of cleanliness in the developer's overflow drain;

4   provision of agitation (in wash tank).

Within limits, raising the temperature of the water increases the washing rate and therefore reduces washing time. Because of this, automatic processors traditionally have required both hot and cold mains water. The two supplies, when combined through a mixing valve (see p. 223), allow water at a preselected temperature to be fed to the processor's washing tank. Fig. 9.15 schematically depicts the wash-water plumbing of a typical processor.

Many newer models require only a cold water mains supply but it should not be assumed from this that specification of the water's temperature is unnecessary or is not implied. The relevant technical data of at least one manufacturer include: (i) a minimum water temperature of $10°C$; (ii) a maximum temperature of $5°C$ below the set temperature of the developer (for example, if the developer's working temperature were $31°C$, the cold water supply should not exceed a temperature of $26°C$). However, these are wide bounds, within which the characteristics of most cold water mains are likely to come.

A few pages since, we considered a cooling coil for the developer. This coil effected a reduction in the developer's temperature by the continual circulation through it of cold water. However, the process is one of mutual benefit and the developer and the wash water help each other. The wash water, as a result of repeated passages through the developer tank, becomes warmer by heat exchange.

WATER CONSUMPTION

During operation, automatic processors tend to be voracious consumers of water. As might be expected, the quantity of water which may be required is usually more for a processor of high capacity than in the case of a small processor, but it is influenced also by the processor's design and the method employed for film washing. A manufacturer may sometimes make economy in the use of water a special marketing feature of his equipment, since a processor's consumption of water is a significant part of its running costs. Usually a processor's technical data include a statement of the quantity of water which it consumes at its peak generating capacity: 2, 3 and 4 litres (0·44, 0·66 and 0·88 gall.) per minute are typical.

Because of these relatively heavy demands, processors are often equipped with a water saver, an automatic electronic device which reduces the flow of water (to about 25 per cent of the peak generating demand), during those periods when films are not passing through the processor. The operation of a standby mode was described on p. 209, with reference to a processor's main drive and economy in electrical power.

WATER PRESSURE

A sustained pressure of water is significant to the operation of automatic processors and a manufacturer's technical data sometimes specify the limits of this pressure: for example, that the processor requires a full flow pressure of 1–8 Kg/cm². This is not an exacting demand and the normal tap supply usually meets the purpose without question. If necessary, the pressure of a poor supply can be augmented by booster pumps.

Fluctuations in water pressure and flow can adversely affect a processor's efficiency: films may appear dirty or may fail to dry; or changes may occur in solution temperature.

Filters are often used in a processor's water circulation system and it is an important element of maintenance that these—and indeed any solution-filter in the equipment—are changed regularly. If such filters are forgotten and receive no regular attention, the outcome for processed films is generally worse than if no filter were present. Accumulations of dirt within the filter effectively obstruct the flow of water or other solution and a variety of ill results may obtain, depending on the solution affected: these include surface artefacts, incorrect image density, failure to dry and film-jams in the processor.

A water supply which contains salts and is very 'hard' is another potential agent of destruction for an automatic processor. Insoluble residues (possibly from reactions with outflowing developer) may accumulate in the processor's drain pipe and block it. The resultant backflow of water through the processor (1) dilutes chemistry and thus destroys image quality, (2) is likely to flood electrical components of the processor and entail their replacement. The occurrence of such episodes is a warning to hospital engineers that the water supply to the processors in the radiodiagnostic department may need to be softened.

WASHING PROCEDURE

The washing process to which films are subjected varies slightly between different processors. In the case of the processor shown in Fig. 9.15, a steady flow of tempered water, at a rate determined by a flow meter ('Sho-flo'), simply enters the wash tank below, through an inlet pipe at one side, and leaves from the top of the tank by an overflow weir on the opposite side.

Other systems include a spray of water through perforated tubes. In one case of this kind, the wash tank is filled by means of external spray tubes, which at the same time give the film a final rinse of clean water as it emerges from the wash rack. In another instance, water enters the wash tank from a side inlet but is pumped from the bottom of this tank into four spray tubes. These are arranged in pairs and their jets impinge on both surfaces of the film as it passes between each couple.

THE DRYING SYSTEM

A film in the dryer of an automatic processor is not really very 'wet'. At entry to the section, a number of squeegee rollers—arranged in opposing pairs—remove excess water from both surfaces of the film, which are then in a damp or moist condition. This is very different from the large amounts of water present when films are taken from the wash tank of a manually operated processor and is one of the reasons why drying in automatic equipment can be completed quickly.

Drying is performed usually through a system of 'air-knives'. These are tubes having a longitudinal slit, through which air is forced at high velocity by motor-driven blowers. The vented tubes are mounted in opposing pairs, the film moving between the 'blades' of air, so that these are drawn simultaneously across both surfaces of the film. Fig. 9.8 shows six pairs of such tubes in the processor's drying section.

In many instances, the air in the system is heated, its temperature being thermostatically controlled at about 50–60°C. An alternative is the use of similarly arranged pairs of infrared lamps (3 in one example) to evaporate water retained in the emulsion. The infrared lamps are associated with cold air in the air knives, the purpose of which is to ensure the removal of water vapour from the film's vicinity.

An advantage of such a system as the one just described is the coolness of the processor during operation. In some hospitals, for various reasons, adequate ventilation of a processing area may prove difficult to obtain and ambient temperatures tend to rise unpleasantly, especially during periods of hot weather. A processor of which the drying section requires no external air exhaust and does not contribute to the warmth of the working environment might be a godsend. (On the other hand, in cold departments on cold mornings, some processors may be as comforting as an electric fire!)

MAINTENANCE OF AUTOMATIC PROCESSORS

Something has already been said of the care of processing equipment and the importance of regular attention to its cleanliness: automatic processors are no different in these respects from their manually operated fellows. However, because automation must introduce greater complexity of operation, inevitably in automatic processors there is 'more to go wrong' and a more elaborate programme of maintenance is needed for them. This should include contracted, regular inspections by the manufacturer's technical engineers but cannot—if it is to be effective—consist only of these.

Faithfully followed, daily and weekly routines for the operation and cleanliness of a processor are the basis of all preventative maintenance. A radiographer, who believes that the intricacies of an automatic processor may be entirely 'left for when the engineer comes', is headed directly for trouble and a succession of service breakdowns, expensive of time and money.

A manufacturer always issues with a processor a manual of instruction to the operator and this should include a statement of daily, weekly and perhaps monthly routines, which are due from the user for the maintenance of the processor in good general working condition. The book probably will include also a section of advice on processing difficulties which may occur and are amenable to simple ways of correction, within the scope of any qualified radiographer.

In attempting to elucidate troubles attributable to the processor it is necessary to remember that what appears to be merely a mechanical fault—for example failure of films to transport through the dryer or to become dry—may have a chemical cause such as incorrect replenishment. The equipment should not immediately be assumed to be the culprit in all circumstances. Examination of the solution-mixing techniques employed by processing staff may show that the chain reaction of disaster was begun outside the processor.

The manufacturer's manual normally indicates relevant checks helpful to be made in a variety of malfunctioning circumstances and is by far the best reference when a problem with a processor occurs. It always repays careful reading and departmental procedures should be instituted which will obey the advice given for the routine care of a processor. The paragraphs which follow cannot be—and are not intended as—a substitute for a manufacturer's own observations about his product. The guidance given here is necessarily of a broad, general nature.

DAILY ROUTINES

Daily good housekeeping routines are designed to keep roller assemblies clean and free of encrusted chemical deposits. The following is a recommended daily procedure which is included in either the starting-up or shut-down routine of many processors.

(i) Remove the crossover roller assemblies or plates. Rinse under warm running water. Wipe dry.

(ii) Wipe down the entrance rollers.
(iii) Wipe off all chemical deposits in the processing section.
(iv) Wipe all top rollers above solution level.

STARTING-UP

Starting-up routines necessarily vary and it is not helpful to give here any account of the steps by which particular machinery is put into operation. However, the following observations should normally be made before radiographic processing is begun:
(i) solution levels in the processing tanks;
(ii) solution levels in the replenisher tanks;
(iii) operation of the replenisher flow-meters;
(iv) water flow-rate and temperature;
(v) developer temperature;
(vi) temperature of the drier;
(vii) two or three test sheets of film to be put through the processor to clean those rollers which are above solution level and may have accumulated particles of foreign material during the shut-down period.

SHUTTING-DOWN

Shutting-down routines usually include an instruction to leave the processor covers slightly open in order to allow chemical fumes to escape which might otherwise cause rust or corrosion in the processing tanks.

Many manufacturers advise emptying the wash tank each night in order to inhibit bacterial growth. This can be done easily if the drain valve is always kept open to a very little extent, enough to permit the tank to empty slowly over a period of time but not to prevent its being filled from its normal supply tap when work is resumed. Alternatively a small permanent hole may be drilled in the drain pipe to provide a similar outlet.

WEEKLY ROUTINES

The procedures listed below are recommended usually as a weekly but sometimes as a fortnightly routine. The latter is perhaps the maximum interval advisable.
(i) Remove crossover rollers or guide plates. Rinse under warm running water (38°C). Work on obstinate chemical stains with a soft brush and the recommended proprietary solution (e.g. Kodak Developer System Cleaner) or the recommended abrasive (proprietary examples are Scotch-

brite and Pako-pad). Rinse thoroughly and wipe dry. The use of chemical cleaners is a matter for caution always: note the warning on page 232.

(ii) Remove solution racks and similarly clean these rollers. Rollers in the washing section may normally darken with use: the stain is not harmful but bacterial growth *is*. Drier rollers also may darken in time. Manipulations of the solution racks require care in order to prevent splashing of the developer and fixer solutions into each other's tank. A movable splash guard to protect each tank in turn as the other rack is lifted may be provided and should be used.

(iii) Operate each rack manually to make sure that the rollers rotate freely, that gears engage as they should and that there are no missing teeth, broken springs, loose chains or screws or any other evidence of trouble.

(iv) While the racks are out of the tanks inspect the developer and fixer solutions for foreign material.

(v) Clean the drier rollers with a damp cloth, removing hard deposits with the recommended abrasive material (Scotch-brite is one example).

(vi) Remove the drier air tubes and clean them by vigorous agitation in warm water; do not allow them to soak in water for a prolonged period.

(vii) Inspect filters and change them as necessary, a supply being kept available in the department. There may be filters present in all or some of the following systems:

 (a) developer recirculation;
 (b) hot water supply;
 (c) cold water supply;
 (d) air-intake of the drier.

It is beyond the scope of this book to give itemized instructions of a how-to-do-it type for the performance of the above: obviously manufacturers' manuals should be consulted in relation to each processor and operators made familiar with the necessary dismantling and reassembly of the specified parts. These tasks are simpler in practice than in print but should be done carefully.

SOLUTIONS

PREPARATION OF SOLUTIONS

The preparation of solutions for automatic processors and their use are important matters which can affect the correct operation of the equipment in ways not always at once recognized. For instance, when developer replenisher is mixed and the solution is stirred, rather than effectively agitated with an up-and-down motion by means of a plunger, the chemicals can form layers which may result in the solution entirely failing to develop exposed film. Sheets of cleared base are delivered at the output end of the processor in place of radiographs with startling effect.

Developer and fixer solutions which are mixed too dilute may initiate mechanical troubles in the processor which do not necessarily become immediately apparent and of course are *not* specifically mechanical. This is because such weakened solutions cannot sufficiently harden an emulsion in the time available.

Softened gelatin may accumulate on rollers and thus halt the transport of films through the processing section; or films may fail to dry because the emulsion is soft and has absorbed too much water during the wet stage of processing.

On the other hand, such troubles may have origins which truly are due to physical unsoundness within the processor, such as transport rollers not being correctly seated in their holders or a fuse having blown in the drier's heating circuit. Radiographers confronted with these situations can more quickly solve their problems if the techniques of the darkroom staff are known to be above suspicion; otherwise, the question of chemical unbalance as the cause of a fault must often be present. Automatic mixers offer advantage in standardizing the preparation of solutions; as well as in avoiding a possibly toxic—and certainly unpleasant—inhalation of chemical fumes.

CHANGING SOLUTIONS

The frequency with which solutions in automatic processors are changed seems usually to be decided by the user's experience. Rapid-cycle machines, especially those operating on a high temperature chemistry, need a solution change rather more often than those with a dry-to-dry interval of $3\frac{1}{2}$ minutes or longer. This applies particularly to the developer solution if fewer than about 150 films are processed for every 24 of the processor's working hours. Any specific instructions in this respect issued by chemical or equipment manufacturers should be followed.

In the absence of such protocol it is usual to change solutions not less often than the following:

every 12 weeks	half-cycle and full-cycle machines;
every 8–10 weeks	rapid-cycle machines;
every 5 weeks	rapid-cycle with low throughput.

It is convenient to combine a change of chemicals with a service inspection of the equipment and in practice this factor often has the deciding influence in determining when solution changes are actually made.

When the processing tanks are drained in order to renew chemicals there is an opportunity to clean them. A manufacturer may supply a proprietary solution for the purpose of cleaning tanks and racks and in this event the appropriate one may be used. The instructions relating to it should be conscientiously obeyed. Not all manufacturers recommend the use of such cleaners as in certain instances the cleansing substance has penetrated the laminations of rollers constructed in this manner and has caused them to warp.

With reference to the cleaning of tanks, some manufacturers publish advice on the general care of stainless steel and the section on p. 200 is also relevant here.

FAULTS

As equipment becomes more intricate the possibilities of its malfunction also increase. So long as there is someone to work in the darkroom, manual processors usually operate. Artefacts on radiographs attributable to manual processing are fewer and generally well recognized (or *are* they, now that so little manual processing is done?). However, when the occupant of the darkroom is an automatic machine a dual potential for trouble exists:

(i) the processor may fail to transport films;

(ii) the processor may function but the films carry artefacts or be otherwise unacceptable by reason of a processing fault.

The second situation has perhaps the greater difficulty, but the more generally automatic processors are used the more familiar are practising radiographers likely to become with the artefacts and defects which may result from their mal-operation or may be initiated by faulty techniques in the darkroom.

The reader of the following pages should bear in mind that a transport fault or a film artefact may occur because of a particular mechanical defect in a particular processor. For instance if we take a heading such as **cocking or twisting of film in the processing section** here are three different diagnoses from three service manuals:

      guide vane bowed or out of place;

      worn crossover roller studs;

      burrs on the guide plates in the racks.

All this book can hope to do as a problem-solving aid is to cover the common ground between a number of processors and provide a few general indications of possible sources of trouble. In the following pages difficulties are listed alphabetically.

ARTEFACTS ON THE FILM SURFACE

Artefacts produced by an automatic processor on the surfaces of a film may have a cause which is simple but remains obscure. The following paragraphs have no pretension to providing a complete reference library of detection: the most they can hope to do is to give a little guidance to the events most likely to have occurred.

In all cases, careful observation of the artefacts themselves should first be made in order to determine whether they possess any or all of the following features:

1 they are at right angles to the path of the film's travel;
2 they are parallel to the path of the film's travel;
3 they so repeat themselves, or have such dimensions that a relation is established with specific parts of a processor (for instance, crystallized chemicals may produce pi-lines, so called because they recur at intervals determined by the circumference of the encrusted roller);
4 they appear on the top surface or the lower surface of the film (the top surface is the side facing upwards to the operator as the film is fed to the processor).

The study of these characteristics is usually rewarding because they may suggest or exclude certain locations as originators of the trouble: for example, crossover guide plates are in contact only with a film's upper surface; and outer rollers in a rack are in contact only with a lower surface.

LENGTHWISE SCRATCHES

(i) Lengthwise scratches on the undersurface of the film are probably from the feed-tray and are caused by too heavy finger-pressure as the film is fed into the processor. Check also the possibility of grit on the tray.

(ii) Any roller held stationary can produce fine dark scratches. Carefully check for any hestitation in the drive system and inspect all racks and gears, including the detector rollers.

Other possible causes are:

(iii) encrusted chemicals on the racks, especially at the levels of solutions;
(iv) roughnesses or uneven spacing of guide plates;
(v) air tubes in the drier out of position.

PRESSURE MARKS

Possible causes of pressure marks on the emulsion are:
(i) torsion springs too tight (if the rollers are spring-held),

(ii) foreign material on the rollers;
(iii) any defective roller.

STREAKS AND MOTTLES

Streaks and spots on the film may occur in the drying section as a result of any of the following conditions:
(i) dirty slots in the air tubes;
(ii) slots incorrectly adjusted for width;
(iii) faulty positioning of the air tubes;
(iv) too high a temperature in the drier;
(v) dirty filter in the air intake;
(vi) squeegee rollers not properly adjusted.

Streaks and mottles can be produced chemically as well. They occur in:
(i) a developing solution which is too weak;
(ii) a developing solution which has too high a concentration of developer.

Dirt on the film surface is very probably due to dirty water. In areas where the water is excessively dirty, frequent changes of the water-filter or filters in the processor become necessary. So long as this is done all remains well. Unfortunately the practical situation is sometimes one in which—from pressure of work on the darkroom or other cause—the filters are forgotten for a while. They may then become so blocked with dirt that too little water is in circulation and consequently films are not properly washed and are sticky and do not dry. Faced with a recurrent trouble of this kind, a manufacturer may paradoxically recommend that if the water is very dirty no filter should be fitted, as—misused—it can cause more trouble than it is worth.

STRIPPING OF THE EMULSION

The reasons for emulsion peeling may be:

(i) mechanical　rollers too tight,
　　　　　　　　　defective rollers;
(ii) chemical　　developer temperature too high,
　　　　　　　　　fixer not properly replenished,
　　　　　　　　　fixer/hardener concentration not correct.

DENSITY INCORRECT OVERALL

The reasons for radiographs emerging from the processor either too light or too heavy in overall density—assuming the exposure of each to have been properly made in the X-ray room—are inevitably numerous. They include:

    incorrect replenishment rate of the developer;

    contamination of the developer (for instance by the fixer);

    exhausted developer;

    incorrect developer temperature;

    incorrect techniques of solution preparation;

    no circulation of the developer solution.

Each of the above situations has several potential causes. Examples are:

    electrical failure in a pump;

    microswitch out of adjustment;

    blocked filter;

    disconnected hose;

    kinked or otherwise obstructed pipe.

Such defects, though possibly simple in origin, are not necessarily quick to elucidate. Radiographers who are required to solve them appear to need a variety of talents which range from a penchant for plumbing to interviewing skills (darkroom technicians' accounts of what they do).

If the fault is not with some mechanical part or system of the processor but is due to an incorrectly prepared developing solution, trouble sometimes arises because the role of the developer-starter is not fully understood. In Chapter 6 it is explained that the function of the starter is not to start but to brake: that is, it decreases the initial energy of the developer when solutions are changed and the developer is fresh. If too much is used the developer will be lethargic and the processed radiographs too light in density; if too little starter is used the restraint on the reducing action of the developer is not strong enough and radiographic densities consequently are too high overall. It is most important that the proportions of developer to starter should be correct.

DRYING DIFFICULTIES

FILMS NOT DRY

Many of the troubles listed in the next section as the causes of films not being transported through the drier may also be agents which prevent it from becoming dry in the interval before it is ejected from the processor. The reader is referred to the conditions which affect transport but the following factors should be eliminated as well:

(i) drier tubes dirty;

(ii) drier tubes improperly located;

(iii) air inlet filter dirty;

(iv) squeegee roller not tight;

(v) squeegee roller wet—because for any reason water level in the washing section is too high;

(vi) insufficient water circulation.

FILMS NOT TRANSPORTED THROUGH DRIER

The following conditions are among those which may prevent films from moving through the drier.

(i) Mechanical defects. Examples: warped rollers; incorrectly seated rollers; hesitation in the drive because the rollers are too tightly or too loosely engaged.

(ii) Film surfaces tacky for any reason, such as the following:

emulsion inappropriate to the processing cycle;

improperly replenished solutions;

improperly mixed solutions;

solution temperatures too high;

wash-water temperature too high;

drier temperature setting too low;

a fault in the drier's heating circuit.

FOGGING OF FILMS

Films which appear to have been fogged in the processor suggest the following situations:

(i) covers not tight on the processing section;

(ii) processor not sealed against the darkroom wall;

(iii) safelight over the feed-tray not safe (check particularly the wattage of the lamp);

(iv) developer contaminated by fixer.

JAMMED FILMS

When a number of films jam, the one which began the trouble is fairly obviously the film nearest the exit of the processor. This is not to say that the fault which originates the pile-up is necessarily at the same site: it could be further back in the system. For instance, too high a developer temperature may cause the surfaces of a film to be tacky and prevent its travel through the fixing or the drying section. It is consequently essential when dealing with a film jam both to inspect the immediate site for evidence of trouble and to think of the possible causes which might be found at any earlier processing stage.

CLEARING A FILM JAM

(i) Unless the film being processed is a roll, do not turn off the power.

(ii) Remove a crossover ahead of the pile-up.

(iii) Remove the jammed films and put them in a dish of water to avoid them sticking together.

(iv) Carefully remove the rack where the jam occurred—if it is a solution rack turn off the circulation pump for that particular solution.

(v) Examine the rack and tank for a possible cause of the trouble, such as sheared gear teeth, warped rollers, stretched or missing springs.

(vi) Replace the rack if it is satisfactory.

(vii) Re-introduce the films lengthwise into the processor as near as possible to the jamming point.

In the case of roll film the power must be switched off and the film cut at the feed-tray before the jammed section can be cleared.

Afterwards the following possibilities should be considered and eliminated in turn.

(i) Two films overlapped or fed one on top of the other.

(ii) Too short a film (less than 10 cm) fed without a leader.

(iii) A damaged or folded leading edge on a film.

(iv) Detector rollers unevenly set.

(v) Warped rollers.

(vi) The feed-tray out of alignment.

(vii) Any crossover, roller or solution rack out of alignment.

(viiii) Solutions not up to level; recirculating pumps not operating.

(ix) Solution improperly mixed.

(x) Solution temperature too high.

(xi) Incoming water temperature too high.

(xii) Drier temperature too low—if the failure occurred in the drier.

(xiii) Rollers and racks dirty.

TWISTING OF FILMS IN THE PROCESSING SECTION

The following conditions are among those which cause films to cock or turn in the processing section.

(i) Any mechanical factor which causes uneven roller pressure at any point. Examples: gear teeth broken; gears not fully meshed but riding on top of each other; warped rollers.

(ii) Chemical deposits on solution rollers which impede or alter their motion.

(iii) Algae or bacterial growth on the wash rack which results in slimy rollers.

(iv) Roughnesses on guide plates or crossovers.
(v) Feed-tray or detector rollers out of alignment.

Transport difficulties obviously are ascribable either directly or indirectly to the automatic processor involved; they do not occur in the course of manual processing. However, when radiographic artefacts are under investigation there is a tendency to put the blame on a complicated component of the darkroom and thus on the automatic processor. It is important at the same time to exclude simple extrinsic causes, for the processor is not necessarily the agent of every trouble. Fogging may be due to defective safelights or lightleaks in the darkroom as a whole; rough handling of film can occur elsewhere than in the equipment itself.

From processing equipment a natural progression takes us to the part of the X-ray department in which this equipment may operate. At one time this area would have been easy to define and describe in terms generally applicable to virtually every hospital: the processing area was a darkroom, with which might be associated an adjacent room or space where processed radiographs were viewed and checked for quality. Even now, in many hospitals this is the case. That it is not the case in all is due to the increasing use of daylight film-handling and processing systems.

DAYLIGHT PROCESSING

The new practices of daylight processing entail either methods for automatically loading and unloading cassettes or equipment which provides for the so-called cassette-less radiography: in this, a sheet of film is fed to an appropriate area beneath an X-ray table, or behind a vertical chest stand, from a magazine and then—after exposure—directly to a processor. (These systems are fully described in Chapter 11.)

A processor used in this way—that is, one which is accessible to films from a daylight system (either cassette-dependent or otherwise), but is not accessible to any other film—is sometimes said to be dedicated. Perhaps a better way of describing it is to say that the processor is integrated with the system. This integration accelerates the availability of the finished radiograph and increases the rate of throughput of examinations in the X-ray room concerned. It offers a highly purposeful and efficient method of handling full-sized sheets of X-ray film, before, during and after exposure.

However, processor-integration is necessarily inflexible. For instance, a fault in the processor or even the 'down-time' required for a routine service prevents use of the whole system during the period concerned. A processor solely dedicated to equipment for daylight-film handling is appropriate to the majority of X-ray departments, only if it is one of a number of other processors.

Daylight film-handling does not inevitably entail the use of an integrated processor. A daylight system may operate by means of (a) film dispensers which can load a cassette with a sheet of film of appropriate size, and (b) an adaptor kit which is installed on a processor and enables it to:

1 unload a daylight cassette;
2 unload a special film-transporter magazine;
3 accept a film manually unloaded from a conventional cassette (implying association with a darkroom).

Nearly every X-ray department must use some materials or equipments, or both, which at present prohibit daylight-handling. These include:

(a) direct-exposure film;
(b) a vacuum pack which encloses a film and an intensifying screen (often applied to 'low-dose' mammography);
(c) a curved cassette, such as that used in equipment for panoramic projections of the jaws;
(d) the magazines from a rapid film-changer.

Thus, an X-ray department which employs some method of handling and processing films in daylight nevertheless requires—and is very likely to possess—a darkroom, or an area which readily may become a darkroom as occasion demands.

Daylight film-handling systems receive a more detailed account elsewhere (Chapter 11). Below, we shall first consider the planning and construction of an X-ray darkroom and then proceed to some account of viewing rooms and open dispensing/processing/viewing areas.

LOCATION OF THE DARKROOM

To the question of the correct siting of the darkroom in the department, the quick answer is that it should be central to the radiodiagnostic rooms which it will serve. Application of this principle results in the darkroom being adjacent to a single radiographic room in a small department, or placed between two radiographic rooms in a rather larger one. In each case the common wall or walls are likely to be provided with a hatch, through which cassettes may be passed on their way to and from the processing room. This system clearly saves time for radiographers as well as such wear and tear as may be associated with walking further than they need while carrying cassettes.

It is obvious that this type of planning is sensible and correct for many small departments and that in the larger one a natural extension of it might be to provide a darkroom for a number of radiographic rooms, in the manner sketched in Fig. 10.1.

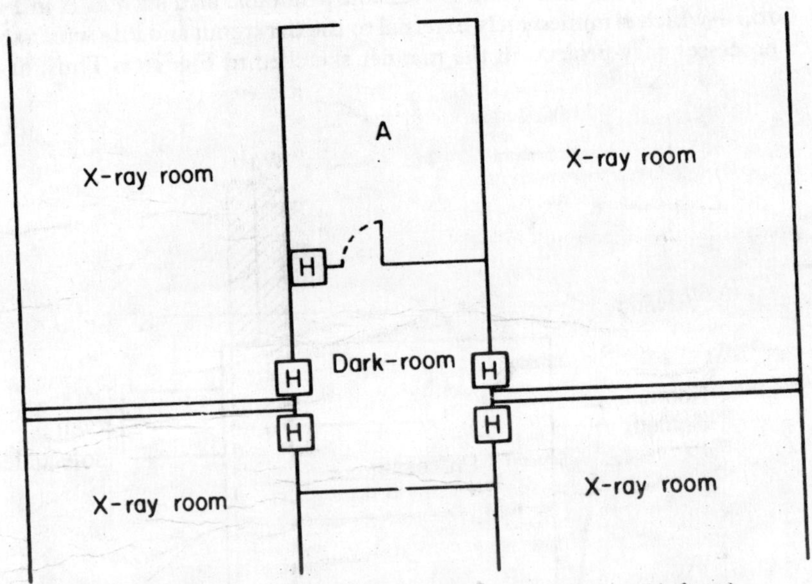

Fig. 10.1. Plan for a possible siting of a darkroom to be directly accessible from 4 radiodiagnostic rooms.
H Cassette hatches
A Adjacent viewing checking area.

In the simplest radiological department which consists of one X-ray room and generator and is staffed probably by only one radiographer, the possibility is that, apart from its actual radiographic exposure, all other work on the film will be done in the darkroom. This means that cassettes will be unloaded, reloaded; films processed, checked and possibly even sorted in the darkroom. This is perfectly satisfactory for the type of department just described.

However, if we imagine this situation scaled two or three times larger, then it becomes obvious that delay will occur because parts of the work cannot be done simultaneously.

Radiographs may not be checked for quality and sorted by one group of people, while others are unloading cassettes or chemically processing, since the first activity requires white light and the second depends on a reduced specialized illumination to which the film is not sensitive. It becomes necessary when the volume of radiographs in a department is above a quite limited level, to break down darkroom procedure into stages of the work which need safelighting and those which do not.

Such a separation is very easy to achieve, if the processor is of the automatic variety and there is available a suitable area such as A in Fig 10.1—which is immediately external to the darkroom and into which the processor may project, in the manner sketched in Fig. 10.2. Thus, dry,

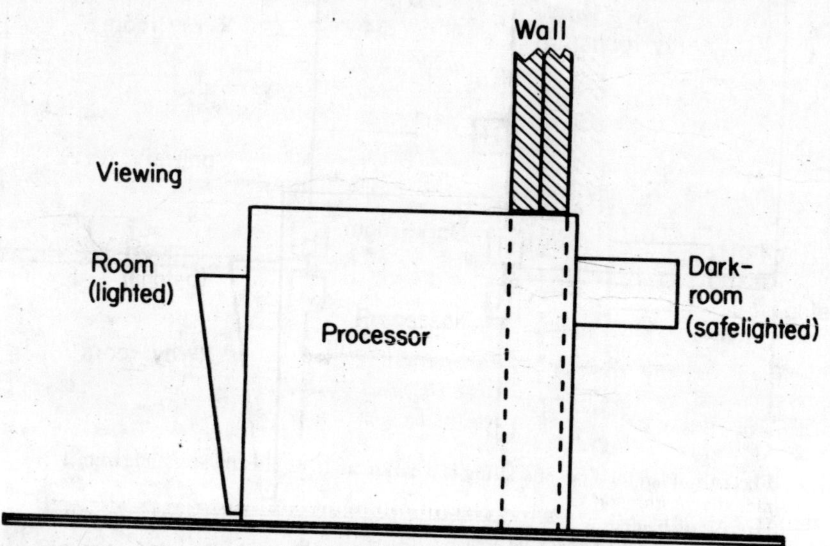

Fig. 10.2. A through-the-wall position for an automatic processor. (Elevation.)

finished radiographs are issued to a lighted room, where they may be viewed carefully, without interrupting other work and without interruption by it. The only tasks occurring within the darkroom are unloading and reloading procedures and the feeding of exposed film to the processor(s).

Manual processors, however, do not so conveniently lend themselves to a through-the-wall arrangement of their work. The situation requires a specially constructed washing tank which the darkroom wall may straddle, similarly to an automatic processor. The tank has a double-ended lid, hinged at a fixed middle section, so that access to each end of the tank is separately obtained on either side of the darkroom wall. The lids are interlocked, for the same purpose as are the doors of a cassette hatch, so that each may be opened only if the other part is closed. The developed and fixed—but not yet fully washed—radiographs, which are mounted in their processing hangers in special racks on runners in the tank, are manually pushed by technicians from the darkroom end of the tank towards the viewing-room end. With the darkroom section of the lid closed and the other part open, radiographers in the viewing room may pull wet radiographs from the tank and check them, without interrupting other processing stages which must be safelighted.

Such an arrangement is neither convenient nor comfortable for the operators but would be useful to a department which combined the use of manual processing with the production of large numbers of radiographs. In the United Kingdom the Department of Health does not recommend manual processing where the throughput is greater than 50 films during any working day, or the X-ray department has more than two radio-diagnostic rooms. Student radiographers working within the United Kingdom are unlikely to become familiar with the special wash tank just described.

In sequence with their processing, the sorting of radiographs has been mentioned. This implies linking each set of films, where necessary to those of a previous examination, and certainly to an envelope and the requisition form and index card of the patient concerned. We see this particular activity becoming allied to the work of the department's record-keeping office and thus the sorting room—whether served by an automatic processor or a manual one—should be within easy reach of the office. A new factor has entered our original idea of correct darkroom planning and if we wish to have several darkrooms we must consider, with *their* position, the situation of sorting areas in relation to the functions of radiographic documentation and of radiological reporting.

Darkrooms which are distant from radiodiagnostic rooms may raise the question of how best to convey to them cassettes or films or both; and equally how best to return loaded cassettes from the darkroom to the locations where radiographers need them. In the past a number of different mechanical systems have been described and used and sometimes were expensive and inefficient. No doubt the most reliable method must be personal conveyance by radiographers or other people, to whom various forms of little cart, even supermarket-type trolleys, may be helpful for the purpose. A modern trend is to take processing to radiographers as far as possible, by the use of daylight systems, cassette-less radiographic equipments and processors in X-ray rooms. Such methods now are recommended for multi-roomed departments, if their use will avoid the provision of the mechanical cassette conveyor or film conveyor.

DARKROOM CONSTRUCTION

In the darkroom many features of equipment and layout must vary with the dimensions of the room, the method of processing and the division of the work. These will be considered in later sections. Certain structural aspects are important for all darkrooms. These include the nature of floor, walls and ceiling; the ventilation and heating; the type of entrance.

FLOORS, WALLS AND CEILING

Many X-ray departments have suffered from darkrooms which are too small, as well as having other faults no doubt: but it is equally possible for a darkroom to be too large for maximum efficiency, if technicians must cover a wide area between, say, the point at which a cassette is unloaded and the processing unit.

To give some 'ideal' size in precise figures is not helpful, for a general assessment cannot take into account the number of people likely to work in a particular darkroom, or the number of examinations made in the department which it serves. Another factor is the type of processing: automatic units make large darkrooms less desirable. All these aspects should be considered when planning the size of a new darkroom. We can say, however, that no processing room which is in constant use should be smaller than 9 m² in area. The ceiling should be not less than 2·7 m in height, and preferably not greater than 3·3 mm if ceiling reflector lamps are to be used.

Particularly if the whole, or the greater part of a processor is within a darkroom, then the nature of the floor's material should be such that:

1 it is non-porous;
2 it is resistant to staining by chemicals or other liquids;
3 it does not become slippery when wet.

An absorbent floor covering cannot easily be cleaned. Chemicals spilled upon it not only will stain the surface but as they remain in the floor's material may possibly contaminate the surrounding air when dry.

Not all impervious materials are equally resistant to stains and some may easily become slippery when wet. Semi-vitreous and non-vitreous tiles are unsatisfactory from the first point of view, and concrete, terrazzo or ceramic tiles have a tendency to the second disadvantage; this can be improved by the inclusion in them of a small amount of abrasive, granular material. Satisfactorily resistant substances are those of a composition which has a high proportion of asphalt: porcelain and natural clay tiles also are good, as well as some varieties of hard rubber and rubber sheet.

Any adhesive material employed to fasten down a floor covering must of course be waterproof, as also should be the floor itself.

In general the previous recommendations apply as much to the walls as to the floor, particularly of course to areas in the neighbourhood of sinks and wet processing equipment which should be protected to a height of at least 1·3 m. A rear splash panel for this purpose is a common accessory to such processing units. Alternatively, or even in addition to it, ceramic or plastic tiles or sheets of Formica or similar material can be applied to adjacent wall surfaces.

Elsewhere on the walls, a durable, good quality paint should give adequate protection if tiling cannot be used throughout. Untreated brickwork which is exposed to constant chemical contamination may undergo a gradual process of destruction which is difficult to arrest.

The decor of a darkroom must not be dark in colour. In fact a gloomy environment is insiduously depressing and unnecessary. A glossy cream or white paint on the walls, for example, would do very well. Orange, yellow, or green, are to be avoided since they will reflect very poorly the light from safelamps of a similar colour.

Modern practice is to obtain as much reflected light as possible in a darkroom. Reflection of the available light provides throughout the room a diffuse illumination which often can be maintained at a surprisingly high value and gives little impression that the place actually *is* dark. Reflected light does not differ in wavelength from the incident light which causes it and consequently offers no greater risk to sensitive materials. It may in fact decrease the number of lamps required in the room and certainly lessens strain on those who must work there.

Paints are sometimes said to be acid-resistant. It is worth noting that, while this description may testify to their behaviour when under fire from fixing solutions, it is no indication at all of what may happen should the splashes be of an alkaline nature; that is, should they have come from the developer and not the fixer.

The type of paint on the ceiling is also significant since it should not be of a character to produce flakes which are likely to fall on sensitive materials or on open cassettes below. It is bad practice to leave cassettes lying open. For the same reason plaster is to be avoided. A good quality, modern emulsion paint is probably a satisfactory material from this point of view. To avoid a similar risk from falling particles, any water pipes, electric conduits or air ducts preferably should be enclosed above a false ceiling. This provides a smooth, intact surface overhead which can easily be kept clean.

Some of the foregoing observations are directed towards the protection of the darkroom from the effects of contact with chemicals. While others remain important, this may have less significance if processing is by automation and virtually the entire processor is on the other side of the darkroom wall. In this case the darkroom, unless it contains as well a stand-by unit for hand processing, becomes in effect a dry working area in which chemicals are not prepared, solutions changed, or wet equipment cleaned.

However, the problem has been moved rather than removed. Resistant materials which we have mentioned as suitable for a darkroom are appropriate also for the adjacent viewing room, at least in the immediate vicinity of a processor: here servicing and cleaning of the equipment and the preparation and storage of chemicals are likely to be conducted.

RADIATION PROTECTION

Darkrooms, or rather the personnel and sensitive materials associated with them, require protection from ionizing radiation, usually—although not necessarily—X rays from adjoining radiographic rooms. Existing situations should be re-examined when new installations are made, particularly when a minor diagnostic unit is replaced by one of greater output. The arrangement of X-ray apparatus in any case should be such that the primary beam is never directed at a wall of the processing room.

Walls are mainly affected but ceilings and floors also should be considered if X-ray generators, or equipment employing radionuclides are in operation on another storey of the building. These remarks apply also to storerooms where reserve stocks of film may be kept, and in this connection some attention should be given to the route along which films are normally taken, either from their point of delivery to the store room, or from the latter when they are moved to the position of current stock in the darkroom.

The structure of a room in which film is stored or handled should have a lead equivalency of 2 mm. For this purpose the following are appropriate materials:

1 A 25 mm layer of high quality barium plaster. (1 part fine barium sulphate; 1 part coarse barium sulphate; 1 part Portland cement).

2 A single brick wall; that is, 225 mm of *solid* brick.

3 A wall which is half a brick in thickness and has in addition a half-inch layer of high quality barium plaster.

4 A 150 mm thickness of concrete.

5 A 250 mm thickness of coke-breeze blocks.

6 Lead 'Plymax' boards with 2 mm of lead.

In using protective materials attention particularly should be given to

obtaining an overlap at points of discontinuity in the wall; for example at
the site of a transfer hatch for cassettes.

It is an accepted part of many codes or guidance notes for good
radiological practice that a qualified physicist, or other competent expert,
should monitor any new room, or modified existing room, in or near to
which ionizing radiations are being handled: this rule naturally will
include the processing room. In the absence of a more accurately made
check, the entry of ionizing radiation into a darkroom can easily be
proved by placing a coin on an envelope-wrapped film and fixing the
latter to the suspect wall of the room; the coin should lie between the film
and the surface of the wall. This can be left for some time, for a week
perhaps but the period certainly should be longer than that for which any
film would remain in the vicinity during the normal occurrences of work:
in this connection the susceptibility of stored film materials should not be
overlooked. In a room which is not sufficiently protected, a faint image
of the coin will be apparent on the test film after processing.

VENTILATION AND HEATING

Owing to its enclosure for many hours of the day adequate ventilation of
the darkroom is extremely important. The space considered necessary for
a patient in a hospital ward is given as 1,000 cu. ft. and this would seem
a fair recommendation for each technician in a darkroom. Unfortunately
much lower figures are sometimes stated and applied. During intermittent
use an allowance of 400 cu. ft. upwards might be tolerated but in most X-
ray departments which employ darkroom staff it is unrealistic to suppose
that these people are not subjected to a confining environment
continuously throughout the day.

It is sometimes recommended that darkrooms should have large
windows which can be opened after working hours or at any other
convenient time. Experience suggests, however, that in a busy department
there is hardly a convenient time, and even the phrase 'after working
hours' may be found in fact to signify those of the night between midnight
and perhaps 8.0 a.m. A better direction of energy is to provide the
darkroom with a fully efficient system of air-conditioning rather than
expend concern if planning is such that it cannot possess a window.

The air in a darkroom should be completely changed at least 5 times
per hour; some authorities have been found to state even up to 10 times
in the same period. The most usual way of doing this is to obtain cross
ventilation by means of an extractor fan or fans situated at a high level in
the room, while air is drawn in from some outside source at a low level.
While many darkrooms possess the amenity of an extractor fan, sometimes

insufficient attention is given to the air intake to the room, reliance being placed simply on what may be drawn through its entrance, perhaps from a reception area or corridor. The air intake preferably should be from the outside and ideally would be filtered to remove dust and other particles.

Suitable apparatus for the intake of air may be either a blow-in fan, or else non-mechanical in kind: that is, a light-proof baffle with a variable aperture which can be fitted in a wall, window or door. Any device which communicates from the darkroom must be light-trapped: this applies equally to a simple louvre and to 'intake' and 'extract' fans. Ideally intake and extraction would be from diagonally opposite points, both open to fresh air. In practice this situation can seldom exist.

An intake fan situated on an outside wall will lose efficiency if the temperature of the room is much greater than that outside; the tendency of the air is to move outwards then, rather than inwards. This will be improved if the incoming air can be warmed by passing it through a radiator. Some fans have a heater attached for this purpose. It is also helpful if the extractor fan or fans can be given greater power than their intake companions. Fans placed outside the building should, as far as possible, be situated in places sheltered from prevailing wind pressures and they must have a cowl for light-proofing and to protect them in bad weather. Many fans have switches which permit adjustment of their speed.

The installation of a good air-conditioning system would be more efficient than cross ventilation by fans and perhaps not enough use is made of it. Certainly it is not found in older institutions.

Darkroom temperatures should be maintained between 65°F (18·3° C) and 68°F (20°C). The relative humidity of the atmosphere should be ideally 40 to 60 per cent.

Proper heating of the darkroom is a lesser problem as a rule than its ventilation. Whatever system is employed in other parts of the hospital is likely to serve also the darkroom. Hot water radiators are very common. If electrical heaters are used they should not be of an open filament type which are dangerous to personnel and an added fire risk to sensitive materials. Furthermore attention must be given to the brightness of any pilot lamps associated with electrical equipment in the darkroom: the light emitted may be of a colour or intensity which will fog X-ray or fluorographic film handled in its neighbourhood.

TYPE OF ENTRANCE

It is of course possible to employ as a means of entering or leaving the darkroom a simple, single door. If only one person is using the room there is unlikely to be any difficulty from lack of access to it during processing procedures.

However, such an arrangement carries other pitfalls. The door should have a latch or lock, if mishaps are to be avoided when someone unknowingly attempts an entrance whilst light-sensitive materials are being handled. The door fastening should be capable of being released from the outside if an emergency arises, especially if the room has no window. Whether or not the lock has such a safety feature, a potentially dangerous situation exists for an operator who is working alone. In the event of an accident or sudden illness, entailing loss either of consciousness or of mobility, it might be a long while before help reached the victim.

In some countries—of which the United Kingdom is one—legislation exists which makes provision for the safety of people at work. Inspections of X-ray darkrooms under the terms of such legislation have led to recommendations that no one should work alone in these circumstances. However, it is unrealistic to suppose that there may always be two or more people in an X-ray darkroom. An 'on-call' duty radiographer, for example, processing films during an emergency examination, is very likely to be alone; additional personnel, who may be on the scene, almost certainly at the time are concerned more with care of the patient than of the radiographer!

A darkroom door should be sound in structure, well fitting and completely light-proof. To this end it may be necessary to fit round the edges a sealing strip of a type sold commercially for the exclusion of draughts. This is better than the suggestion sometimes made of hanging a curtain across the door: to be effective such a curtain must reach and overlap floor level and it becomes inevitably not only a light trap but one for dirt and dust as well.

However, in the interests of safety or if a number of people have to use a darkroom, it is better to provide an entrance which is able to eliminate problems inherent in a locked door and to function independently of any processing need. Practically, there are two ways of doing this: (i) by the employment of double doors arranged on either side of a small vestibule; (ii) by the construction of a continuous passage made like a labyrinth.

DOUBLE DOORS

Figure 10.3 shows one possible scheme for the use of double doors; each door should be sturdy in structure and well fitting, so as to prevent the admission of any light when it is closed.

The double door system is economical of space. If the door nearer to the darkroom opens into the room and the outer doors open outwards,

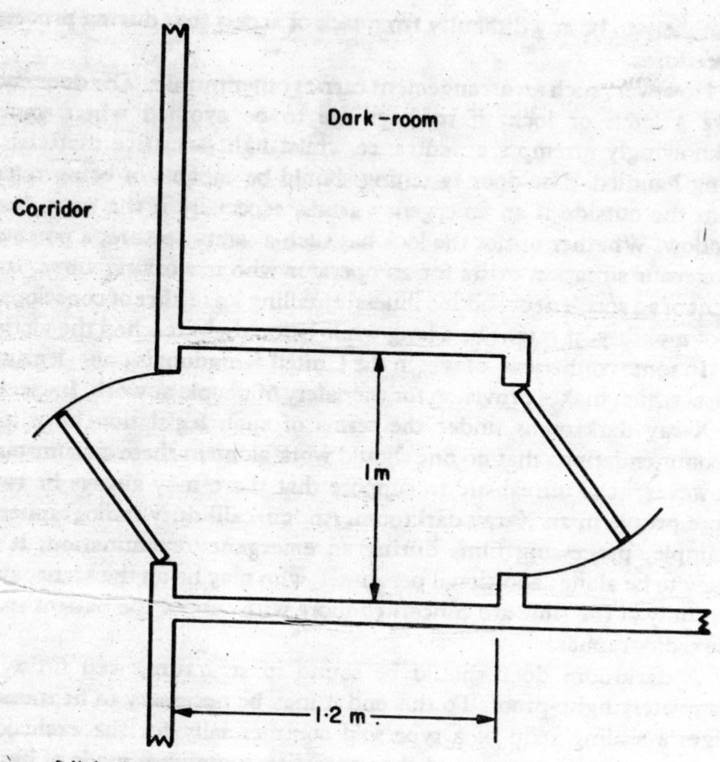

Fig. 10.3. A light-lock entrance to a darkroom, using double doors.

(as in Fig. 10.3) the dimensions of the vestibule between them can be—and sometimes are—very small indeed: the space may be no larger than is required to accept one adult of average build (while breathing out?). Sometimes darkroom planning may allow the inner door to be of the sliding type: this will save space in the darkroom. A light-lock which depends on double doors has the disadvantage of being not fully foolproof since there is certainly a chance that someone may emerge from the inner door simultaneously with the entrance of someone else through the outer. An electrical interlock can be fitted which prevents either door from being opened unless its fellow is closed. Such a sophistication inevitably is subject to failure at some time or another and the occasional disaster to films can occur.

Human disasters also may occur as we have seen (p. 249). In the interests of greater safety it must be possible to override the door-interlocks or to use a master key to obtain entrance to the darkroom.

A variation on the double-door theme is to have a revolving door, similar to that found in some hotels or other public buildings. In this case, when bulky equipment must be conveyed to the darkroom, a means of folding away the wings of the door is essential, to provide unimpeded access to the room. It is perhaps not a convenient form of entrance to anyone who is carrying a number of film cassettes.

LABYRINTH

A typical labyrinth for a darkroom consists of two parallel passages and a facing wall. Such an arrangement is shown in plan form in Figure 10.4. In principal, the design of a labyrinth should be such that light is reflected at least three times between the external area and the darkroom; more accurately, the required process is not reflection but absorption, since the aim is to diminish the intensity of light to a harmless level. In this action, a labyrinth's effectiveness will be greater if:

1 a matt black paint is used for the interior of the passages, the central baffle and the facing portions of room walls;
2 the vertical height of the entrance is limited to 2 metres;
3 the length of each passage is not less than 3 metres;
4 the width of each passage is not more than 700 mm.

If required for the assistance of staff entering the labyrinth from relatively bright surroundings, safelamps, or a white or luminous line at eye-level, may be fitted along the passageway.

The only real disadvantage of a labyrinth is that it requires relatively more space than other entrances. Its advantages are:

(a) it provides easy and instant access to the darkroom at all times;
(b) it offers no hazard to a single-handed operator;
(c) it may effectively participate in the ventilation of a darkroom if the air beyond is reasonably fresh;
(d) it is adaptable, as—if sufficient space is available—the principle is suitable for a number of differing architectural designs.

DARKROOM ILLUMINATION

Electric shock is a potential hazard in the darkroom owing to the proximity of electrical equipment to water and the possibility that persons using this equipment may have damp hands and be standing on a floor possibly wet.

Any light or illuminator situated near the site of wet manipulations, and preferably *all* lights in the darkroom should be operated by a pullcord switch. Electrical points should be of the three-pin shuttered type and both these and any hand-switches of insulating material should be

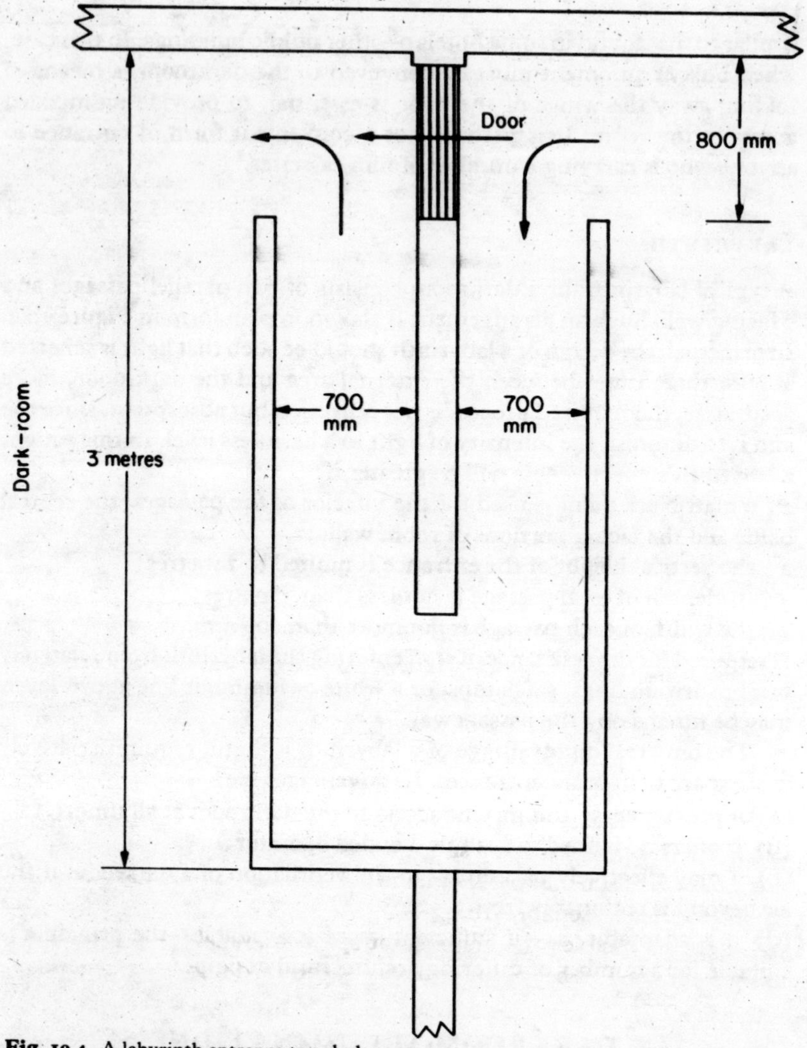

Fig. 10.4. A labyrinth entrance to a darkroom.

waterproof. Non-current-carrying metallic items, such as the case of an electric interval-timer, should be earthed.

Darkroom illumination is in two categories. These are:

1   general white light;
2   safelight.

To this we may add in some instances:

3   viewing equipment.

GENERAL WHITE LIGHT

Usually white light will conform with normal hospital practice. It should be placed close to the ceiling to avoid strong shadows.

White light is necessary to the darkroom to enable work which does not involve sensitive materials to be properly performed; for example, cleaning of the room and processing equipment, and the inspection of intensifying screens. A reasonable strength of light obviously is required but if it is dazzlingly bright technicians may suffer loss of visual accommodation which will be disadvantageous to them.

If the room is large enough to warrant more than a single central ceiling fixture, one should be placed over each main working area.

SAFELIGHTING

A darkroom's safe illumination need not—and consequently should not—be less than the maximum level of brightness permitted by the most sensitive material which is being handled in it.

The term 'safe' to some extent is misleading in so far as it is not absolute: it implies only a degree of safety. No emulsion is completely insensitive to light, even to a darkroom lamp of the colour described as safe for its handling. We can say (a) that its response is related predominantly to wavelength or colour, but that also significant are (b) the intensity of the light and (c) the duration of the exposure.

In the X-ray darkroom (a) is a readily established factor if the correct colour of safelight is chosen; (b) is controlled by attention both to the wattage of the lamps used and their distance from any point at which sensitive material is handled; (c) is bound to be a variable, depending on the technician's method and speed of work. Overlong exposure to safelight is a possibility which is always present and no one responsible for any processing should permit sensitive materials to remain unprotected: it is very bad practice to unload a large number of cassettes and stack their contents along a bench prior to putting all the films collectively into the processor. If films must be accumulated in this way, a fitted light-tight drawer or container, deep enough to allow hangers to stand vertically within, should be provided.

In a general radiographic darkroom there is no necessity to work in a red light. Fluorographic and other orthochromatic materials require special consideration and are discussed in Chapter 16. Apart from these the spectral sensitivity of X-ray film, whether it is to be used with intensifying screens or intended for direct exposure, does not extend beyond the blue bands of the spectrum. It can therefore be manipulated for a limited period in brown or olive-green lighting and one of these is generally employed: they represent the region of the spectrum for which we have greatest visual sensitivity at low levels of illumination.

Lacquered bulbs or those of coloured glass are not a satisfactory form of darkroom lighting. The first are very likely from wear to suffer cracks in their coating and become unsafe for sensitive materials; the second do not provide a sufficient range of colour to be useful.

Safe illumination commonly takes the form of a lamp fixture of special design. In this an ordinary pearl bulb of not more than 25 watts is used and a coloured filter placed in front of the bulb will tint the light to the required hue. This makes it quite simple to alter the colour of the safe-lighting should it become necessary, or to renew any filters that are damaged. Safelighting can be either direct or indirect.

DIRECT SAFELIGHTING

Direct illumination is local in nature. A lamp of this kind is shown in **Fig. 10.5.**

The lamp has a circular filter 14 cm (5½ in.) in diameter and it may be either suspended from the ceiling or fixed to the wall above a bench, processing unit or other working point. It should be placed so that

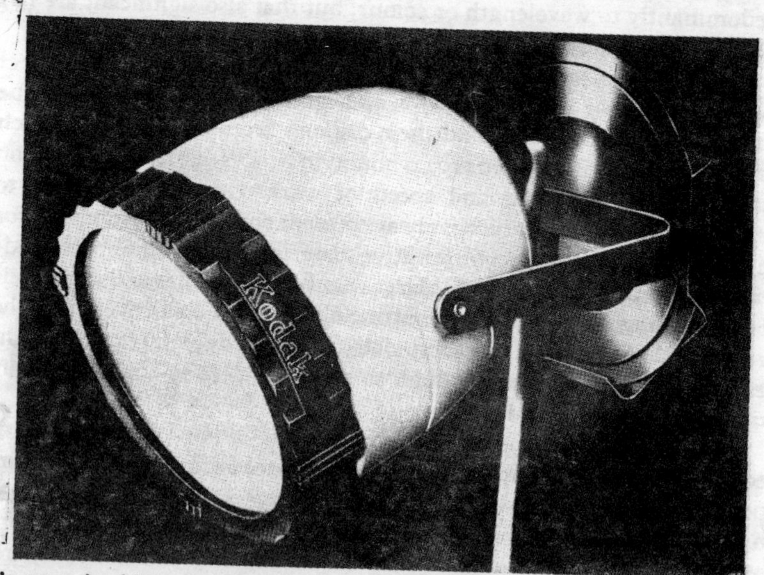

Fig. 10.5. A safelamp for direct lighting. It may be fixed to the wall or be ceiling-suspended. *By courtesy of Kodak Ltd.*

sensitive material is normally handled no nearer to it than 122 cm (4 feet) and it should be situated the same distance from any similar lamp placed in another working area of the room.

Films should not be held close to safelamps. To do this is to expose them to an uncontrolled intensity of light to which quite probably they are sensitive. This situation is most likely to arise if the radiographer attempts to assess a radiograph's quality during wet processing by removing it from the developer and holding it against the light from a neighbouring safelamp.

Safelamps are often situated near a manual processing unit; the implication sometimes is that this lamp is needed for the inspection of films during development. Whether or not this is its intended purpose, it is often unfortunately the use to which it is put. There *are* arguments for placing lamps near the processing unit: it is a major working area and may not otherwise be adequately illuminated, but in principle these safelamps should always be suspended overhead.

Often a safelamp is sited in a darkroom above the feedtray of an automatic processor and is operated by the processor. The lamp illumines the working area during the introduction of a film but is circuited so that the light goes out as soon as the processor has accepted the film. The reappearance of the light after an interval indicates the processor's readiness for the next sheet of film. This darkroom lamp is never the only such signal of the processor's cycle. There is usually a pilot lamp on the processor itself functioning in a similar way; and sometimes a brief audible indication as well is given as soon as the processor may receive another film.

The use of any direct illumination is not recommended for fast orthochromatic or panchromatic materials.

INDIRECT SAFELIGHTING

Indirect safelighting is intended to provide general illumination of the darkroom. In this case the safelamp directs the light towards the ceiling which reflects it back into the room. When lighting is used in this way some standardization of the reflective abilities of the ceiling clearly is needed. It should not have a dull surface but should be painted a glossy pale cream or white. Its height should be within 2·7–3·3 metres. If a high ceiling cannot be avoided then it is necessary to hang white reflectors at least 1 m² above each safelamp and these are more efficient if their surface is convex.

Fig. 10.6 shows a safelamp which has filters on both its upper and lower surfaces and is thus suitable for providing both indirect and direct

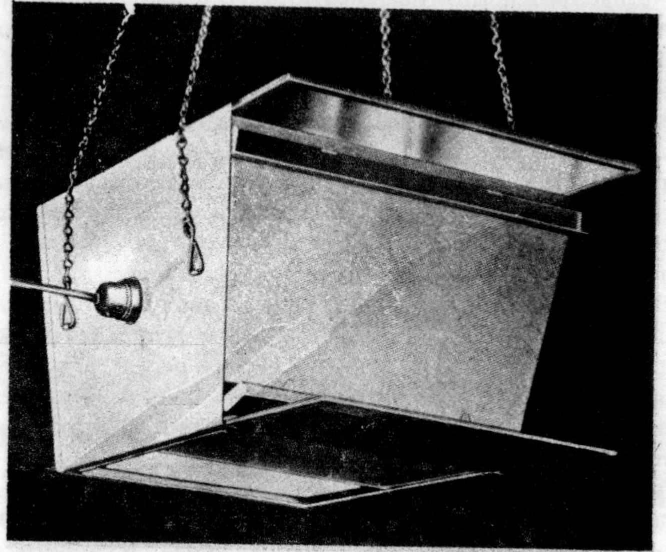

Fig. 10.6. A safelamp for both direct and indirect illumination. *By courtesy of Kodak Ltd.*

illumination simultaneously. One of these may be allowed for every 6·5 m² of floor space. The lower edge of the lamp should be not less than 2·1 m above floor level.

SAFELIGHT FILTERS

The filters used in safelamps are usually a sheet of gelatin dyed to the appropriate colour and for protection sandwiched between two sheets of glass. The glass incidentally also helps to diffuse the light but this is a minor function.

The gelatin will deteriorate if it is subjected to extremes of heat and moisture. Assuming that the design of the lamp is efficient in keeping it cool, the most likely cause of overheating of the gelatin is the use of an electric bulb of too high a wattage. It is very tempting to try to improve darkroom illumination by replacing a 25 watt lamp with another of greater power but this must never be done.

If the level of safe illumination appears to have diminished in a darkroom it may well be because cleaning is overdue. Safelamps and filters require regular attention in this respect: they readily attract dust and loss of efficiency from this cause can be insidious and unnoticed. The suspension of hanging lamps should be such that they can readily be taken down if necessary. There is usually provision for easy removal of the filters.

SAFELIGHT TESTS

Safelights should not be trusted implicitly or indefinitely. From time to time tests are necessary to ascertain that the illumination employed in fact is safe. These may be required in any of the following circumstances.

1   The darkroom is a new one.

2   Safelights have been changed or additions made to them.

3   A technique or method of work has been altered. For example, the introduction of a faster type of emulsion, or of a multi-film cassette such as that of the Schonander rapid changer, may each entail intervals of exposure to safelight which have become unsafe; the first because the emulsion is more sensitive and the second because the time required fully to load a cassette is naturally longer.

4   A particular lamp is suspect as the cause of fogging, perhaps because of deterioration of the filter, or less probably erosion of metal parts.

There are several ways of making a check on the safety of darkroom illumination. The following is one recommended procedure.

1   A cardboard holder to take the film in making the test should be previously prepared. This holder should be of a size to accomodate the film. In use, the two edges of the holder are folded over so that the side-edges of the film each have a narrow strip which is covered by a folded edge of the cardboard holder and thus shielded from exposure to the safelighting as the test is made. (See Figs. 10.7 and 10.8).

2   The film selected for the test should be of the fastest speed which is in use and is processed in the darkroom.

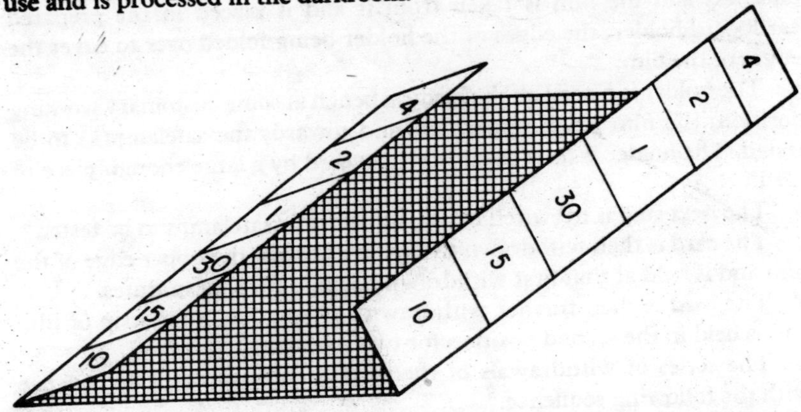

Fig. 10.7.

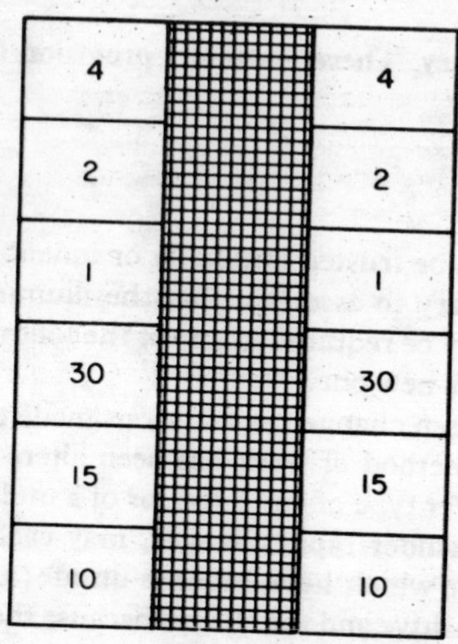

Fig. 10.8.

3   The selected film is taken in a cassette to an X-ray room. A sheet of lead is used to cover half of the cassette lengthwise so that the area of film beneath this mask receives no X-ray exposure. The other half of the film in the cassette is given a slight exposure to X rays sufficient to produce on development a density of 0·8. Exposed films are more sensitive to light than those which have had no exposure and in the darkroom films in either state will be handled under safelights, as cassettes are unloaded and reloaded. So it is worth having both unexposed and exposed areas on the film to be used for the test.

4   In the darkroom, all lights are turned off. The cassette is opened in darkness and the film is taken from it and is placed in the prepared cardboard holder, the edges of the holder being folded over to cover the edges of the film.

5   The holder is placed on the loading bench at some customary working position, the film being uppermost and towards the safelamp(s) to be tested. The holder is then completely covered by a large enough piece of card.

6   The next step is to switch on the safelamp or safelamps to be tested.

7   The card is then withdrawn to expose a strip at the upper edge of the film and is held at that first withdrawn position for four minutes.

8   The card is then further withdrawn to expose another strip of film and is held in the second position for two minutes.

9   The series of withdrawals of the card is constituted in accordance with the following sequence.

1st withdrawn position maintained for 4 minutes
2nd withdrawn position maintained for 2 minutes
3rd withdrawn position maintained for 1 minute
4th withdrawn position maintained for 30 seconds
5th withdrawn position maintained for 15 seconds
6th withdrawn position maintained for 10 seconds.

10   When the last strip of film has been exposed for 10 seconds, the film is again completely covered with the piece of cardboard. The series of exposures to the safelighting has been as follows, from the shortest to the longest.

Strip 6   10 seconds
Strip 5 $10+15 = 25$ seconds
Strip 4 $10+15+30 = 55$ seconds
Strip 3 $10+15+30+60 = 115$ seconds $= 1·9$ minutes
Strip 2 $10+15+30+60+120 = 235$ seconds $= 3·9$ minutes
Strip 1 $10+15+30+60+120+240 = 475$ seconds $= 7·9$ minutes

11   The safelamps are turned off and the film is processed in darkness. It is then examined for the results of the test.

It will be realized that the surface area of the film (see Fig. 10.9) can be divided vertically into four separate regions. Area A had no pre-exposure to X rays (it was shielded in the X-ray room) and no safelight exposure (it was shielded by the folded edge of the holder). Any density

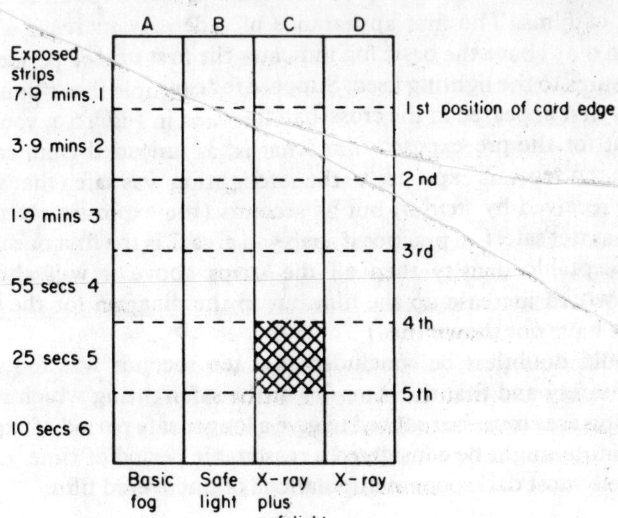

Fig. 10.9.

in this area is basic fog. Area B has had no X-ray exposure (it was shielded in the X-ray room) and has received a controlled series of increasing exposures to safelighting; its reaction to these is the reaction of unexposed X-ray film with which cassettes are loaded in the darkroom. Area C has had a slight exposure to X rays in the X-ray room plus the controlled exposures to safelighting in the darkroom; its reaction to the safelighting is that of exposed films being processed in the darkroom. Area D has had a slight exposure to X-rays but no exposure to safelighting because it was covered by the folded edge of the holder.

In examining the processed film with the aid of a densitometer, the area D can be used to establish that the pre-exposure to X rays was about right in giving a density of 0·8. The area A can be used for the measurement of the basic fog. The areas C and B are then carefully examined for the first appearance (as the eye travels up the film from its bottom to top edges) of a density increase which is more than 0·05 above the basic fog.

If no such density appears, then the tested lighting is safe for up to almost eight minutes both for the exposed and for the unexposed X-ray film which has been used for the test. This certainly would be a time-interval long enough for all the usual darkroom practices and might be considered to be much longer than was necessary. The safelighting could be increased in intensity to give more illumination for the darkroom workers and the test would then be repeated to establish that the new safe period of exposure was nearer to the time actually required for the handling of films. The first appearance of a density increase which is more than 0·05 above the basic fog indicates the first unsafe period of the test exposures to the lighting used. Suppose for example that this increase in density first appeared in the cross-hatched area in Fig. 10.9, you would know that for the pre-exposed film (that is, as unloaded from cassettes after use) ten seconds exposure to the safelighting was safe (that was the exposure received by strip 6) but 25 seconds (the exposure received by strip 5) was not safe. (In practice if strip 5 in area C is the first one to show the unacceptable density then all the strips above it will also show densities which increase up the film but in the diagram for the sake of clarity we have not shown this.)

It would doubtless be concluded that ten seconds was too short a period of safety and that the intensity of the safelighting which reached the working area must be reduced to give a longer safe period of exposure. Half a minute might be considered a reasonable period of time in which to complete most darkroom manipulations of uncovered film.

VIEWING EQUIPMENT

In a small department where the darkroom must contain all stages of manual processing provision is necessary for the assessment of wet radiographs.

For this the minimum requirement is a single illuminator wall-mounted above the processing unit, possibly on a shelf but preferably attached directly to the wall. In principle this illuminator should be situated above the washing compartment of the processing unit and it is very susceptible to splashing: rust and corrosion of metal parts are bound to develop sooner or later.

As far as possible an illuminator used in this way should be protected. A wet film attachment is helpful. This is a sheet of clear Perspex which has the same area as the illuminator and can be suspended in front of it by special fixtures at the top; the free lower end is formed into a curved drip tray. The efficacy of this arrangement will be increased if the illuminator can be supported at a very slight forward angle to bring its lower part out of the line of falling drops.

A special design of illuminator for darkroom and other wet use is wall-mounted in a completely enclosed shell of translucent plastic material. This is very serviceable and should be preferred to modifying a conventional illuminator. Any illuminator employed for wet viewing must be operated by a pull-cord switch. It is bad practice to use in the darkroom an illuminator discarded from elsewhere and operated by the usual form of toggle or variable control rotary switch.

SWITCHING OF LIGHT CIRCUITS

White-light switching should be arranged to reduce the possibility of its being switched on accidentally while films are under manipulation. If the safelight and normal light circuits are separately controlled at wall points in a 'dry' area of the room, the switches should be placed at very different heights, the one for the white light being put out of normal reach: for example the safelight switch might be 1·5 m from the floor and the whitelight switch 2 m.

It is recommended practice to have a cord-operated master control for both circuits positioned near the door of the darkroom. This is often combined with a cord-operated change-over switch which will give either white or safe lighting and this should be situated near a working area: there can in fact be more than one switch for this purpose, for example near the loading bench and another above the processing unit. If the room has several white lights this arrangement may operate only the central light or all of them, if desired.

Another system sometimes used is to provide a separate pull-cord switch for every white light and to situate this near the light. The method does not exclude the provision of a master control near the entrance but there seems little to recommend it from the point of view of convenience.

A drawer- or door-operated switch in series with the white lights is a useful safety device which can be fitted to a hopper or container used for the storage of unexposed and largely unprotected sensitive materials. Should it be opened when the white lights are on in the room this switch will operate to extinguish them.

Another common practice is to fit an indicating lamp, usually red or orange, outside the darkroom door. This is wired in parallel with the safelights and provides visible warning whenever they are in use. Such a device becomes less desirable, and no doubt is unnecessary if the entrance to the darkroom is by means of a continuous light-trap without the use of doors. Safelamps placed in the latter type of entrance for guidance preferably should not be associated with the safelights of the room. They are better operated by a master control switch for all circuits placed near the point of entry, from which one at least of these lamps should be visible.

DARKROOM EQUIPMENT AND LAYOUT

The work to be done in an X-ray darkroom (a) involves the handling of dry film materials and (b) may include processes which depend on chemical solutions and consequently are wet in nature. Cassettes, intensifying screens and unexposed film—all costly items—become unservicable when damaged by stains and splashes. A radiograph contaminated similarly prior to processing, or during or after drying, may be useless because of lost image quality. It is clear that overlap between wet and dry operations in a darkroom should be avoided.

A well planned darkroom should have the following characteristics.

1   Effective separation of wet and dry operations, if both occur in the room.

2   Orderly sequence of successive stages of the work.

3   Neat layout of the equipment in adequate space.

4   Clear 'traffic lanes' so that technicians are not in each others' way if more than one is working in the room. We will return later to these four points, having some knowledge of the appliances concerned.

In broad terms we can say that the equipment necessary to an X-ray darkroom is (a) a bench upon which to unload cassettes, prepare films for processing and reload cassettes; (b) apparatus in which processing is performed; (c) certain essential accessories. When we examine these headings in more detail we find that some of their practicalities depend closely upon whether the method of processing is automatic or manual. These methods and the instruments for each have been described in the previous chapter and need not be discussed now. We will consider for the moment what other equipment is required in a darkroom where the processor is of an automatic variety.

THE DARKROOM WITH AUTOMATIC PROCESSING

THE LOADING BENCH

Perhaps the first requisite of a darkroom's loading bench is that it should provide enough space. It should be long enough to allow 3 or 4 of the largest cassettes to be placed upon it side by side without an overlap if they are opened. At least 2·5 m per operator is the recommended allowance in length and 600 mm the minimum width of such a bench. It should be not less than 900 mm high and preferably mounted on a plinth which will allow the operator a toe space of 75 mm.

The top of the bench should be a hard wood, such as teak. Very often now it is covered with some material which can be easily cleaned. Thick linoleum is a very good choice because it is hard wearing, sound-deadening and anti-static. Theoretically any such covering should be of a kind which will not readily acquire a static electrical charge, such as linoleum. Formica, another substance which is sometimes used, is *not* non-static and consequently as a rule is not recommended. However, in practice it appears to give little trouble under general working conditions, if technicians devote reasonable care and do not handle film with haste and roughness.

The darkroom requires storage space for:

(a) unexposed films ready for immediate use;

(b) a further stock of unexposed materials for use in the near future, perhaps a week's supply.

FILM STORAGE

Hopper. Unexposed films intended for immediate use in reloading cassettes are most conveniently kept in a hopper under the loading bench. This device roughly is a cone-shaped drawer hinged at its lower edge. Its appearance and a plan showing a possible arrangement of films are sketched in Fig. 10.10. This inside of a film hopper should be painted black.

Usually the hopper has about four compartments, the first and deepest of which will accept the two largest sizes of film, for example a box of 35 cm × 43 cm and another of 35 cm^2; the next slot may house the 30 cm × 40 cm films; the third compartment will have 2 smaller sizes together; and the last space may be occupied by narrower films, such as 15 cm × 40 cm.

Whatever the particular sizes or varieties of film in use in a department, or their actual dispositions in the hopper, it is clear that this is a useful piece of equipment in providing orderly storage with ready access. Each box of films should be opened. The contents should be unpacked down to their folder wrappers, if any, and replaced in the box so that the folded edge of such covering is uppermost; that is, in the position it usually occupies when dispatched by the manufacturer. The box itself is then put into the hopper, both as a protection to the films against dust and to prevent the likelihood—particularly as depletion occurs—of films becoming curved under their own weight when standing vertically in a free space.

It is suggested that in reloading the hopper, the new box should go in with the new supply of films. This will assist determination of the emulsion serial numbers should any of a batch of films be found to be technically faulty. Manufacturers' representatives consulted about such occasional defects are in a poor position to give assistance if the films are in the wrong box.

The hopper must be well made and completely light-tight. It frequently includes the following additional features.

1   On the outside a prominent printed warning that it should not be opened in white light. It is well to keep this notice fresh and readily visible.

2   A lock of the 'Yale' type to enable the hopper to be left secure in the absence of trained staff.

3   A switch which breaks the white light circuit should the hopper be opened.

(3) is often considered as alternative to (2) though it is not necessarily so: if the darkroom has a window or if the darkroom door has been left open, only the lock may save the films from exposure to daylight.

Drawers. In place of a hopper a number of shallow light-tight drawers could be used; one is needed for every size and variety of film required in the department. Preferably these drawers should be plainly labelled in regard to their contents. While singly they require less space, their sum demand—if an adequate number are to be provided—is perhaps greater

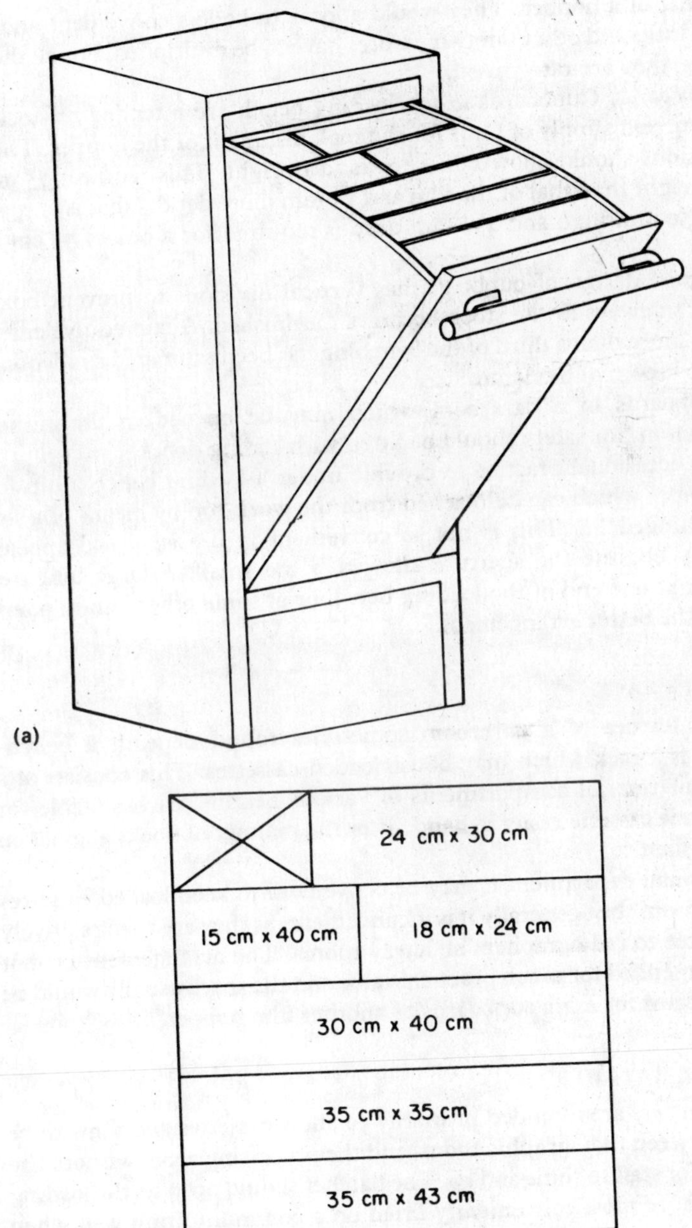

Fig. 10.10. (a) A film hopper.
(b) A plan for the arrangement of different sizes of film within a film hopper.

than that of a hopper. They would appear to be less convenient and of course locks and other safety measures have to be multiplied. For all these reasons, they are rarely used.

Cupboards. Cupboards in the loading bench are intended to stock a small current supply of films for the replenishment of the hopper. Their dimensions should allow boxes to stand upright. This requires 75 mm more height than that of the film and 75 mm more depth; that is, a space some 550 mm high and 430 mm deep is required for a box of 35 cm × 43 cm.

A good design of cupboard has vertical divisions to prevent boxes tipping sideways as the stock becomes diminished. A run equivalent to slightly more than a third of the benching has been estimated as adequate for a darkroom of moderate size.

Cupboards in a darkroom which may be opened in diminished illumination, for safety should be fitted with sliding doors.

It is occasional practice to provide under a loading bench a bin for waste paper which can be reached from the work-top by means of a slot with a hinged lid. This is not so convenient in use as would appear, generally because the aperture allowed is too small. A large bin, free standing at one end of the loading bench or at some other handy point, is often the better arrangement.

CASSETTE RACK

Another feature of a darkroom sometimes found beneath a bench-worktop is a rack which may house loaded cassettes. This consists of a number of vertical compartments of various heights, each suitable for keeping one cassette easily to hand, after the manner of books aligned on a library shelf.

In a small department it may be convenient to keep loaded cassettes in a darkroom; but generally it is inconvenient, as they are then relatively inaccessible to radiographers in X-ray rooms. The arrangement cannot be recommended for much practical value and the space usually would be better utilised for extra cupboards or another film hopper.

CASSETTE HATCHES

Cassette hatches are intended primarily to allow cassettes and films to be passed between radiographic rooms and the processing room without the necessity for staff to come and go. The hatches should open on the loading bench and are most conveniently fitted on a communicating wall when X-ray rooms and darkroom can be adjacent. However, if the darkroom serves several X-ray rooms it is obviously cannot be next door to all of them. In these circumstances and if no mechanical system of film transport is available, hatches placed in a wall accessible from a corridor or hall-way and near to radiographic rooms are beneficial. They enable work to flow easily into the darkroom and provide lodging for cassettes which have been reloaded and are ready for use.

In simplest terms a transfer hatch is an opening in the wall, of similar design to the domestic pattern so often found between dining room and kitchen. However, a cassette hatch, if it is to be practical, must have certain special features as follows.

1   An interlocking device is necessary in order to prevent both doors of the hatch from being simultaneously opened and thus admitting white light to the darkroom at some unwanted moment.

2   The hatch must be light-proof in structure.

3   If its situation is between radiographic room and darkroom, the hatch must be proof also against X rays; this is usually ensured by incorporating lead in its composition. Some hatches are all metal in construction and others are made of plywood on either side of a layer of lead.

4   There must be some means of distinguishing beyond doubt between exposed films entering the darkroom for processing and reloaded cassettes passing from the darkroom. This most commonly takes the form of a division into two compartments, one being labelled 'Exposed' and the other 'Unexposed'. Each legend must be repeated so that is is apparent from either side of the hatch.

Various slightly different designs of cassette hatch are in general use and students may be acquainted with a number in their own departments. One type, for example, consists primarily of a vertical drum which can be rotated. Another pattern may have a lower horizontal compartment for exposed materials and two vertical sections above for outgoing cassettes. Alternatively, perhaps in a large department, the whole of a hatch may be allocated to arrivals and other separate hatches to departures: in this case it is probably wise to give a rather larger number to the outgoing reloaded cassettes than is required for materials entering the darkroom for processing.

THE DARKROOM WITH A MANUALLY OPERATED PROCESSOR

Where the processor is of a manually operated type (a so-called 'wet' processor), the darkroom requires additional equipment—rather than different equipment—relative to automated processing. Like its auto-mated counterpart, the darkroom with a manual processor must contain the following features which we have described on pages 263 to 266:

1   a loading/unloading bench, with provision for film storage;

2   cassette hatches.

In addition to these, the darkroom with the 'wet' processor should have:

3   storage space for processing-hangers;
4   a hot and cold water supply and a suitable sink;
5   storage space for packs of chemicals and mixing equipment;
6   a drying cabinet.

The darkroom will also need a silver recovery unit of a low current-density variety.

HANGER STORAGE

The most usual arrangement for hanger storage is to provide wall brackets above the loading bench. These brackets are grouped in pairs to support a supply of clean, dry hangers ready for use. For convenience, the hangers should be arranged on the brackets so that only one size of hanger occupies any particular pair of brackets.

A typical metal bracket for this purpose projects about 230 mm from the wall when mounted and holds about 12 hangers. The end of each bracket is slightly upturned to lessen the risk of hangers falling from their perches and damaging cassettes, intensifying screens or films which may be contemporary occupants of the bench beneath.

When these brackets are being fixed to the wall, the two making up a pair should be placed 360 mm apart from each other. A reasonable space between each pair would be approximately 100 mm and a suitable height above the bench—for most people—would be 750 mm.

THE DARKROOM SINK

The 'wet' darkroom requires a general purpose sink. With the processor itself, this constitutes the 'wet' section of the room. Whilst there may not be a completely free choice of site for equipment which requires a water supply, it is important not to place the sink or processor in a position continuous with the loading bench. The 'wet' and the 'dry' should be along opposite walls of the darkroom.

The sink should be deep, about 250 mm, and about 750 mm × 450 mm in its other dimensions. For comfort the top of the sink should not be less than 750 mm from the floor. Hot and cold water should be supplied, the taps being placed at least at a sufficient distance (about 400 mm) above the sink to allow the introduction under them of a bucket or Winchester bottle without difficulty. An anti-splash device should be fitted to each tap.

Draining boards are useful on either side of the sink if space allows.

Good quality stainless steel or teak are suitable materials for these. It is sometimes suggested that a drainage area for wet films can be formed by placing the sink between the processing unit and the drier but this space is seldom large enough to be really useful. Furthermore racks over a sink for the drainage of films are above eye level in order to be out of the way: this results in water running down the technician's arms when hangers are put in position and naturally the arrangement is unpopular.

There are of course other good reasons for placing the sink and the processing unit adjacent to each other. Such a situation makes for compactness in the wet section of the room and facilitates cleaning of the processing unit, since a hose can readily be run from the taps to the latter.

Cupboards under and near the sink should be provided. They are needed for the storage of equipment for cleaning and for mixing chemicals, and of chemical stocks.

DRIER

There are various types and sizes of equipment available for drying processed radiographs which use the same simple commodity—hot air. Moist air exhausts from these driers and it should not do so into the darkroom. If the unit is situated there, a duct must be provided for the air's removal.

The traditional form of drier is a free-standing metal cupboard, usually finished in enamel or lacquer. In this, films of assorted sizes can be hung in their hangers, or by means of suspension bars and clips, from slotted racks; generally a double row of racks is fitted but if the cabinet is small it may have only a single one. A drip tray is often provided beneath and sometimes an interior safelight to facilitate use of the drier in the darkroom.

The cabinet has a fan for circulating the air and heater elements to warm it; these are sometimes separately switched. Doors should not be kept open when the heater is on and some units have a thermo-switch which will break the heater circuit in these circumstances and prevent excessive rise of temperature in the electrical elements.

Certain rapid driers are available which depart altogether from the older washing-day conception of hanging films to dry in hot cupboards. Basically, these driers are the drying section of an automatic processor.

The operator feeds the film to an input tray whence it is taken through squeegee rollers and so through other assemblies of rollers. As it travels, hot air is blown on to the film through tubes directed at both emulsion surfaces. The air is filtered to ensure that it is clean and warmed by a 1 kW heater and fan, the temperature being electronically controlled.

In a manner similar to the assemblies of complete automatic processors, the rollers can be easily removed for cleaning; the filter is accessible for replacement. The materials used in the construction of the drier are mainly stainless steel and modern chemically resistant substances such as PVC (polyvinyl chloride); the bearings on the unit are nylon.

The drier is compact in design and is suitable for bench or table mounting. It can be operated from a 13 ampere or 15 ampere wall socket. A drip tray receives the small amount of water discharged during use of the drier and this can be drained by means of a clamped tube.

A drier of this kind is very much more rapid than any of the cabinet type and its adjustable rate of operation gives a through-put of between fifty and ninety 24 cm × 30 cm films/hour.

By way of summarizing this discussion of darkroom equipment the student is referred to Fig 10.11 which shows an outline plan of a room which uses a manual system of processing and includes all its stages.

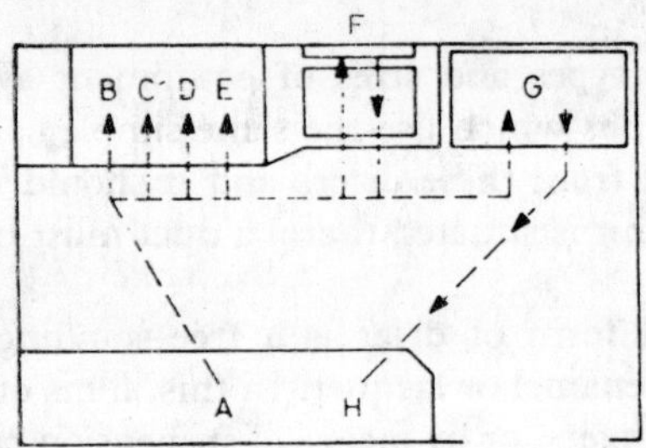

Fig. 10.11. Simple plan of a small darkroom. *By courtesy of Kodak Ltd.*

A...H	Dry bench.	F	Sink with draining-rack above.
B,C,D,E	Processing.	G	Drier.

The student should look at this in relation to the four points which we first considered. These were:

1 effective separation of wet and dry sections;
2 orderly sequence of events;
3 neat layout;
4 clear traffic lanes.

THE X-RAY VIEWING ROOM

The viewing room of a modern radiodiagnostic department is the area where an automatic film-processor will issue its finished products. If the processor is hand-fed in a darkroom, then it is obvious that the viewing/receiving area must be a room or lobby immediately on the other side of the darkroom wall, which is the one containing the processor.

If the processor is associated with daylight loading and is free standing, then the function of the viewing room is expanded and may comprise:

1   a film-dispensing area;
2   a processing area;
3   a viewing area.

The immediate adjacency of such a room to a darkroom becomes less significant. Nevertheless, a safelighted area is nearly always necessary, however an X-ray department may handle the majority of its work. Such an area may be provided in a number of ways and the choice of any particular plan is influenced by the department's needs. Any of the following considerations may be important.

1   A processor integral with a cassetteless or other daylight radiographic system may not need a darkroom near it, unless the associated film-dispensing equipment requires safelight loading.

2   At present in general diagnostic X-ray departments, few processors are solely dedicated to a film-handling system but must accept, also, films from other than daylight cassettes and possibly some direct-exposure (non-screen) film.

3   Film dispensers have been known to jam. A rescue operation—if it is not to result in an unjustified wastage from fogged packs of film— must take place in safelighting or in no light at all, should it become necessary to open the dispenser.

As distinct from conventional darkrooms with processors, such as we have described on earlier pages of this chapter (pp. 240 to 270), perhaps the commonest plan for providing a safelighted area is to equip a dispensing processing/viewing room—or part of it—with sliding partitions. These can be arranged so that their closure will produce a light-tight area of some suitable extent, which will include the processor and can be safelighted, thus offering a darkroom facility whenever it is needed.

Fig. 10.12 is a plan for a processing area in a department where a daylight radiographic system serves a pair of radiodiagnostic rooms. Sliding partitions, fitted in each of the two indicated positions, would provide the means to create a darkroom round the processor when temporarily necessary. The reader should note, however, that such a darkroom would not be suitable for any but occasional use: radiographers may still use the film dispensers unimpeded, but exposed materials have no ready access to the processor, nor may radiographers easily view the results of their work. It would be an unsatisfactory mode of operation if it were to continue for long.

We must now consider in greater detail each of the operational parts of a viewing room, beginning with its viewing function and progressing

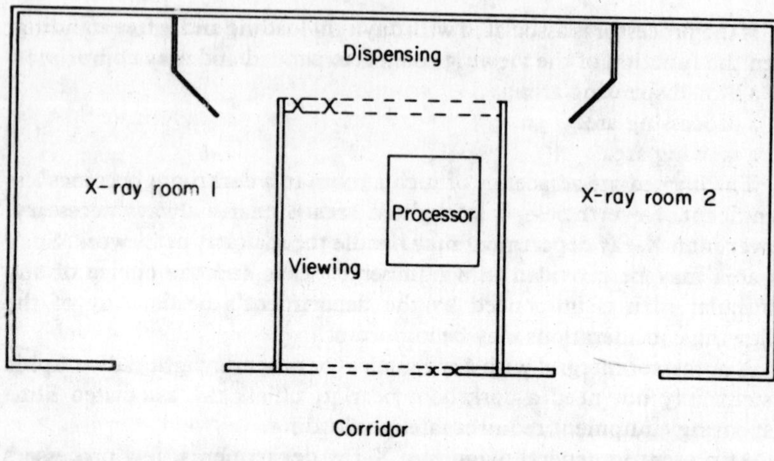

Fig. 10.12. A plan suggesting how a daylight processing area might become a darkroom by the use of suitably placed folding doors.

from this to those processing and dispensing functions which it may include.

THE VIEWING FUNCTION

The activities which normally occur in a viewing/receiving room are the viewing and checking of processed radiographs, very often their sorting as well and in some instances their immediate reporting.

A number of factors will influence the inclusion of a reporting function, which perhaps are little relevant to the present topic. If reports are regularly to be made and transcribed as films emerge from the processor, one essential is the almost continuous availability of radiological and secretarial staff, virtually to sit at the processor's end to carry out this operation. Other considerations also are significant, such as the availability of previous radiographs, the speed of documentation of current films and the possibly distractive effects of noise and movement in the area. Instant reporting in the viewing/receiving room has a necessarily limited application and does not greatly affect our present discussion of the design and material equipment of the space concerned, apart from the observation that the area may include a reporting cubicle.

What size a viewing area properly should be is not an easy question to answer. Much will depend upon the number of X-ray rooms which the processor serves. A recommended ratio is one automatic processor for each whole pair of radiodiagnostic rooms, in a department of six rooms or more; three- and five-roomed departments are recommended to have two automatic processors. (These figures do not include processors which are integrated with a film-dispensing system.) The throughput of films and the number of people (clerks, radiographers and possibly radiologists) who have to work in the area also may be significant determinants of an ideal size.

The simple answer to the question of its size is that the room should be as large as possible, since there can be no doubt that it is a major nerve centre of any X-ray department and is crucial to the department's organisation and communications. All the work ordinarily performed in a viewing/sorting room requires concentration and none should be skimped or carelessly attended because of inadequate space, because of pressure from other people attempting to prevail with their own tasks and because of a crowded, frenetic ambience. Hospital planners, however, are seldom aware of such factors and are usually more generous in allocating space to radiodiagnostic rooms than to a radiographic checking/sorting function. A dispensing/processing/viewing area which might be sandwiched between two radiodiagnostic rooms and was about half the size of each room (that is, 18·5 m²) would be appropriate.

THE RADIOGRAPHIC WORKBENCH

The most important furniture in a viewing/sorting area is a radiographic workbench which should provide the means to:

1   illuminate and view processed radiographs;

2   file checked radiographs—for a short period, of hours at most—in an orderly sequence so that they are readily available for clearance;

3   provide similarly organised rallying points for all associated documents, (these are film envelopes, requisition cards and typed flimsies which may accompany the cards).

This workbench can be designed in any of several styles to meet constraints imposed by architectural and other peculiarities of a site. For instance, if the room is large, the workbench may perhaps be centrally placed and accessible from either side. This is usually a sensible arrangement, given that the area is great enough to allow a free traffic-flow round the bench.

More often, however, the space allotted to viewing/sorting is cramped to a degree and is more efficiently utilised if the workbench stands along a wall.

Whatever may be its particular other features, the essentials of the workbench are that it should include:

1   inset, lit, panels on which radiographs may be placed for transillumination;

2   vertically partitioned shelving above.

The different sections of this shelving should be alphabetically indexed so that a patient's radiographs and their partnering documentation, as these are accumulated, may be filed there under his name. If space permits, a few extra sections without permanent labelling are very useful as they may be allocated at need to a category of work which requires assembly on its own: for example, in order to gather together for a consultant radiologist a group of barium or angiographic studies which he has performed and on which afterwards he must report.

The length of the workbench is largely dictated by the space available. Dimensions of the lit panels necessarily are less flexible, since none must be smaller than the largest film processed. At least two adjacent such areas are required: 35 cm × 43 cm would be a suitable extent for each, in the case of a general radiodiagnostic department. It is preferable if the panels are separately switched, for reasons both of power economy and to avoid dazzle whenever only one is in use.

The working surface of the bench may be horizontal or sloped, but in the latter case should have a raised edging to prevent films, papers and items such as pens and paper clips from falling off. Cupboards underneath offer useful storage space, which may be required not only for stationery (labels, envelopes and so on), but for short term occupancy by processing chemicals and perhaps unexposed film materials, if the area is associated with a daylight film-dispensing system independent of a darkroom. Each of these supplies needs well-defined, separate storage; to stuff everything together in one cupboard is impractical and invites more problems than it solves.

The siting of the workbench within the viewing area not only may be influenced by the amount of space generally available but should be considered in relation to the position of the processor. Radiographs emerging from the processor should not have to be carried far, before a radiographer has the means to check their quality. Because of this, it may sometimes be better if immediate radiographic assessments are made on standard X-ray illuminators which are near to the output end of the processor(s). These illuminators, of which there should be at least two, should be wall-mounted at a height of 150 mm above a conventional worktop. The workbench becomes then solely a site for film sorting and documenting. Sometimes, film-sorting may be moved to another area from viewing/checking, for instance to be near reception and records. If the department is large and many films are being processed there may be several reasons for such a separation of these functions: the topography of a department might be one, for example; and another might be that there are several processors, each serving a particular colony of X-ray rooms and physically distant from the others. Students are likely to find a variety of arrangements within the departments where they work and may like to consider the merits and demerits of each plan.

THE PROCESSING FUNCTION

Processing features of the radiographic viewing area usually include equipments which provide for solution replenishment and silver recovery, but also may include the processor itself if a daylight film-handling system is in use. Each of these equipments are described elsewhere in this book. In the context of room planning and design, the most important thing to be said is that—even without the processor—the first two need good ventilation and ample space. An operator should be able to work at the equipment (whether chemical storage tanks or a unit for silver recovery) without distress and without impediment, either from structural features of the room or because other people continually are passing close at hand.

A CENTRAL CHEMISTRY ROOM

In some large departments a different plan is applied. This is to provide a single, special purpose room in which processing solutions are prepared, held in large reservoirs and fed through supply pipes to a number of processors throughout the hospital, some of which may be at relatively remote sites: distances up to 150 m have proved easily manageable. The solution room may also contain any equipment concerned with the recovery of silver from used fixer solutions (see Chapter 7).

The arguments for a room of this kind are several.

1 A central solution room allows the manipulation of chemicals—which in some degree produce acrid and unpleasant odours—to take place in well ventilated isolation, away from the department's busy areas.

2 Centralising solution-replenishment and silver-recovery facilitates some concentration of responsibility for these functions. A single darkroom technician may readily supervise the chemistry of a whole department.

3 When large quantities of developer replenisher and fixer replenisher are each mixed and provided to a number of processors, the employment of automatic mixers has a better cost-effectiveness.

4 A single source of chemistry in an X-ray department assists the control of image quality.

A central chemistry room may have a disadvantage when it is necessary to renew the chemistry in a remote processor, as staff may then have to transport several gallons of fresh solutions from the central replenisher tanks to wherever the processor in question is situated. The problem could be overcome by the introduction of other supply lines through which a suitable pumping station, installed in the chemistry room, would drive the required quantities of solution wherever and whenever needed.

The ideal size of a central chemistry room must be influenced by the number of processors involved but an area of 9 m² should be sufficient for a large department. Its site must entail consideration of the distance to the furthest processor, but the room and the processors should all be on the same floor, if possible. Chemical routes should be so planned and designed that replacement of interconnecting tubing (which should be plastic) is relatively easily effected, if this becomes necessary at any time. An efficient system for air ventilation/extraction is of first importance.

A central chemistry room should contain the following:

1. two large tanks, one each for developer and fixer replenishing solutions;
2. water-mixing valves if automatic processors require them;
3. water filters;
4. silver recovery unit(s);
5. a sink;
6. solution-mixing equipment, preferably automatic;
7. space for the bulk storage of concentrated chemicals.

If the X-ray department has no central facility for mixing and dispensing replenisher solutions, then features 1–7 above will be present in the processing section of the viewing area. Again, it is to be noted that good ventilation of the area is extremely important.

THE FILM-DISPENSING FUNCTION

Figure 10.13 is a sketch plan of a self-contained area which communicates directly with two radiodiagnostic rooms and in which a daylight film-handling system allows radiographers to load cassettes, process exposed films and finally view these as they emerge from the processors.

On the wall of the staff corridor are seen four film-dispensers, each dispensing a different size of film. These dispensers are shared by the two X-ray rooms and are within easy reach of either room. Although the diagram shows an arrangement of four dispensers, in practice the number may be any for which space is available and the rooms concerned have need. When a daylight system is to be employed and the usages of radiodiagnostic rooms are considered—whether only one room, or several which are to share the system—it is important to determine what may be the minimum number of different sizes of sheet film with which each

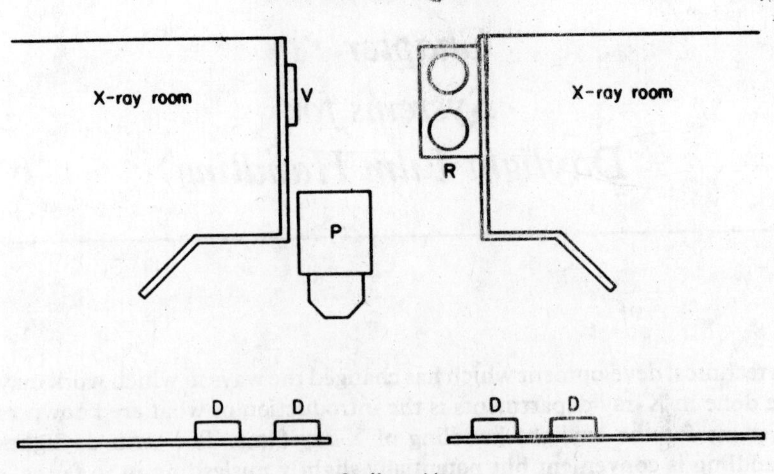

Fig. 10.13. A plan for a dispensing/processing/viewing area to serve 2 radiodiagnostic rooms.

room may adequately operate. Film dispensers are expensive and should not be needlessly proliferated throughout a department.

In Figure 10.13, dispensers which deliver a single sheet of film are illustrated, but a floor-mounted centralised dispenser, supplying a number of different sizes of film, would be equally appropriate to the area.

The arrangement shown, of course, is not the only permitted one but is typical of a present trend in planning. The concern is to avoid old difficulties of cassette or film conveyance by manual or mechanical means, from the X-ray room to some central processing facility. Daylight film-handling systems are more fully discussed elsewhere in this book (see Chapter 11), but in effect all types achieve the same purpose of bringing the processing of radiographs closer to where it is really needed, in or very near to the X-ray room itself.

A single film dispensing/processing/viewing area can be planned on lines similar to those of Figure 10.13 so that as many as four radiodiagnostic rooms are served. Overall, arrangements of this kind accelerate the availability of radiographs after an examination and allow radiographers to check their work, without going far from the X-ray room and from a patient who may on the table.

Chapter 11
Systems for
Daylight Film Handling

A technical development which has changed the ways in which work may be done in X-ray departments is the introduction of what are known as systems for the daylight handling of X-ray films. The term daylight-handling is convenient but potentially slightly misleading in so far as it may give to the uninformed an impression that daylight is essential for these systems. This impression is entirely erroneous for if the systems would not operate equally well under artificial light, in windowless rooms and in the dark night hours, they would obviously be of very little use to most X-ray departments!

In fact the term daylight film-handling means that as the film goes from exposure in the X-ray room to its viewing as a finished radiograph in the reporting area, it need not progress through a darkroom at any stage. The equipments of the systems can be installed in areas where the lighting is unspecialized, being the ordinary light of day or artificial sources: no safelighting is needed. So these methods might be called film-handling systems which can operate in actinic light but we must admit that to call them daylight systems is much more convenient.

It is not difficult to see what are the advantages of such daylight systems. Possibly one of the most important is that radiographers who work alone in X-ray departments (as they so often do when answering emergency calls) are able to remain in contact with their ill and injured patients and are not required to close themselves away in safelit rooms in order to process films and to reload cassettes. There is in fact no need to coop anybody in a darkroom, so working conditions are improved, time is saved and skilled staff are more efficiently used. X-ray rooms do not need to be close to darkrooms and so there is greater scope in departmental planning. The automated handling reduces the risks of damage to films and intensifying screens.

These systems have no disadvantages which seriously outweigh the gains but there are some aspects which should make planners pause before they install them. The questions to be asked are as follows. How much space do the items of equipment need? What happens in the event of breakdown? Can the high costs of purchase and installation be met? What arrangements are to be made for processing films which cannot be handled through the daylight system? Examples of these are dental radiographs (intra-oral), orthopantomographs, some mammograms and any radiographs for which a curved cassette is required.

Daylight film-handling systems can be classified in the following two categories.

(i) Systems which provide automatic unloading and reloading of cassettes in ordinary lighting. They may be linked with an automatic processor, either directly or by means of a portable film-transporter, so that the finished radiograph emerges without having been in a darkroom. Such procedures imply cassettes which are particularly designed for their systems. It is therefore not possible to use in the systems other specialized cassettes or films which are radiographically exposed in light-tight paper packs and this explains why the radiographs mentioned above cannot be part of a daylight system.

(ii) Systems which have been described as cassetteless radiography. In these the films are passed from containers which hold them prior to the radiographic exposure into an exposure position, whence they proceed to the processor, either directly and automatically conveyed or carried by hand in a transporter which receives them from the exposure position in the equipment.

DAYLIGHT SYSTEMS USING CASSETTES

Daylight systems which handle cassettes perform a series of operations for which the following items of equipment are necessary:
(i) a cassette which in normal room lighting can be automatically loaded before radiographic exposure, unloaded afterwards and then reloaded with film in readiness for the next exposure;
(ii) a film dispenser or cassette loader which will load cassettes in normal room lighting;
(iii) a printer or identification camera which, while the film is still in the cassette, records on it required information about the patient and the X-ray examination of which the radiograph is a part;
(iv) a cassette unloader which will unload the cassette in normal room lighting;
(v) an automatic processor into which the films can be fed.

THE CASSETTES

The cassettes for daylight systems may be end-loading. Such a cassette is unlike a conventional one which has a back and hinges on one edge so that the actions of opening and closing the cassette are similar to those of handling a book. The end-loading cassette has a slit along one edge which can automatically be opened for the insertion or removal of the film and automatically closed.

Fig. 11.1 shows the components of a daylight system and the item

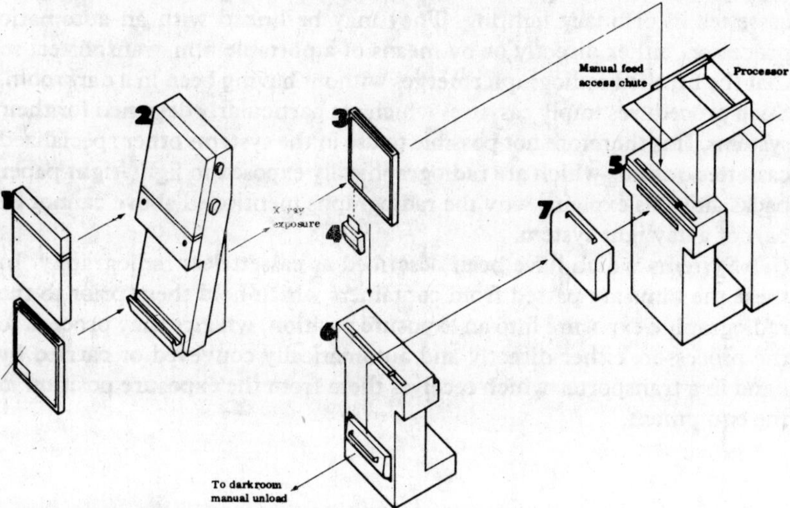

Fig. 11.1. Daylight system.

numbered 3 is the end-loading cassette which is used. Such end-loading cassettes are often adaptable to manual unloading and loading in a conventional darkroom with safelights.

However, the cassettes used in all daylight systems are not bound to be end-loading. Equipment has been devised which mechanically reproduces the manual actions of opening and closing cassettes. It is this sort of equipment which is the heart of the system illustrated in Figs. 11.2 and 11.3.

Cassettes for use in these systems usually have an indication to show that they are loaded with film.

IDENTIFICATION CAMERAS AND PRINTERS

Clearly any system for handling films in ordinary lighting must include a procedure for identifying radiographs. There must be some way of

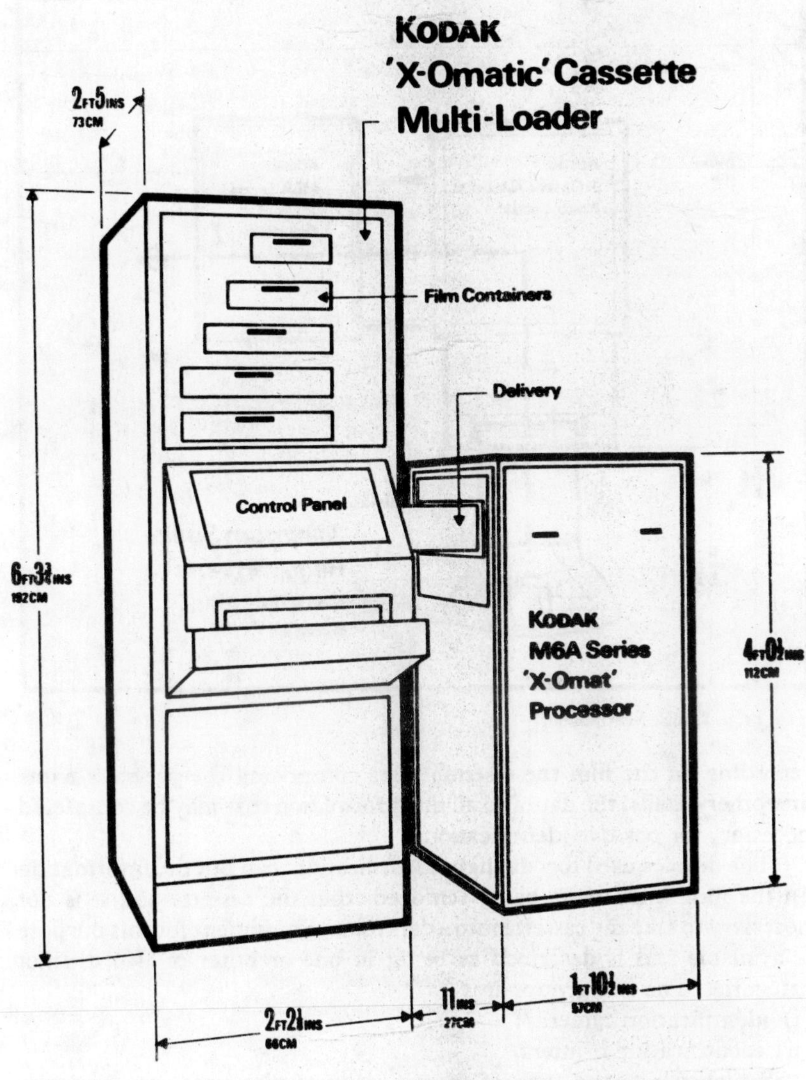

Fig. 11.2. Kodak Multiloader.

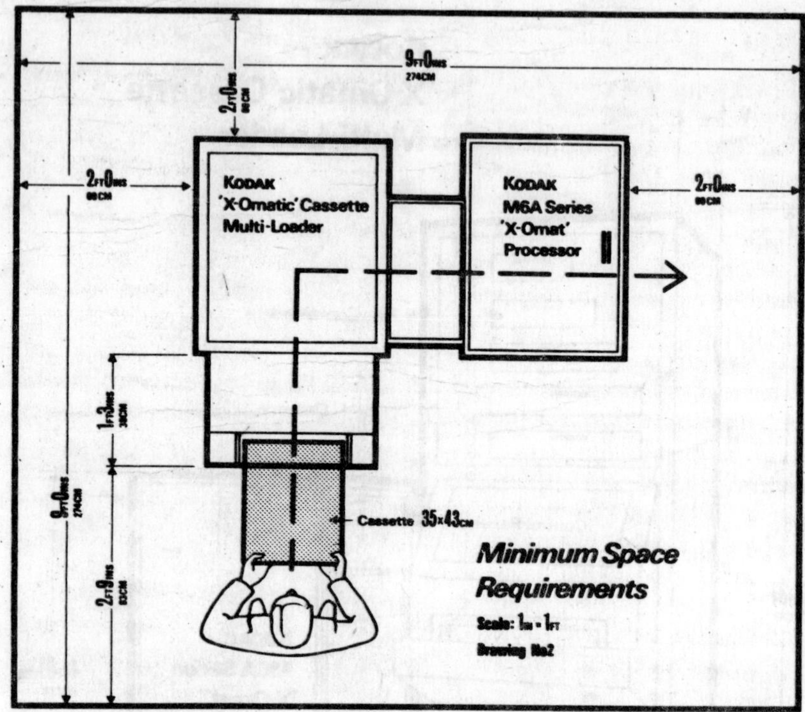

Fig. 11.3. Kodak Multiloader.

recording on the film the essential data comprising the patient's name and other details, the date and all the information that may be considered necessary for positive identification.

The devices used for 'daylight identification' can put the information on the film without its being removed from the cassette and it is not necessary to take the cassette into a darkroom. Equipment for this purpose is available and is described as being in one or other of two distinct categories. The two groups are:

(i) identification cameras;

(ii) identification printers.

Whichever is the type of identification device used, the cassettes which are part of the daylight system include a small lead-screened area which protects the film from the X-ray exposure. The location of this area is obvious from the outside of the cassette: it can be seen indicated in the cassette at 3 in Fig. 11.1. The shielded unexposed, rectangular area on the film beneath this part of the cassette front is available for the photographic recording of the required identifying information.

IDENTIFICATION CAMERAS

Identification cameras used in daylight systems do not essentially differ much from photographic markers used in X-ray darrooms on films which have been taken out of cassettes under safelights and are about to be processed. These markers which operate as cameras and include a lens are described in Chapter 14 on page 414.

The information to be recorded is written or typed on a card which is illuminated when it is placed in the photographic marker or identification camera. Through the agency of mirrors and a lens the image on the card is photographed on the X-ray film when that is inserted in its appropriate place in the marker. An identification camera operating in this way can be part of a daylight system, being usually adapted to deal with cassettes which contain the film to be marked (in contrast to dealing with the film when it is out of the cassette and under safelighting in a darkroom). The identification camera of a daylight system may function in one or other of the two following ways:

(i) it may be part of a cassette unloader which thus identifies *and* unloads film into a carrying magazine or directly into an automatic processor;

(ii) it may be a complete unit on its own which operates only to put the information on the film while it is in the cassette. The cassette then is taken to an automatic unloader or to a darkroom for manual unloading.

When the identification camera deals with films in cassettes, the cassettes need a window over the shielded area of the film on which the identifying information is to be recorded. This window is normally closed by a shutter. When a cassette is placed in the identification camera the shutter is automatically withdrawn and the window is open. The information can then be photographed on the X-ray film. The writing is white on a dark ground.

IDENTIFICATION PRINTERS

Identification printers used in daylight systems are small, handheld devices which record information on the X-ray film while it is still in the cassette. The method used is that of contact printing and not of photography through a lens system as in the identification camera. Such an identification printer is seen marked 4 in Fig. 11.1 and another is sketched in Fig. 11.4. The illustrations indicate that the printer has a light-plate which projects from the end of it and in use is inserted in a slit in the edge of the cassette at the place where the shielded area of the X-ray film is located. This light-plate is a luminescent panel which lights

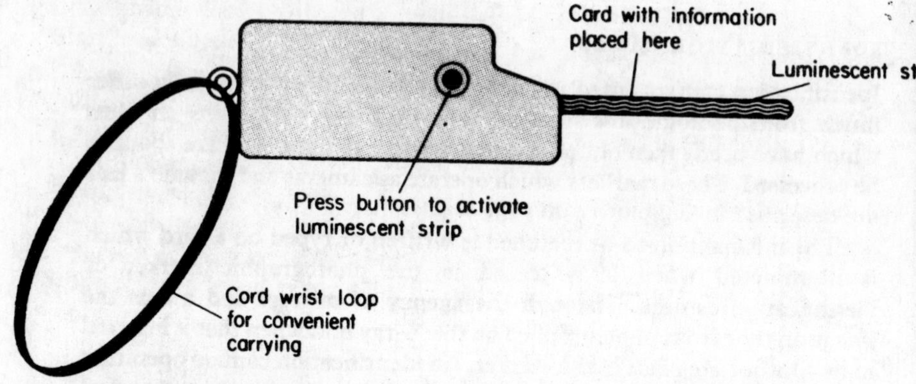

Fig. 11.4. Handheld printer.

when a button at the side of the printer is briefly depressed. The power source is a little 12 volt battery inside the printer.

The identity-information is written or typed on a strip of paper or card which is thin enough to be translucent: opaque card is of no use. This strip of paper is put in close contact with the light-plate and both are inserted into the cassette. When this is done and the button is depressed, the luminescence of the panel behind the paper strip prints the image of the lettering on the film with which the paper strip is in contact. The writing is white on a black ground.

FILM DISPENSERS AND CASSETTE UNLOADERS

FILM DISPENSERS

The film dispenser or cassette loader is a piece of equipment which holds packs or magazines containing X-ray films of conventional sizes. From these stocks it automatically loads films into cassettes which are placed in it at the appropriate loading place. In Fig. 11.1 the film dispenser is numbered 2; this is designed for wall-fitting. Numbered 1 in Fig. 11.1 is the film pack which contains 100 sheets of notched film. This pack is placed in the upper part of the film dispenser, this operation being carried out in daylight. A separate dispenser is required for each film size to be used.

In Fig. 11.1 the cassette is shown immediately below the film pack. When the cassette is correctly placed in the channel at the foot of the film dispenser as indicated in Fig. 11.1, it is automatically loaded with one film from the pack above it, the film passing into the cassette through the slit which has opened along its upper edge. There is a signal which shows that this happened and features of the design eliminate possible double loading of the cassette.

A film dispenser which can be charged with a pack of films in daylight is not bound to be a part of all such systems. In some of them the cassette loader carries a number of magazines, there being a separate magazine for each film size to be used from the loader. These light-proof magazines must be taken to a darkroom and under suitable safelights they are charged with up to 100 sheets of film of the size appropriate to each magazine. Replaced in the cassette loader, the magazines provide the stocks from which the cassettes are automatically loaded in daylight conditions. The equipment illustrated in Fig. 11.2 is of this type and carries 5 magazines or film containers to hold 5 different sizes of conventional X-ray films. These are dispensed appropriately and singly into each cassette coming into the equipment.

All film dispensers or cassette loaders must of course maintain the film protected against actinic light and against ionizing radiation. They must be easy to operate and quick in functioning so that they can handle many cassettes in an hour. A film dispenser which was tiresome to use and slow to load cassettes would produce such a bottleneck in a busy X-ray department as to vitiate many of the advantages of having a daylight system. Any automatic cassette loader must be able to improve on the performance of a pair of human hands! Film dispensers/cassette loaders are usually placed in central work areas so that they may serve more than one X-ray room: for example, two or three rooms.

CASSETTE UNLOADERS

Daylight systems must include procedures for automatically unloading cassettes so that the exposed films which they contain may be passed on to the next stage in the production of the finished radiograph, this next stage being chemical processing.

In the daylight system shown in Figs. 11.2 and 11.3 the same piece of equipment first of all unloads and then loads cassettes. It is connected directly by a delivery channel to an automatic processor and the exposed film which has been removed from the cassette is automatically passed through to the processor, whence it emerges as a finished radiograph. So in this system the same piece of equipment is both a cassette loader which charges the cassette with film and a cassette unloader which passes the film on for processing, the whole operation taking place in daylight conditions.

So that is one way of doing it: making the same piece of equipment act as a cassette loader and unloader and connecting it directly to its own automatic processor which it is designed to feed and very close to which (27 cm in Fig. 11.2) it must be sited. It is possible to put films into the automatic processor *only through* the cassette unloader/loader of this system; not from any other cassette unloader or by hand. The two units would be placed in a central area serving more than one X-ray room and the loader/unloader can deal with up to 240 cassettes of different sizes every hour.

The X-ray department which uses this system still needs a darkroom with safelights under which the film containers of the loader unit can be charged. A darkroom is necessary also for the processing of those films which are not to be put through the unloader/loader and its associated processor: for example, dental films and orthopantomographs.

However a unit which combines the functions of cassette loading and unloading is not the only possibility for the daylight extraction of films from cassettes and their forwarding for processing. The system illustrated in Fig. 11.1 has a different arrangement.

In Fig. 11.1 the piece of equipment numbered 6 functions in daylight to unload a cassette which is placed as the vertical arrow indicates into an entrance slit on its top surface. The film taken from the cassette is automatically loaded into a rotary magazine: this is seen inserted into the lower part of the cassette unloader and is also seen at 7 in Fig. 11.1 removed from this station. The unit numbered 6 thus functions to unload cassettes and load the rotary magazine. This magazine holds up to 25 films of mixed sizes and is used to transport films by hand to an automatic processor.

This then is another way of doing it: providing a station which is a cassette unloader and a magazine loader and is intermediate between the radiographic exposure to the film and its subsequent entry to an automatic processor. The transporting magazine is used to carry the films from several cassettes to an automatic processor.

This can be a versatile system, for these intermediate stations which in daylight can unload cassettes and take the films into carrying magazines can be set up as convenient in several working areas, with film dispensers close at hand so that the emptied cassettes can be reloaded. From these areas the films are conveyed by hand to a central automatic processor which serves all the areas.

In Fig. 11.1 an automatic processor is seen at the extreme right of the diagram. The piece of equipment at number 5 is a special cassette unloader which is fitted to the front of the processor. In daylight conditions this unit can unload a cassette which is placed in it as the vertical arrow indicates, passing the film into the processor. Such cassette unloaders usually provide a visible indication when the film has left the cassette. The unloader can also accept the transport magazine as Fig. 11.1 indicates and in daylight conditions can unload all the films from the magazine, passing them singly into the processor.

Fig. 11.1 also shows that the cassette unloader fitted to the front of the automatic processor gives access through a chute to the entrance slot of the processor for anyone feeding films by hand, after manually removing them from cassettes or magazines. To use manual feeding through the access chute it is of course essential for the processor to be in a conventional darkroom with safelights.

DAYLIGHT SYSTEMS WITHOUT CASSETTES

CASSETTELESS SYSTEMS FOR CHEST RADIOGRAPHY

Daylight systems for automatically handling X-ray films without putting them into cassettes are in use especially for radiography of the chest. If an X-ray department has a work-load which requires the exposing and processing of more than 100 full-size X-ray films a day in examining chests then it is worthwhile to consider installing such a system.

The important features of the equipment are as follows:

(i) a loading section or a magazine to hold the films protected from light and radiation before exposure;

(ii) a means to charge the loading section in daylight with a number (say 100–125) of unexposed films if the system is to be independent of a darkroom and safelights; or the provision of a removable magazine to be taken from the unit and charged with films in a darkroom under safelights;

(iii) an exposure area in which each film in turn is compressed between intensifying screens and held for the exposure as in a conventional cassette;

(iv) push-button control to give automatic transport of each film in turn from the loading section or magazine into the exposure area;

(v) the automatic recording of identification details for the patient and the examination when a card containing the information is inserted appropriately in the unit;

(vi) an automatic processor directly joined with the unit by means of a communicating channel along which each film in turn is passed from the exposure area to the entrance slot of the processor;

OR

(vii) a removable transporter into which the exposed film is automatically passed and in which it may be conveyed by hand to the processor. Such a transporter holds several films and may simply be a carrying case which is opened by hand in a darkroom under safelights, the films being fed by hand individually into the processor; or it may be a combined transporter and feeder which can be attached to an automatic processor and can feed the films into it one by one.

Fig. 11.5 is a sketch diagram to show how in such a daylight system for chest radiography the elements might be combined for a functioning arrangement. This diagram is not to be taken as an exact representation of a daylight system from any particular manufacturer although it is based on equipment which is commercially available.

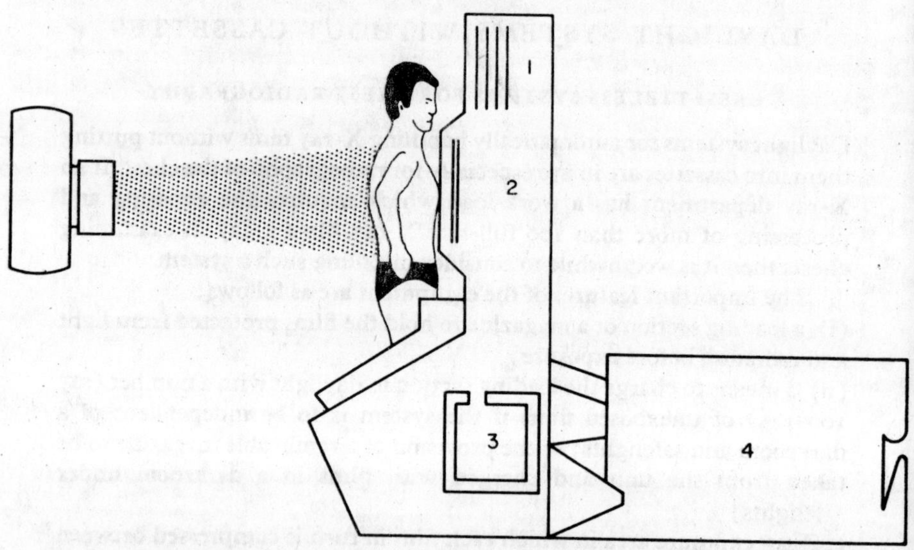

Fig. 11.5. Sketch of a cassetteless daylight system for chest radiography.

In the diagram the loading section is seen numbered 1 at the top of the piece of equipment; a pack containing 100 films can be loaded there in daylight. From the loading section, the film is dropped downwards into the exposure section, which is numbered 2 in the illustration. There the film is compressed between intensifying screens and moved into a forward situation close to the patient, being held there for the radiographic exposure. After the exposure has taken place, the film and the intensifying screens between which it is clamped are moved into the previous retracted position (at the numeral 2 in Fig. 11.5). The film is then released from between the screens and drops down to 3 in the diagram. This is a container which can hold up to 50 films, can be removed from the apparatus in daylight and is used to transport the films to the automatic processor.

The container may be simply a transporting case which is taken to a darkroom where the processor is and opened under safelights; the films are then removed by hand and fed into the processor. Or it may be a transporter-feeder which can be attached to an automatic processor which is standing in daylight and used to feed the films automatically into the processor. The system is then independent of a darkroom and the whole procedure, from unexposed film to finished radiograph is completed in daylight conditions. Fig. 11.5 unrealistically combines two incompatible possibilities for it shows at 4 an automatic processor directly connected to the equipment by means of a communicating channel along which the films can be automatically passed. In this case, of course, the transport container shown at 3 would not be required. The system is again independent of a darkroom and furthermore is completely automatic.

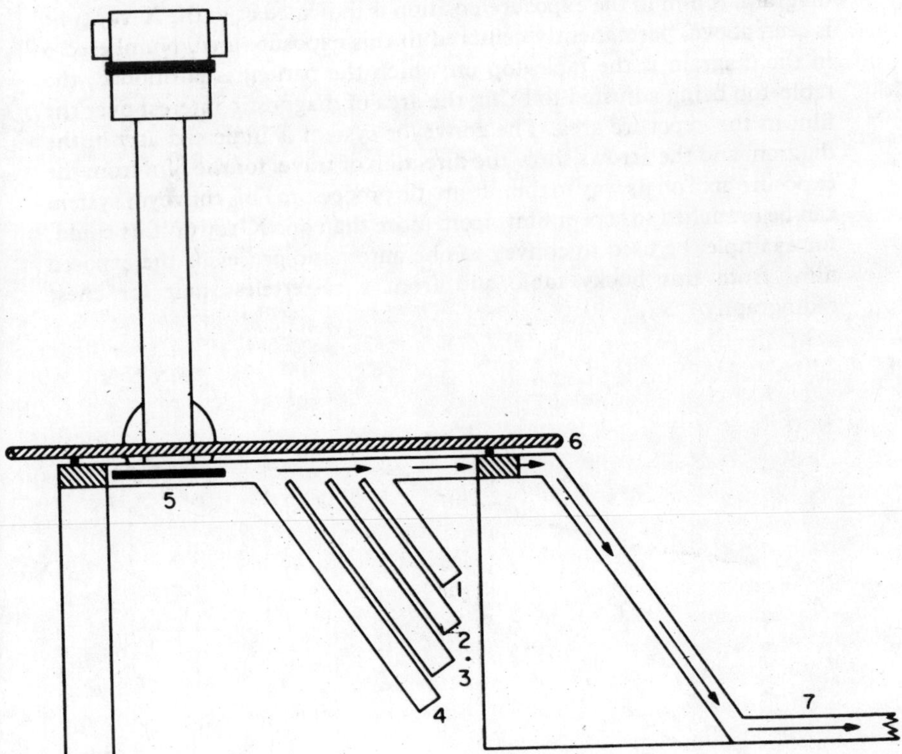

Fig. 11.6. A cassetteless daylight system for general radiography.

The need for hands as transporters of the film-transporter to the processing site (whether under safelights or in daylight) has been eliminated.

A CASSETTELESS SYSTEM FOR GENERAL RADIOGRAPHY

Equipment is available which uses a cassetteless system for general radiography. The automatic bucky table has beneath it four magazines, each for a different film-size and holding up to 100 films. Push-button control achieves automatic transport to the exposure position for a selected film. In the exposure area the film is held compressed between intensifying screens for the purposes of the exposure. Immediately afterwards it is moved automatically into a conveyor system which takes it into the attached processor.

Fig. 11.6 is a sketch diagram to indicate the arrangements. The magazines which hold the stocks of films are numbered 1, 2, 3 and 4 in the diagram. A film in the exposure position is indicated at 5: the X-ray tube is seen above, permanently centered to this exposure area. Numbered 6 in the diagram is the table-top on which the patient is positioned, the table-top being adjusted to bring the area of diagnostic interest over the film in the exposure area. The conveyor system is indicated at 7 in the diagram and the arrows show the direction of travel for the film from the exposure area on its way to the automatic processor. This conveyor system can be branched to accept films from more than one X-ray unit. It could, for example, be used to convey to one automatic processor the exposed films from this bucky table and from a cassetteless unit for chest radiography.

Chapter 12
The Radiographic Image

The student now understands how a radiographic image is produced by radiation transmitted in varying amounts through the subject to activate silver halide grains in an emulsion and produce black deposits of silver. The action of X rays (or of the X rays in combination with the light from intensifying screens) is amplified many times by chemical development, the object of the processing cycle being to produce a permanent image which can be viewed by transmitted light. In the present chapter certain features of this image and factors affecting it are further considered. Fig. 12.1 sketches the components in a radiological examination.

COMPONENTS IN IMAGE QUALITY

The varying transmitted radiation may be considered as a certain amount of information (or an invisible and inaudible signal) which must be changed into another form: in the case of a radiograph this other form is a visible image. The quality of this image is its ability to reproduce in a visible pattern the varying transmission of X rays through the object radiographed: the image is of the highest quality if the reproduction is exact and clear, without omissions, additions, distortions. The sole object in producing the image is that it should be *seen* by a human eye. In order that it may be seen it must have:

(i) sufficient sharpness of out-line (or an acceptable degree of unsharpness);

(ii) sufficient contrast (difference in brightness between various parts of the visible image);

(iii) sufficient resolution (or distinctness).

There are therefore three important features of the image to be distinguished as follows:

(i) unsharpness in outline;

(ii) contrast;

(iii) resolution.

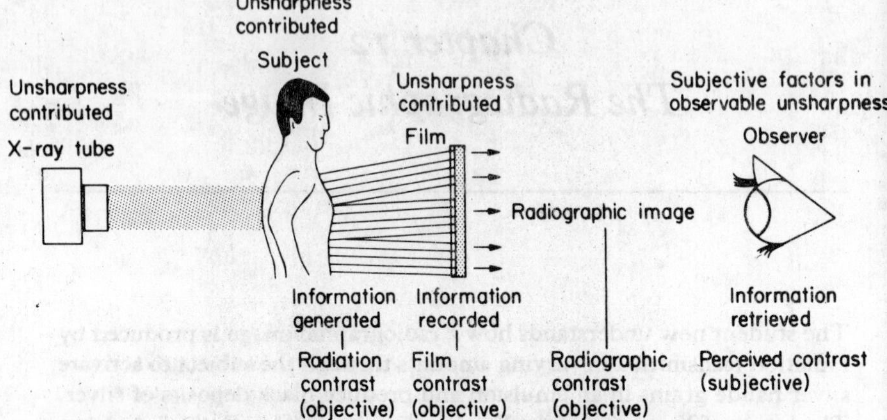

Fig. 12.1. Radiation contrast is expressed as the ratio of transmitted intensities for different areas.

    Film contrast is expressed as the average gradient of the characteristic curve.

    Radiographic contrast (or image contrast) is expressed as differences in density between different areas.

    Radiographic contrast depends on (i) radiation contrast and (ii) film contrast.

These are the three quantities to be considered in assessing the quality of the image for they can be measured and evaluated to compare the qualities of imaging systems.

The subject consists of a number of elements which form it: for example, the trabecular structure of bone is a series of small bone elements. These structural elements are the *detail* of the subject and they are of course separated by very small distances, being closely compacted together.

The resolution of the image is its ability to reproduce as separate images structural details which are separated by very small distances. The resolution depends upon both sharpness of outline (or degree of unsharpness) and difference in brightness (contrast). However lacking in unsharpness, the image of a black cat in a dark cellar has no resolution since it has no contrast; similarly an image of a man in black on a snowfield will not be resolved if he is moving on skis at a speed which makes all his outlines a blur.

It is important for the student to appreciate about these three quantities in the image that:

(i) unsharpness and contrast are two entirely separate and unrelated quantities;

(ii) resolution is a function of unsharpness and contrast;

(iii) where images are of equal unsharpness, the one with the higher contrast has the better resolution;

(iv) where images have the same contrast, the one with the less unsharpness has the better resolution.

(v) all three quantities can be measured objectively and values given to them.

MEASUREMENT OF UNSHARPNESS

What does the expression 'sharpness of outline' mean? It is the breadth of the boundary between two areas of different density, and it can be measured by means of a special densitometer known as a microdensitometer.

Fig. 12.2 shows two areas of different density, A and B. A recording

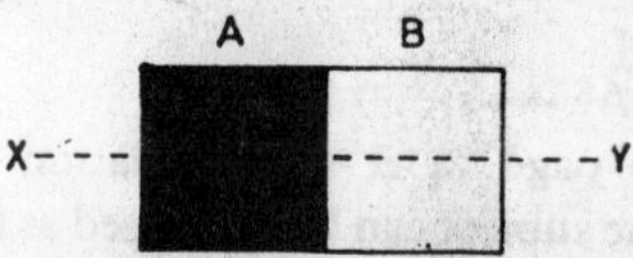

Fig. 12.2.

densitometer can be used to record the densities measured along the horizontal line XY, and a graph can be made in which density is plotted against points on the line (millimetres). If the boundary between the two areas is sharp in outline, the graph will show a vertical drop between A and B as in Fig. 12.3. If the boundary between A and B is not sharp but is diffuse, the graph will show a sloping fall between A and B as in Fig. 12.4. The breadth of the boundary indicates the degree of unsharpness.

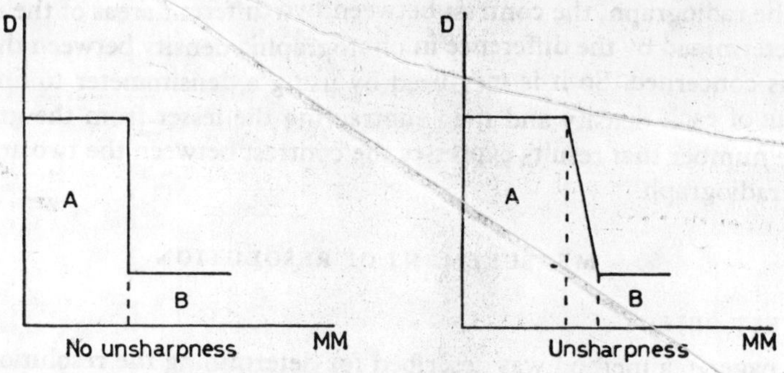

Fig. 12.3.   **Fig. 12.4.**

MEASUREMENT OF CONTRAST

As Fig. 12.1 and earlier parts of this book (see page 74) show, there is more than one form of contrast to be considered for a radiologic examination. Fig. 12. 1 shows the following:

(i) radiation contrast (in the subject);
(ii) film contrast (in the material);
(iii) radiographic contrast (in the radiograph);
(iv) observed contrast (in the viewer's perception).

The first three are objective quantities and can be measured. The last one is subjective, variable between individuals and in the same individual between different conditions for observation. Clearly the first three are all components in the observed contrast but the observer adds to them an individual and unmeasurable component. So observed contrast cannot be evaluated as a numerical quantity.

RADIATION CONTRAST

As was indicated on page 74 et seq., radiation contrast between two different regions of the subject can be expressed as the ratio of transmitted intensities (number of X-ray photons) for the regions considered: or as the ratio of transmitted exposures for two different areas on a photographic film which is recording the image.

FILM CONTRAST

As explained in Chapter 3, film contrast is expressed as a quantity by the average gradient of a characteristic curve.

RADIOGRAPHIC CONTRAST

In the radiograph, the contrast between two different areas of the image is determined by the difference in photographic density between the two areas concerned. So it is measured by using a densitometer to find the value of each density and then subtracting the lesser from the greater. The number that results expresses the contrast between the two areas in the radiograph.

MEASUREMENT OF RESOLUTION

A TEST OBJECT

On page 26 a method was described for determining the resolution of a photographic image and expressing the resolving power as the number of line pairs per millimetre which can be distinguished as separate lines. Resolution in a radiologic image can be similarly expressed by means of a test object composed of a series of lines which are alternately radiopaque and radioparent (compare with the black and white lines in the photographic test). The radiologic test could use a set of radioparent lines (they might just be slits, for example) set in a plate which was radiopaque: or the other way round, as would be achieved by setting lead strips in perspex.

MODULATION TRANSFER FUNCTION

Another method used to test the resolving power (ability to reproduce detail) of a radiologic imaging system is to determine modulation transfer functions for the system. This is a parameter also used for examining images produced by optical systems in general photography.

Modulation transfer function is a difficult concept for many of us to understand. In trying to explain it, we suggest that the reader looks again at Figs 12.2, 12.3 and 12.4. Here was depicted a boundary between two areas of different density: a contrast boundary.

In Fig. 12.2 along the line XY, at the boundary between the dark area and the light there is a big change from the one to the other: you should imagine A and B as areas of different density in a radiograph which are transmitting light to the observer's eye. Area B will transmit many more light photons than area A and there is a big change in photon density at the boundary. As you move from A to B there is a rise in photon density and this is a steep rise as the boundary is narrow. If the boundary is broad as in Fig. 12.4 the rise in photon density between A and B is less steep. So at any contrast boundary there is a photon density gradient. By a special analysis known as Fourrier analysis, such gradients can be expressed by means of a set of components which are sine functions. The theory of Fourrier Analysis states that any pattern of fluctuations can be broken down into sine waves. The sine waves have various frequencies and phase relationships. As a form which can be used to test the qualities of images, the sine wave has the advantages of being simple, describable in mathematical terms (which means admirably exact descriptions for people who have mathematics as a second language!) and (very important) capable of showing slight degrees of degradation in an image.

In a radiologic examination we are concerned firstly with a radiation image: this is an image formed of a series of photon densities (X-ray photons) emergent from the subject as the X-ray beam is attenuated and transmitted in various ways by the structures within the subject. The radiation image then is a pattern of fluctuations and has sinusoidal variations associated with it.

The radiation image is to be converted to an optical image (an image for the eye to view) by whatever recording system is used. We are considering here a radiographic record made on film, usually in conjunction with intensifying screens. The perfect screen/film imaging system reproduces the sinusoidal variations of the radiation image as an optical image with the same sinusoidal variations for its photon densities (light photons). When we say that the sinusoidal variations of the radiation image are reproduced as the same in the optical image we mean that the reproduction is faithful: without distortion in amplitudes, alteration in frequencies, disturbance in phase relationships.

In real life the perfect imaging system does not exist and one or more of those parameters (amplitude, frequency and phase relationship) can be untruthfully reproduced. For the recording systems used in radiography, the most important limitation to resolving power is distortion in amplitude for these sinusoidal variations. Distortion of frequencies (harmonic distortion) may be significant at extremes of density and thus is not important for most general radiographic images and phase distortion derives mainly from optical systems which use lenses. So it is distortion in amplitude at which the knowledgeable are to look when they concern themselves with the modulation transfer functions of the screen/film recording systems used in radiography.

To study the modulation transfer function of the imaging system is to study its sine wave response and in the case of the screen/film imaging system with which we are concerned the sine wave response is studied with particular reference to amplitude. Answers are sought to questions such as the following. When the fluctuations of photon densities in the radiation image and the fluctuations of photon densities in the visible light image which is the radiograph are converted into the sine waves of Fourrier analysis, are the sine waves of corresponding amplitude? Is the sine wave amplitude response of the screen/film system maintained as the sine wave frequencies increase? A high sine wave frequency corresponds to an image with a great number of line pairs per millimetre (there are a large number of black-white and white-black boundaries in a short linear space). If the amplitude response is maintained at close to 100 per cent up to a high frequency, the resolving power of the imaging system is high. A fall in the amplitude response indicates a limit to the resolving power of the imaging system. In practice, for example, at a frequency of 1 cycle per millimetre, amplitude response might have fallen to 85 per cent with high resolution intensifying screens and to 75 per cent with very fast screens. These figures show clearly that the resolving power of the high resolution screens is higher than that of the fast screens.

LINE SPREAD FUNCTION

For radiographic imaging systems and screen/film combinations, modulation transfer function can be determined through study of the line spread function. We have seen that the required conversion is that of a radiation image to an optical image (the radiograph). If the conversion is perfect a point in the radiation image is rendered as a point in the optical image; if the conversion is less than perfect the point in the radiation image is spread over an area in the optical image. So the quality of the converting system (the imaging system) could be directly assessed by studying its point spread function; this would answer the question: how much does it spread a point?

In practice it is easier to deal with the spread of a line rather than a point in the image. The image of a line can be scanned by a microdensitometer and its spread observed. This spread is the line spread function of the imaging system and the line spread function can be converted to the modulation transfer function.

UNSHARPNESS IN THE RADIOGRAPHIC IMAGE

In fig. 12.1 various parts of a radiologic examination are sketched as being divisible into 3 sections as given below:

(i) generating information;
(ii) recording information;
(iii) retrieving and interpreting information.

We have already emphasised that in the ideal process, the information generated in the first stage would be retrieved in the third stage without degradation. In real life the ideal is not available. All we can hope to do is to minimize the degradations which occur and are to be understood by radiographers. In our radiographic techniques we aim for a retrieval of information which is matched as nearly as possible to what was generated.

Unsharpness in the radiograph is a degradation which is inescapable. As indicated in Fig. 12.1 it arises in regard to the information both at its generation and its record. In its retrieval by an observer there are subjective factors in the degree of unsharpness which he perceives or fails to perceive. These personal factors are widely variable and interesting but we deem them beyond the scope of this book. We intend to limit our considerations to forms of objective unsharpness which arise in generating and recording the information eventually to be retrieved.

The total objective unsharpness is composed of unsharpnesses arising as follows:

(i) geometric unsharpness, the geometry concerned being that of shadow formation;

(ii) unsharpness introduced by the subjects being examined;

(iii) unsharpness introduced by whatever system is used to convert the radiation image into a visible one and to record it (intrinsic unsharpness).

GEOMETRIC FACTORS OF UNSHARPNESS

Geometric unsharpness in the radiographic image has three origins. These are (i) the size of the X-ray source, (ii) the distance between the subject and the recording surface, which is the film, and (iii) the distance between the X-ray source and the subject being radiographed. The total degree of geometric unsharpness is determined by the relationship existing between these three factors when the image is made.

THE X-RAY SOURCE

The importance of the size of the X-ray source or the focal spot of the X-ray tube can be demonstrated by a simple diagram of the geometry of image formation. In Fig. 12.5 diagram A represents image formation

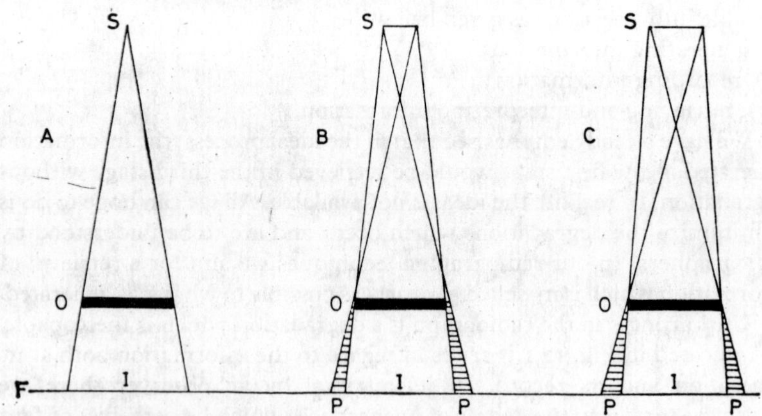

Fig. 12.5. Geometric unsharpness
S   X-ray source
O   object
I   image or true shadow of the object
P   penumbra or half-shadow surrounding the image
F   film

from a point source. It shows that the shadow cast by the object, although larger than the object's true size owing to the spread of the image-forming rays, is nevertheless sharp in outline.

Diagram B shows an image formed by a source which has a certain size; radiation now reaches the object not from a point but from an area. Each part of the object intercepts radiation from all parts of the focal spot, and as a result of this points in the image cease to be points, and become blurred by areas of half-shadow round them. This area of half-shadow is called the *penumbra*, and as the penumbra increases in size the true shadows in the image become more and more diffuse in outline. In diagram C is shown the increase in penumbra resulting from a larger X-ray source. Sharpness of outline is therefore influenced by the size of the X-ray source in this way: the smallest source gives the least penumbra (if other factors are constant).

It is perhaps worthwhile to consider in more detail the implications of the expression 'the size of the X-ray source'. What is its meaning? In the X-ray tube, X rays are produced over the area of the target receiving electron bombardment. The size of this area covered by the electron beam is determined by the shape and size of the filament, the measurements of the focusing slot in the cathode in which it is set and the characteristics of the associated electric field. This area of electron bombardment is termed the actual focus of the X-ray tube, and is the real size of the X-ray source.

In the formation of the image the 'size of the X-ray source' refers not to the real size, but to the size that the source *appears* to be when it is viewed from the film. This apparent size of the source is the projection of the actual focus and is called the effective focus of the X-ray tube. The earlier statement might more precisely be reworded: the smallest effective focus gives the least penumbra.

The actual focus of the X-ray tube is foreshortened by angulation of the target face. A rectangular area of electron bombardment projects as a square when viewed from a point directly below the centre of the anode at 90° to the long axis of the tube. If an observer imagines himself looking up at the anode from this point (A in Fig. 12.6), he will perceive the focal area as a square. If he then moves from his vantage point, goes a little towards the anode end of the X-ray tube, and looks up from there (B in Fig. 12.6), he will find that the focal area is now further fore-shortened, and its vertical dimension appears smaller than it did from the first viewpoint. If he takes another walk back to the first viewpoint, and then an equal distance away from it towards the cathode end of the X-ray tube, he will find on looking up from there (C in Fig. 12.5) that the focal area is now less foreshortened, and its vertical dimension appears longer

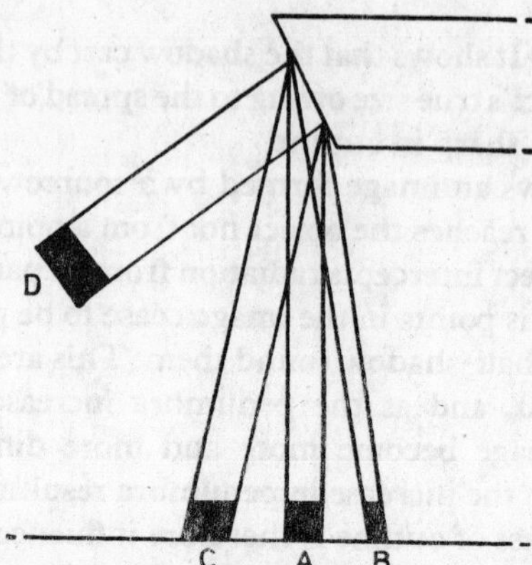

Fig. 12.6. Variation in the apparent size of the focal spot along the axis of an X-ray tube. A, B, and C are three apparent focal areas. D is the actual focal area.

than when he viewed it first. This series of viewpoints and their effect on apparent size of the X-ray source are shown in Fig. 12.6.

This means that in the image less penumbra is produced in parts of the subject under B than in parts under A, and in parts of the subject under A than in parts under C. The image is not equally sharp in outline at all points along the long axis of the tube. This effect is demonstrable in special conditions and is likely to be most noticeable with large focal spots when the X-ray beam is used to cover a big film area at a short distance. In general departmental practice it is usually disregarded, being not perceived when radiographs are viewed.

THE TUBE-SUBJECT DISTANCE

The penumbra produced by an effective focus of a certain size becomes smaller as the distance between the X-ray tube and the subject under examination (the object) is increased. This is shown in Fig. 12.7, where diagrams A and B should be compared. The effective focus is the same in both, but in B the source to object distance is greater and it can be seen that the resulting penumbra is less in size. It can therefore be stated that long tube-subject distances reduce penumbra.

THE SUBJECT-FILM DISTANCE

The effect of the distance between the film and the subject being radiographed is shown in diagram C in Fig. 12.7. Here the effective focus is again the same size as in A and B and the tube-film distance is the same

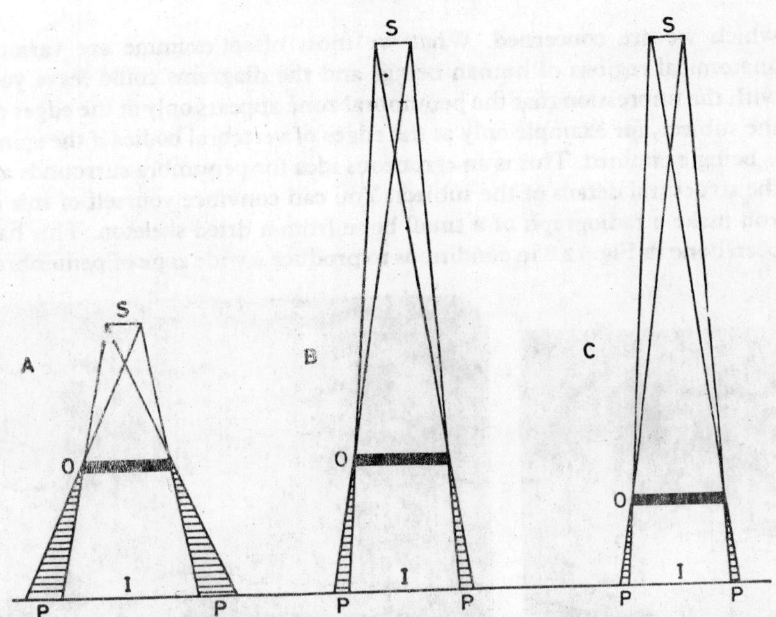

Fig. 12.7. Geometric unsharpness.
S   X-ray source
O   object
I   image or true shadow of the object
P   penumbra or half-shadow surrounding the image.

as in diagram B, but the subject is much closer to the film. It can be seen that the penumbra is again reduced in size.

These dimensions which contribute to geometric unsharpness are closely related to each other and to penumbra in the image in this way.
(i) The smaller the effective focus, the smaller the penumbra.
(ii) The longer the source to subject distance the smaller the penumbra.
(iii) The shorter the subject-film distance the smaller the penumbra.

The increase in penumbra resulting from a larger effective focus, a shorter source to subject distance, or a longer subject-film distance can be offset by adjustment of the other two factors to reduce it. The principles appear simple, but their application to medical radiography involves compromise. This will be discussed in detail when other sources of unsharpness in the image have been examined.

CALCULATING EXTENT OF PENUMBRA

It must be emphasised that the diagrams in Figs. 12.5 and 12.7 are somewhat misleading when you try to relate them to the 'objects' with which we are concerned. What we most often examine are various anatomical regions of human beings and the diagrams could leave you with the impression that the penumbral zone appears only at the edges of the subject, for example only at the edges of vertebral bodies if the spine is being examined. This is an erroneous idea for penumbra surrounds all the structural details of the subject. You can convince yourself of this if you make a radiograph of a small bone from a dried skeleton. This has been done in Fig. 12.8 in conditions to produce a wide zone of penumbra.

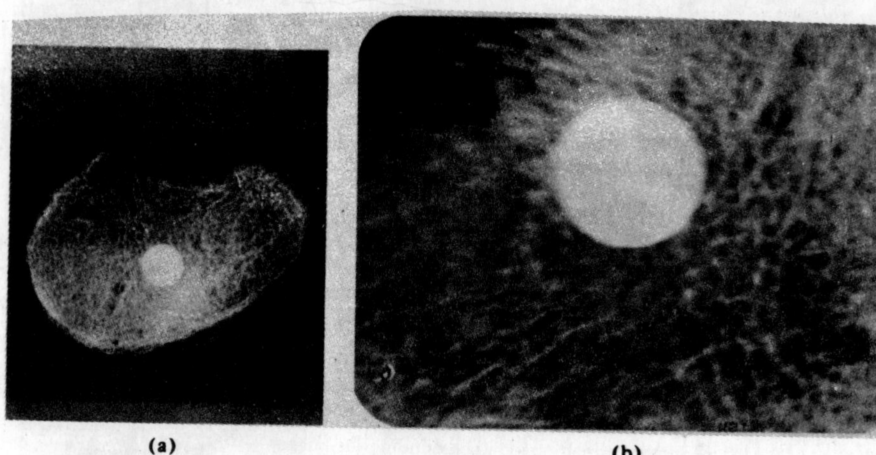

(a)   (b)

Fig. 12.8. Radiographs of a small bone with lead shot embedded in it.

   At (a) the conditions were set up to produce the least penumbra.

   At (b) the object-source distance was decreased and the object-film distance was increased. It can be seen that all the details of the object are less sharp in outline. (There has also been an increase in the magnification.)

It is clear that *all* the bony details in the vertebra are unsharp in outline and not merely the edges of the vertebra itself.

   The width of the penumbra surrounding the structural details can be calculated. The following relationship is used.

$$U_f = F \times \frac{d}{D}$$

U_f is the width of the penumbra.

F is the width of the focal spot.

d is the distance between the object (the structural details in the subject under examination) and the point where the unsharpness is measured (the film).

D is the distance between the focal spot and the object.

   This relationship shows that the penumbra will be wider with (i) larger focal spots, (ii) greater distance between object and film, (iii) shorter distance between focal spot and object. It shows also that (this being important in radiographic technique) an increase in penumbra arising from any one of these three factors can be reduced by appropriate adjustment of one or both of the others.

In practice, of course, radiographers hardly concern themselves with the focal spot to object distance; in applying radiographic techniques, they specify, consider and adjust the distance between the X-ray tube and the film. This is a significant measurement in relation to the film density resulting from any given set of exposure factors. So it is a practical quantity for radiographers to use, whereas knowledge of the tube to subject distance is valueless in most radiographic procedures. It is clear, however, that when a radiographer uses a long tube to film distance in a particular radiographic technique, a long focal spot to subject distance is implied. We aim always to have a subject to film distance which is small (except in the case of special techniques for macroradiography) and thus increase in the tube to film distance increases the source to subject distance.

UNSHARPNESS INTRODUCED BY THE SUBJECT

Certain forms of unsharpness in the radiographic image come from the subject being examined. These forms of unsharpness can be differentiated as arising from three separate sources as given below.

(i) The facts that the subject is at a distance from the film, that the focus of the X-ray tube is not a point but has a finite width and that the focus is not infinitely remote from the subject all come together to give rise to the geometric unsharpness which we have already considered. The subject most usually examined in medical radiology is an anatomical part or region of a patient and clearly the distance which separates it from the film varies with the subject and with features of a radiographic technique.

For example, when the subject is the terminal phalanx of a finger it can be brought very close to the film and penumbral zones in the details of the image will be narrow in width. When the subject is the lumbar vertebrae of a thick-set patient to be examined in the lateral projection (with the cassette in a bucky tray and perhaps a floating table-top) the distance separating the bony structures from the film is much greater. So also is the width of the associated penumbra for the structural details of the image.

(ii) A certain unsharpness arises because the subject by its very nature has not sharp outlines. Let the reader contrast the sharpness of outline presented by the gall bladder or the kidney of a living patient with that shown by the blade of a knife. Those whose concern it is closely to examine and test the quality of radiographic images should be aware of this disparity. The fact is that an index of the resolving power of a system may be misleading if the real subject is very different in form to whatever test object may be used to obtain the index. For example, the test object described on page 295 for measuring resolution is entirely different from the subjects who present themselves for our daily attentions in diagnostic X-ray departments. To use such a test object to indicate the resolving power of our radiologic imaging systems may be to take the road to some wrong conclusions.

The search for sharpness of outline in the image of an unsharp subject which is to be viewed by the inadequate human eye sometimes makes us think of a blind man in a dark cellar looking for a black cat that is not there!

(iii) Some unsharpness can arise because of movement.

So long as the subject is alive some degree of movement during the exposure is always a possibility, with certain types of subject it is a probability, and with certain fields of examination it is a certainty if the exposure lasts long enough. It must be remembered that, apart from the patient's capability in stopping voluntary movement, there are involun-tary movements over which he has no control. Peristaltic action in the abdominal viscera and the heartbeat are examples.

A sufficient degree of motion blurs the shadow outline. A point within the subject is recorded not as a point in one place on the film, but in more than one place on the film and therefore as a blur. The degree of unsharpness produced by motion depends on the rate at which movement has taken place, the extent of movement, and the length of time the exposure lasts. It is also influenced by the focus-film distance and the distance between the moving structure and the film. If the exposure time is sufficiently short, if movement is sufficiently slow in relation to it or small in extent, if the focus-film distance is great and the structure to film distance is small, then movement unsharpness in the image is minimal.

It is common knowledge that photographs of moving objects can be made with cameras allowing short exposure-times. Horses can be shown going over obstacles on a racecourse, golfers can be shown at the height of their 'swing' with all motion apparently arrested. This principle can be applied in radiography. By the use of short exposure-times satisfactory radiographs can be made of body parts where movement is likely or certain.

Some estimate can be made of the probability of subject-motion in regard to any radiographic examination. The radiographer's first assessment will be of the type of subject and his degree of ability to co-operate, taking into account age and physical and mental state. The next assessment takes note of the field of examination, and the presence or absence within it of involuntary movements which it is beyond the patient's will to stop.

This informed assessment is a part of radiographic technique and detailed discussion of it not within the scope of this book. Here it may simply be said that unsharpness due to subject movement is more likely in some instances than in others; it will vary in degree with the rate of movement, the extent of the movement, and the duration of the exposure; it can be reduced by the use of short exposure-times. There are other factors which influence degrees of motional blurring—for example whether the moving part is near the film or remote from it, near the X-ray source or remote from it, moving transversely or otherwise in relation to the beam. These factors are somewhat theoretical and beyond the practical sphere of the radiographer, so they will not be discussed. Difficulties connected with the use of short exposure-times will be considered again in a later section when all the factors of unsharpness are related to each other.

UNSHARPNESS INTRODUCED BY THE RECORDING SYSTEM

We have seen that in the production of radiologic images the basic process which takes place is that a radiation image is converted to a visible one. This is true however the visible image may be displayed or permanently recorded. In diagnostic radiology as we know it today the visible radiologic image is commonly displayed on fluorescent screens and television monitors and is commonly recorded on films, xerographic prints and videotape. When the conversion to a visible image takes place, some unsharpness is introduced by the system employed for the display or the record whatever that may be. This introduced unsharpness has been called intrinsic unsharpness because it is inherent in the system used.

The present chapter concerns itself with radiographs. These radiographs with which we mostly deal are records on film materials which have an emulsion layer on both sides of the base. These films are most often exposed to radiation while held between a pair of intensifying screens in a cassette (although they may be exposed held in light-tight holders without the use of intensifying screens). Let us consider what forms of intrinsic unsharpness such a system introduces.

It is easy to see that since this system comprises only two components, namely the film material and the intensifying screens, the forms of unsharpness which are introduced could be listed in two categories:

(i) unsharpness arising from the intensifying screens and
(ii) unsharpness arising from the film material which is used.

INTENSIFYING SCREENS

When intensifying screens are used in combination with film to make the record, they contribute a factor of unsharpness which is much greater than that contributed by the film. Thus the unsharpness arising from these screens is the most significant one in the recording system. Such sceens are fully discussed in Chapter 5.

The salt screens commonly used are made of crystals each of which fluoresces as a separate entity under the action of X rays. The image is therefore produced by many separate sources of light. These separate light sources result in images with a certain diffusion of outline. The extent of this diffusion depends on the size of the light-emitting crystal, and also upon the distance of the crystal from the film since there is divergence of screen light.

Screens made of larger crystals and consisting of deeper layers of crystals are faster than screens made of very small crystals spread in thin layers—that is they allow of greater reduction in exposure-time. They inevitably result in greater screen-unsharpness in the radiographic image. Screens of very fine grain, that is made of a thin layer of small crystals, are usually termed 'high definition' to draw attention to the fact that they are designed to give a minimum amount of screen-unsharpness. They cannot be expected to be fast enough to allow of very short exposures, since the two qualities—speed and minimal unsharpness from crystal size and distribution—are incompatible.

Where screens are not used at all this factor of unsharpness of course does not exist in the image. Students can see this for themselves by radiographing a specimen bone both by direct exposure and with the use of screens, and then comparing the results.

When screens are used it is extremely important that both screens in a cassette should be in close and complete contact with the film situated between them. This contact must be evenly maintained over the whole area of the surfaces in apposition. Where the contact is poor a marked degree of unsharpness appears in the image.

EMULSION SOURCES OF UNSHARPNESS

When photographic materials were discussed in Chapter 2, reference was made to a phenomenon known as *irradiation*. This was described as a sideways spread of light in the emulsion, and it is a source of unsharpness in the image. A similar effect occurs in radiographs, a sideways spread in the emulsion both of X radiation and of the fluorescence of intensifying screens. In the case of X rays there is scattering within the emulsion not only of the X-ray quanta but also of electrons released in absorption processes. These electrons can make developable silver halide grains which have not been reached directly by an X-ray quantum. The contribution of these effects to the total unsharpness may be regarded as very small indeed in most diagnostic radiography on medical subjects.

With very high energy X rays the film unsharpness resulting from electron scattering will be greater, since the more energetic quanta can energize more electrons. It has been said that for X rays produced at 1,000 kV each quantum absorbed accounts for 80 grains being made developable. The unsharpness resulting from these effects would be measurably greater in a radiograph taken with a supervoltage therapy set than in radiographs made at conventional diagnostic kilovoltages.

In regard to the resolving power of photographic materials, grain size was mentioned in Chapter 2 and the phenomenon of graininess was discussed. The size of the grains in emulsions used for radiography makes no significant contribution to the unsharpness of the image. It has been shown that there are many factors resulting in such degrees of unsharpness that grain size and its effect on resolving power can be neglected in conventional radiographic images.

PARALLAX

Parallax refers to the fact that when near and distant objects are seen from different viewpoints, their relationship to each other seems to change and is not perceived as it truly exists.

Fig. 12.9 shows a dark circle immediately beneath a light circle, and when viewed from position A they are seen to be superimposed. In Fig. 12.10 they are seen from two other positions. An observer in position B would find the dark circle towards his left hand and the light circle towards his right. An observer in position C would find the dark circle to his right hand and the light circle to his left. This apparent change in relationship is called parallax.

X-ray film has an image produced on both sides at once, and thus there are really two separate images at a distance from each other which is the thickness of the base plus the thickness of each emulsion layer. When the film is wet and the two emulsions are swollen by moisture, the images have appreciable separation. As they are viewed by an observer, one is closer to him than the other; the one image might be termed a near object, the other a more distant one.

This separation of the images gives rise to a parallax effect or an error in superimposition of the two images. As a result the final image viewed does not have outlines as sharp as those seen in an image which is truly a

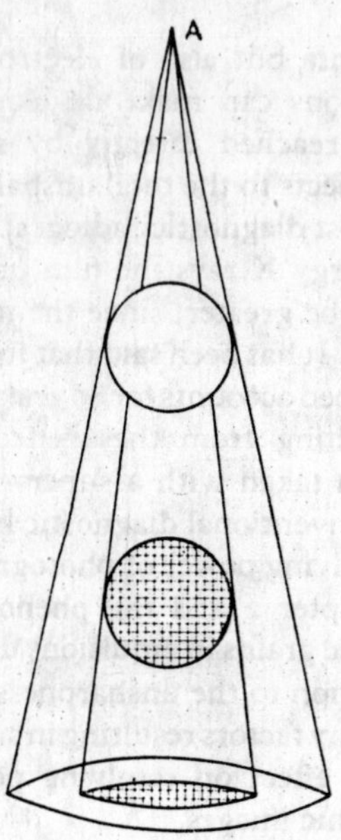

Fig. 12.9.

single one. This degree of unsharpness is greatest when the film is wet and it is negligible when the film is dry. Even in a wet film it is not necessarily noticeable, but it is one of the reasons why radiologists prefer not to make final reports on radiographs which they have not viewed dry.

GEOMETRIC, MOTIONAL AND INTRINSIC UNSHARPNESS IN RELATION TO THE RADIOGRAPHIC RESULT

Consideration of all factors together, and of the degree of unsharpness actually present in a radiograph, leads straight to the heart of the radiographic problem. Students can soon appreciate the dilemma if the previously indicated sources of unsharpness are taken in turn, and thought is given to making the contribution of any one of them absolutely minimal.

What would reduce geometric unsharpness? Clearly the answer is a short subject-film distance, long tube-film distance, and small effective focus for the X-ray tube. Very short subject-film distances may be impossible to obtain. The heart, for example, is lodged within an incompressible thoracic cage and the patient's measurements may provide additional distance beyond the radiographer's control.

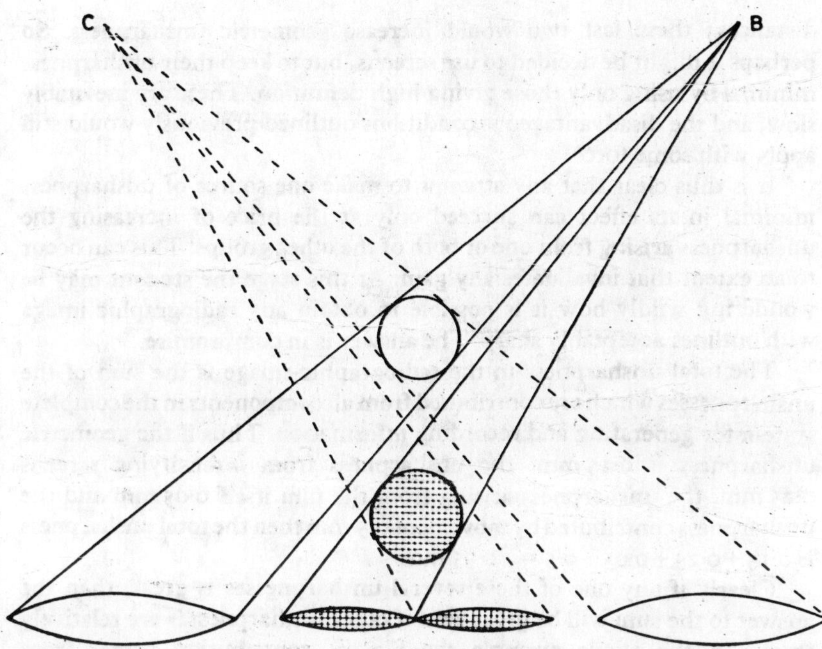

Fig. 12.10.

It may be easy to arrange for the X-ray tube to be remote from the film, but if this is done exposure factors must be increased. This requires long time-intervals or greater electrical loads on the X-ray tube, and perhaps a combination of both. The greater electrical loads require larger focal areas because of the heat generated, so the use of a small effective focus becomes impossible. The longer time-intervals may increase motional unsharpness. If it is decided to use the smallest possible focus, then long tube-film distances cannot be used for the reasons shown above.

What would reduce motional unsharpness? The use of short exposure-intervals. This requires high electrical loads, which demand large focal areas; or less electrical load combined with shorter tube-film distances. Both these factors increase the unsharpness of geometric origin.

What would reduce unsharpness from factors which are intrinsic to the recording systems (film-screen combinations) which are generally used? The most significant improvement would be given by refusal to use intensifying screens. This would demand for thick body parts exposures many times greater than those in use with screens. Longer time-intervals would be necessary (with increase in motional unsharpness), higher electrical loads (with need for larger focal areas), and shorter tube-film distances; these last two would increase geometric unsharpness. So perhaps it might be decided to use screens, but to keep their unsharpness minimal by using only those giving high definition. These are inevitably slow, and the disadvantageous conditions outlined previously would still apply with some force.

It is thus clear that any attempt to make one source of unsharpness minimal in its effect can succeed only at the price of increasing the unsharpness arising from one or both of the other groups. This can occur to an extent that invalidates any gain. At this stage the student may be wondering wildly how it is possible to obtain any radiographic image with outlines acceptably sharp. The answer is in compromise.

The total unsharpness in the radiographic image is the sum of the unsharpnesses which are contributed from all components in the complete system for generating and recording information. Thus if the geometric unsharpness is 0·15 mm, the unsharpness from intensifying screens 0·25 mm, the unsharpness arising from the film itself 0·05 mm and the unsharpness contributed by movement 0·5 mm then the total unsharpness is 0·15 + 0·25 + 0·05 + 0·5 = 0·95 mm.

Clearly if any one of these several unsharpnesses is great, then the answer to the sum will be great even if other unsharpnesses are relatively small. In the above example the biggest contribution comes from movement. This *could* be reduced at the cost of increasing the contributions from others but the *total* unsharpness might be smaller as a result: the increase in others would be worth accepting as the price to be paid for making the movement unsharpness smaller and thus achieving a result in which the total unsharpness had been reduced to an acceptable level.

For example, the use of fast screens and a broader focal spot which takes a higher loading (the fast screens and the higher loading are both chosen to reduce the exposure times to be used) might give a screen unsharpness of 0·4 mm and a geometric unsharpness of 0·25 mm. The film unsharpness would remain at 0·05 mm. The use of a very much shortened exposure time could reduce movement unsharpness virtually to zero. Then the total unsharpness would be 0·4 + 0·25 + 0·05 = 0·7 mm.

Such reduction in total unsharpness achievable by adjustment of the several contributions forms the basis for selection of technical factors in any given radiographic examination.

The thickness of the body part, the probability or certainty of movement, the rating of the X-ray tube, the size of the focal spot and permissible levels of electrical load, the radiographic output required to give adequate film density at a given tube-film distance—all these are balanced and selected to give an optimum result in each case. The radiographer may be said to work with an informed empiricism. If the student will mentally review familiar radiographic techniques, and consider fully the effects on unsharpness of changing one or more of the factors, it will doubtless be possible to appreciate how the contribution from each of the sources are balanced so that the total unsharpness shall be as small as possible.

Certain examinations naturally present little difficulty. For example, when X-raying one finger the radiographer has every assistance in trying to obtain a sharp image. The body part is small, the subject-film distance is short, total immobility can be secured in most cases, little radiographic output is required from the X-ray tube so small effective focus and short time-intervals can be used, and screens are not necessary. In obstetric radiographic examinations, the problem is very much greater and is solved only by accepting some elements of unsharpness in order to prevent others from producing intolerable diffusion in the image.

THE CONTRAST OF THE RADIOGRAPHIC IMAGE

It was explained in Chapter 3 that radiographic contrast is a function of radiation contrast in the subject and the contrast available from the material being used to make the record. This is true, but as well as these important factors there are others which influence the contrast of the image. The topic will now be given fuller consideration.

The contrast of the radiographic image can be distinguished as having separate elements.

(i) Objective radiographic contrast. This can be calculated and given numerical form since it is the difference in density in various parts of the image. As shown in Chapter 3, density can be measured with instruments. If a certain area of the film has density D_1 and another area has density D_2, then the objective contrast between them is $D_1 - D_2$.

(ii) Subjective perceived contrast. This is visual contrast, the difference in brightness between areas of the film as it seems to an observer. It is clearly not measurable since it is an individual assessment, variable between observers and for one observer at different times.

Factors affecting objective contrast influence also subjective contrast, but there are factors affecting the contrast as it seems (for example, viewing conditions) which have no effect on the computable objective contrast. In the present section subjective contrast will not be considered, since its proper place is in relation to the distinctness with which the image is made visible—that is the resolution of the image as it was earlier stated. Subjective contrast is discussed again on page 322.

While it can be stated that the outlines wanted in a radiograph are usually the sharpest possible, it is by no means so easy to express what is wanted in contrast. Radiographs are produced to be viewed and used by all too human observers, and radiographers soon learn that variations are possible in individual judgements on what constitutes a 'good radiograph'. These individual judgements turn on differences in density and contrast, not upon differences in sharpness about which people are usually agreed.

It can be said that the highest possible contrast is not the most useful diagnostically, and very low contrast can fail to make structures visible. Between these two extremes is a level of contrast which is satisfactory and gives good visibility of structures. This 'satisfactory' contrast will not be the same for all types of radiographic examination. The student can appreciate this by comparing as examples a barium meal study, a cholecystogram, a plain film of the renal area, a posteroanterior view of the skull. It may be difficult to be content with these vague statements, but it is a fact that no one can give a simple and quantitative answer as to what satisfactory contrast will be.

The factors which influence objective radiographic contrast can be divided into three main groups. These are (i) radiation factors, (ii) film factors, and (iii) processing factors.

RADIATION FACTORS IN OBJECTIVE CONTRAST

Radiation factors altering contrast are twofold and result from (i) the quality of the primary radiation and (ii) the scattered radiation reaching the film.

QUALITY OF THE PRIMARY RADIATION

The student is by now familiar with the facts that the quality of primary radiation is altered by change in the kilovoltage across the X-ray tube and that raising the kilovoltage makes the beam more penetrating. A change in penetration by the X rays alters radiation contrast within the subject.

If a certain stepwedge is radiographed at low kilovoltage there will be a big difference in the intensity of radiation transmitted through its two ends; this means greater image contrast. The same step-wedge radiographed at higher kilovoltage gives a changed picture. There is less difference in absorption between the two ends of the wedge, the harder beam being better able to penetrate the thick end of the wedge, so that more radiation than previously is transmitted through this part.

Fig. 12.11 shows a step-wedge radiographed at seven different kilovoltages, and the picture obtained with 40 kV on the left edge of the figure should be compared with that given by 100 kV on the right edge.

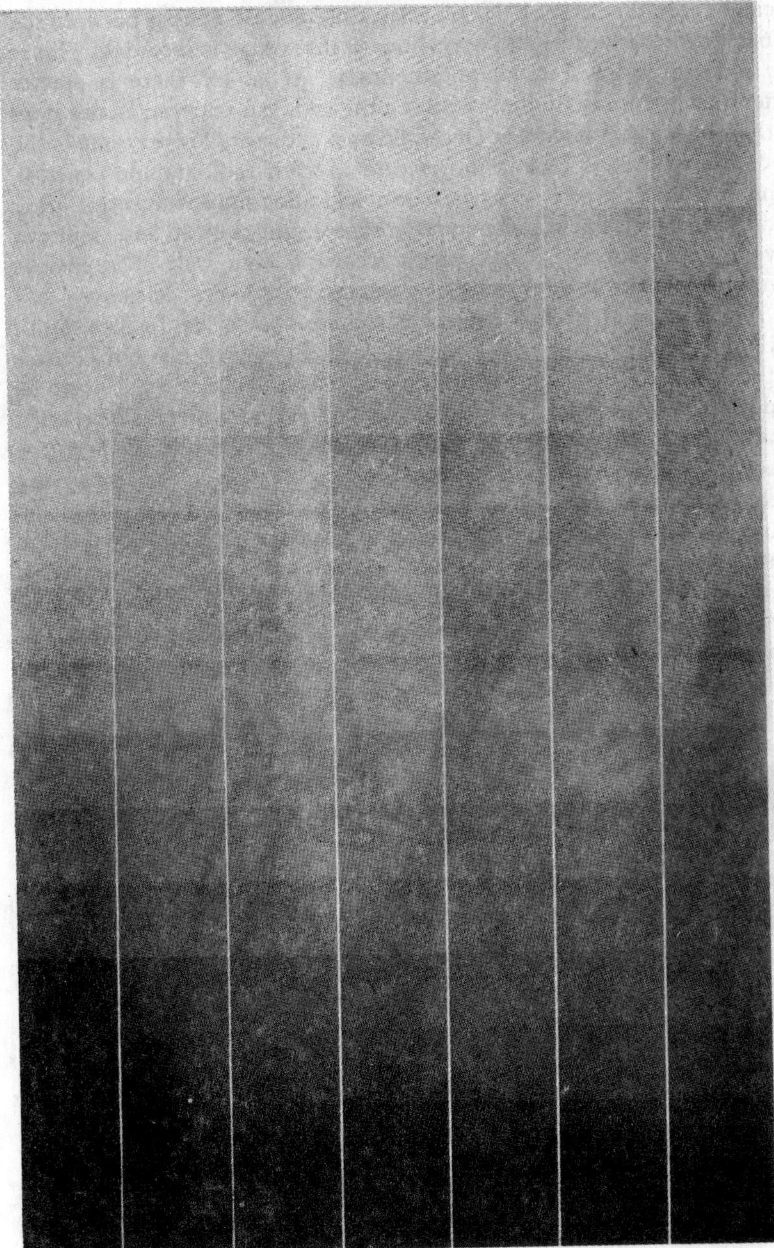

Fig. 12.11. A stepwedge of 17 different thicknesses of aluminium exposed at 7 different kilovoltages. *By courtesy of Kodak Ltd.*

It can be seen that at 100 kV there is less difference in density between the two ends of the wedge, and every step in the wedge is recorded. This is the picture of low radiographic contrast. At 40 kV there is greater difference in density not only between the ends but between all the steps of the wedge that can be seen; it should be noted that not every step of the wedge is recorded. This is the picture of high radiographic contrast. What is true of the step-wedge is true of all radiographic subjects; higher kilovoltage levels out absorption differences in the subject, and results in lower image contrast. Low contrast records a long scale of intensities (every step in the wedge); high contrast records a short scale only.

A certain value of objective contrast is not, however, the first aim of radiographers selecting radiation quality since other factors limit choice of tube voltage. Leaving aside 'high kilovoltage techniques', it may be said that radiographers select kilovoltage for particular radiographic examinations with adequate penetration of the subject as the basis for selection; the alteration in radiographic contrast is an accompanying effect which is accepted. In certain cases when selecting kilovoltage the radiographer *does* use knowledge of the resultant changes in radiation contrast within the subject. For example, in an anteroposterior projection of the dorsal spine choice of higher kilovoltage (by flattening absorption differences) enables the relatively radiolucent upper parts and the relatively radiopaque lower parts of the subject to be successfully recorded together.

Choice of kilovoltage, whether based on the need for penetrating the subject or consideration of radiation contrasts within the subject and their effects upon the image, is not an exact process. It is made empirically by the radiographer on the basis of experience.

EFFECTS OF SCATTERED RADIATION

The student has learned by now what happens to X radiation when it passes through the human body; some is transmitted, some is truly absorbed, some is scattered. In diagnostic radiography a proportion of scattered radiation can reach the film if no preventive measures are taken. On the film it creates a density which in the main is not image-forming. This has a most significant effect on the contrast of the resultant radiograph.

When it is remembered that objective contrast is difference in density, and that density is an expression of the light-transmitting ability of areas of the film, then it can be seen that an overall added density which decreases light transmission over the whole radiograph is bound to affect contrast. Since the scattered rays do have some projective action, their effect is also to decrease slightly the sharpness of the recorded detail, but it is their effect on contrast which is most significant in the general deterioration of the image.

When the kilovoltage across the X-ray tube is increased, the scattered radiation becomes more penetrating than that produced by a primary beam generated at lower kilovoltage and a bigger proportion of it goes forwards. These changes in scattered radiation are most important results from the use of higher kilovoltage.

If no measures are taken to control the effect on the film, the loss of contrast is most marked. Since thick body-parts require higher kilovoltage for adequate penetration and give rise to more scattered radiation by reason of the greater volume of tissue irradiated, loss of contrast will be most severe in these cases. It is a fact that without means to control scattered radiation it would be quite impossible to secure good radiographs of thick parts of the body; the images would be entirely unacceptable because of the low level of contrast.

In practical radiographic technique this loss of contrast is controlled through two approaches. These are (i) to reduce the formation of scatter, and (ii) to prevent scattered radiation from reaching the film.

Reduction in the formation of scatter. This will result from (i) the use of lower kilovoltages and (ii) limitation of the volume of irradiated tissue. It has been explained that the need for adequate penetration of the subject determines choice of kilovoltage, so this is not available as a method of controlling scatter. Much more important and useful is the reduction in scatter made by limiting the volume of tissue which the beam irradiates.

Compression of compressible body parts and the use of beam-limiting cones and diaphragms achieve this limitation. The student may be assured that the improvement in contrast which follows is not just a piece of textbook theory. It really works, as will be evident by comparison of radiographic results. The student should take opportunity if available to compare any of the following examples: a cholecystogram on a corpulent subject done with and without compression and beam limitation, an anteroposterior view of the lumbar spine of a similar subject in the same conditions, a lateral pelvimetry projection taken with and without a cone, or any similar examinations where the part to be demonstrated is very thick. (This is *not* a suggestion that such radiographs should be produced experimentally with a view to comparison).

Preventing scattered radiation from reaching the film. This is done by the use of a secondary radiation grid interposed between the patient and the film. Lead strips which compose part of the grid absorb oblique scattered rays, while the useful image-forming primary rays pass through radiolucent elements in the grid. Modern grids perform very effectively their task of screening the film from scattered radiation, and are an essential accessory for X-ray examination of thick parts of the body. They provide the means to obtain radiographic contrast which is not merely adequate but can be brilliant.

Since the grid inevitably absorbs some primary rays as well as the scattered radiation, exposures must be increased when a grid is used. This means increase in dose to the patient. This increase in dose is insignificant when it is realized that to make the radiograph without a grid would result in a valueless image and thus exposure of the patient to a dose of radiation which would certainly be smaller but also quite useless.

As well as being scattered by a patient's body, radiation is scattered from other structures such as the X-ray table. Some effort can be made to prevent access to the film by this radiation. It is therefore common practice to make the backs of cassettes and exposure-holders radiopaque. When direct-exposure film is used in its paper envelope, a piece of lead-rubber can be put behind it to absorb radiation scattered back towards the film from the table; this takes the place of the radiopaque backing to a cassette.

FILM FACTORS IN OBJECTIVE CONTRAST

It was explained in the last section of Chapter 3 that two important factors in radiographic contrast are (i) radiation contrasts within the subject and (ii) the film contrast. If the film contrast is low, the radiation contrasts within the subject are not amplified and the resultant contrast in the radiographic image is poor. Radiation contrasts in the subject are often very slight and film of low contrast cannot give good results. On the other hand film material of high contrast amplifies radiation contrasts in, the subject and results in an image of good contrast which is acceptable. Films used in radiography now have a contrast which rather more than doubles the radiation contrasts within the subject when they are recorded in the radiographic image.

The contrast of the film material is not a factor for the control of contrast in the image which can be manipulated by the radiographer. It is inherent in the material, is characteristic of it in the conditions of development used, is standardized in manufacture and remains a most important factor in the contrast of the image. Images seen on fluoroscopic screens not only are markedly less bright than those viewed on radiographs, but are much lower in contrast. The lack of contrast results from absence of the help given to radiographic images on film by the inherent contrast of the materials in present use.

Faster materials tend to have lower contrast, and screen-type film exposed to direct radiation has less contrast than when exposed between screens. This is a fact demonstrable by D log E curves and plain observation of results, but perhaps it is not of much importance to a radiographer who is not driven by some failure in supply to make the experiment. Certainly in emergency screen-type film has been used without screens to radiograph extremities, when the marked loss of speed is immaterial with results that were acceptable though slightly lacking in contrast.

PROCESSING FACTORS IN OBJECTIVE CONTRAST

Processing factors in objective contrast relate almost solely to factors of development.

There are many aspects of a developer and the technique of its use which can influence the contrast obtained. These may be listed as follows.

(i) Type and constitution of developing solutions.

(ii) Temperature of developer and time of development.

(iii) Freshness of developer.

(iv) Agitation of the film in the developer.

The aim in radiographic processing is to standardize as many of these as possible, and one of the benefits of automatic processing is that standardization of all can be achieved.

TYPE AND CONSTITUTION OF DEVELOPING SOLUTIONS

A great number of different developing formulae have been devised for general photography, even although the number of basic solutions is relatively small. Different formulae achieve different results, and the composition of the developer markedly influences the time required to reach a given contrast. The limit on the contrast which can be achieved is set by the film material used and the conditions of development.

The number of available X-ray developers is small, and they are all Metol-hydroquinone or Phenidone-hydroquinone solutions. These function to give good contrast in a standard development time at a given temperature.

The various ingredients in developing solutions have different functions to perform, and the developer will vary in performance if its ingredients are not all present, or are present in proportions which are not correct. Thus the amount of actual developing agent present, the Metol-hydroquinone and Phenidone-hydroquinone ratios, alterations in the amounts of alkali and of restrainer present, and the concentration of the solution as a whole, are all factors which influence the length of time required to reach a given contrast.

TEMPERATURE OF DEVELOPER AND DEVELOPMENT TIME

A family of D log E curves is shown in Fig. 12.12. These are the result of developing X-ray films for different lengths of time in a developing

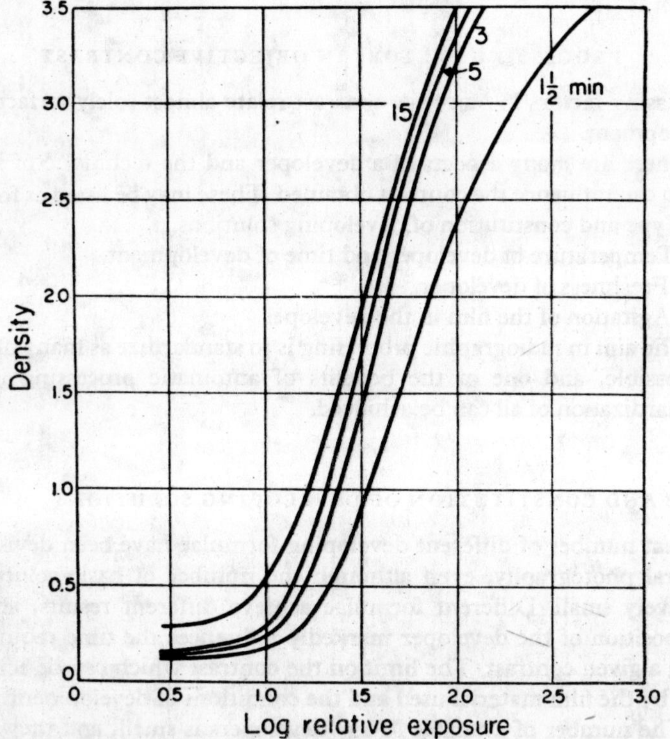

Fig. 12.12. Characteristic curves of a typical screen-type X-ray film, developed for a series of times at 68°F.
By courtesy of X-ray Sales Division, Eastman Kodak Company, Rochester, New York.

solution at a standard temperature. It can be seen that the slope of the straight-line part of the curve at first increases rapidly with development time but does not appreciably change after 5 minutes' development.

This demonstrates that the contrast of the film increases as development continues through its early stages, but that soon a point is reached beyond which contrast does not increase although development time is extended.

Fig. 12.13 shows another family of D log E curves made to demonstrate the effect of developing films for the same length of time at different temperatures. Such curves show an increase in contrast between about 55°F and 68°F and later (80°F) a reduction in contrast. There is a point around 65°F beyond which no increase in contrast is achieved by increasing temperature.

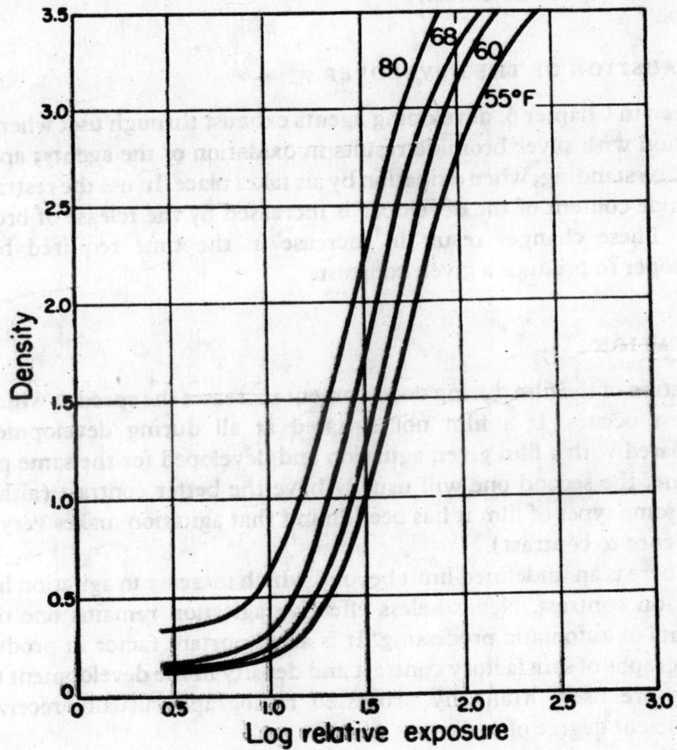

Fig. 12.13. Characteristic curves of the film of Fig. 12.12 but developed for 5 minutes at a series of development temperatures.
By courtesy of X-ray Sales Division, Eastman Kodak Company, Ltd.

In conventional manual processing the standard conditions of time and temperature have been set at 4 minutes (in the U.S.A. 5 minutes) development at 68°F (20°C). In automatic processing the technique of development is different, and development times are much shorter. Success depends on the use of special developing solutions suitable for working at a raised temperature, together with other factors. Whether manual processing or automatic methods are used, the object of the standardized technique is the same—to provide an image of satisfactory contrast in a period of time which is short enough to avoid fogging by action of the developer on unexposed silver halide grains. The effects of time and temperature may be summed-up by saying that slight prolongation of time increases contrast, but that long extension decreases contrast, and that in general development at extremes of temperature results in impaired contrast.

EXHAUSTION OF THE DEVELOPER

As seen in Chapter 6, developing agents exhaust through use, when their reaction with silver bromide results in oxidation of the agents; and also through standing, when oxidation by air takes place. In use the restraining bromide content of the developer is increased by the release of bromine ions. These changes result in increase in the time required by the developer to produce a given contrast.

AGITATION

Agitation of the film during development increases the speed at which the process occurs. If a film not agitated at all during development is compared with a film given agitation and developed for the same period of time, the second one will usually have the better contrast (although with some types of film it has been found that agitation makes very little difference to contrast).

There is an undefined limit beyond which increase in agitation has no effect on contrast. Nevertheless effective agitation remains one of the benefits of automatic processing. It is an important factor in producing radiographs of satisfactory contrast and density in the development times which are used. Manually processed radiographs usually receive an insufficient degree of agitation.

THE DISTINCTNESS OF THE RADIOGRAPHIC IMAGE

The distinctness with which the detail of the subject is made visible in the image is affected by all those factors which govern radiographic contrast (differences in density) in the image. These features are objective and can be measured.

Distinctness is governed also by factors which are not objective. These subjective factors can be stated, but they are variable and cannot be measured; they include elements which are external to the image, for example the conditions in which it is viewed. It may fairly be said that distinctness is a visual quality and has more subjective than objective components. While not measurable these components can be listed and their effects assessed; this will be done in the following paragraphs.

FACTORS AFFECTING DISTINCTNESS

IMAGE FACTORS

Important factors in the distinctness of the image are (i) the degree of unsharpness and the objective contrast as already discussed, and (ii) the degree of exposure. Where boundaries are sharp, it is possible to perceive differences in density which are very slight indeed; there is good definition even when the objective contrast is very low. If the difference in density is very great, structures can be clearly perceived even when the boundaries are not very sharp; resolution is good even when the detail sharpness is not the best that can be obtained.

The student may care to consider practical radiographic examples of these phenomena. In certain examinations differences in density *are* slight and maximum sharpness of outline results in satisfactory resolution; for example the demonstration of foetal parts in early pregnancy, and visualization of the bile ducts in intravenous cholangiography. Equally it is possible to consider instances where the difference in density is very great, and the resolution is acceptable even although the outline is not sharp. This fact is sometimes a comfort to radiographers when they view the radiographs of a recalcitrant child with a coin in his stomach. (At the same time it is on record that a straight pin has been made to disappear because it was moving; its image had no sharpness of outline, and resolution was not obtained even although contrast existed.) It is clear that resolution does not depend upon sharpness only or upon contrast only, but is determined by the two in correlation.

The degree of exposure significantly alters contrast in the image as it seems to an observer. Where overexposure exists, densities overall are increased but objective contrast (unless overexposure is gross), is not altered; differences in light-transmission through various regions of the film are in fact there and could be measured. It is simply that the eye cannot perceive these differences if the densities in general are so great that the light of the illuminator is not transmitted through them. The observer finds therefore that visual contrast is diminished by over-exposure; this visual contrast is subjective contrast and it cannot be measured since it is an impression received by the eyes of an individual viewer.

Underexposure results in lack of density. The developed image does not have the full range of densities produced in it, and there is thus deficiency in contrast both objective and subjective. The light from the illuminator coming through the film diminishes apparent contrast further, for the bright light in areas of low photographic density reduces for the eye small differences that exist.

VIEWING FACTORS

The importance of viewing conditions to distinctness in the image is their effect upon subjective contrast. Viewing factors can be considered under two headings. These are (i) those relating to the illumination, and (ii) those relating to the eyes of the observer.

The illumination. The viewing illumination can vary in colour, intensity, and uniformity. Modern X-ray illuminators are fluorescent-strip lighting not groups of electric bulbs, and they give a uniform blue-white light. This colour of light and its uniformity result in an improvement in visual contrast, enabling the range of densities in a well-exposed and correctly processed radiograph to be perceived as they actually exist.

In overexposed radiographs, increasing the brightness of the light improves subjective contrast. It allows the viewer to appreciate differences in density that he could not previously see. For an underexposed image, decreasing the brightness of the light improves visual contrast up to a certain point; there is an obvious limit here, for eventually the light would become too dim to penetrate the denser parts of even a weak image.

Illuminators may be equipped with a control for altering brightness so that conditions can be adapted for viewing a variety of radiographs. It is common practice also to have available in the reporting room a source of bright light (this may be just a single light bulb of sufficient wattage conveniently placed) against which regions of high photographic density can be viewed.

The level of illumination in a room where viewing is done also is significant in its effect upon apparent contrast. If the room is brightly lit the subjective contrast will be diminished. The effect of a shaft of sunlight illuminating the radiograph by reflected light can be to reduce to nil the apparent differences in light transmitted through the image from the X-ray illuminator. It is customary for reporting rooms to have their windows covered by curtains or screens so that the illumination in the room is low, and there are no unshielded bright lights when reporting is in progress. It is unnecessary, however, for radiographs to be viewed in a room from which all light apart from that of the viewing illuminators is entirely excluded.

The eyes of the observer. Image contrast as it seems to the eye is affected by the level of illumination to which the eye is adapted, and by the extent to which dazzle is present. An eye adapted to a bright light is unable to perceive differences in the deeper density range, and beyond a certain level all the densities look black, the eye being unable to perceive detail in these regions. If the eye is dazzled by bright light coming through parts of the image which have little density, there is again lack of ability to perceive detail.

It is possible to prevent dazzle by masking areas from which bright light is coming. For example if a radiograph of 24 cm × 30 cm size is being examined against an illuminator which is 38 cm × 45 cm, a piece of black card to cover the illuminator with an aperture cut in it can be placed as a surround to the radiograph. This will exclude extraneous light. It is customary to view industrial radiographs against very bright illuminators which have a means of confining the light to certain areas of the film.

This importance of the viewing situation to distinctness in any radiographic image is well recognized by radiologists, who would not consider basing a report on appearances which had been viewed against a window or before a ceiling light. While his clinical colleagues may sometimes regard viewing conditions more casually, the radiologist will give to these so that they may be exactly favourable as much care as he devotes to other aspects of radiological technique. It is of little value to expend time, effort, and money in the production of first-class radiographs if they are to be viewed in conditions which vitiate their quality.

SIZE, SHAPE AND SPATIAL RELATIONSHIPS

So far in this chapter we have considered in regard to radiographic images their lack of sharpness, their contrast and their resolution: these are all seen to be important, measurable entities. We have not as yet provided answers to this question: do the structures examined appear as images which are truthful in regard to the sizes, shapes and spatial relationships of the different structures? We know that shadows can mislead on all three of these, so perhaps it is no surprise to find that radiographic images (which are subject to the geometry of shadow formation) can be similarly false.

The term radiographic distortion refers to incorrectness in the proportions of structures recorded radiographically, and to lack of truth in their apparent alignment and relationship to each other. The most truthful result is obtained when a structure being radiographed rests with its principal planes parallel to the film, and the X-ray beam is aligned so that the central ray is at right angles to these planes and to the film, and is passing through the area of main diagnostic interest.

The student should compare two such examples as these: (i) a lateral view of the lumbar spine, the patient lying correctly in the true lateral position and the vertical X-ray beam centred at the level of the third lumbar vertebra; and (ii) a lateral view of the same region in a subject with a broad pelvis who has been allowed to sag at the waist towards the table so that the long axis of the spine is not parallel to the table, and the central ray is not vertical to it. In the first case the bodies of the vertebrae are seen as they are, distinct and separate from each other, with radiolucent structures occupying the spaces between them. In the second case the vertebral bodies overlap each other, and do not appear to be separated in space at all. If knowledge of them rested solely on such radiographic appearances, one would assume that in parts they overlie each other. The second image is a distorted one.

In dental radiography it is very easy to produce a similar effect by incorrect alignment, and to cause teeth to overlap each other, thus failing to render truly their relationship. It is equally easy to distort their true proportions, and produce images which are elongated or foreshortened in shape.

In general, radiographic technique is directed to restricting to a minimum distortions due to projection, but in some cases such alterations in apparent alignment and relationship are made with intention. It can be a useful technique for separating from intrusive structures some particular region which is to be visualized. The student can doubtless think of several examples; separation of the two sides of the mandible in lateral-oblique projections; the 30 deg. occipitomental view of the facial bones which by this technique are cleared of structures in the posterior fossa of the base of the skull; displacement of the clavicles from the apical regions of the lungs in examinations of the chest.

Exact knowledge of the distortions producible in radiographs is thus part of the radiographer's armoury, whether the effect being sought is their avoidance or their deliberate production.

The next question to be considered is: are radiographic images life-size for the structures which they represent? The simple answer is that they are not, the falsity being most usually that of magnification: the image is somewhat larger than the structure it depicts.

This enlargement occurs because the X-ray beam diverges from its source, spreading out so that it becomes greater in cross-section. This results in radiographic images which may truly be said to be larger than life (Figs 12.8 and 12.14).

The degree of enlargement that occurs is not a constant. It is determined by the distance separating structures being examined from the X-ray source and the distance between the X-ray source and the film which records the image. Magnification becomes greater for structures which are close to the source and for short source-film distances; it becomes less for structures which are far from the source and for long source-film distances.

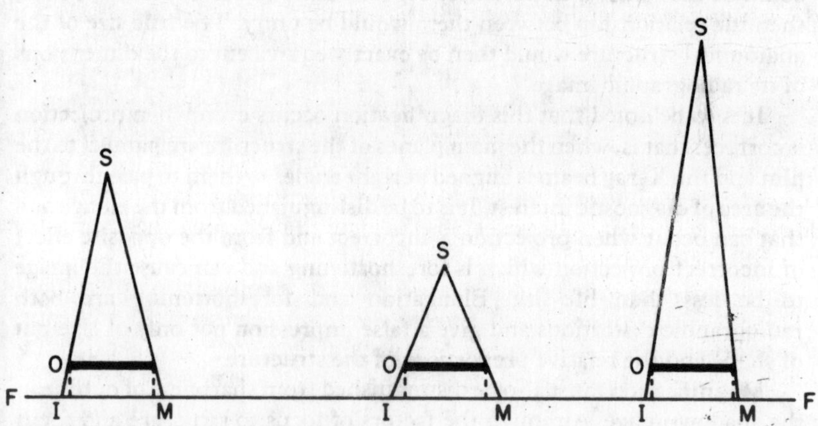

Fig. 12.14. Enlargement in the X-ray image.
S   X-ray source (assumed to be a point).
O   object.
IM Size of image.
F   film.

With an anatomical structure parallel to the film and the central ray at right angles to the film, the true dimensions of the structure can be calculated from its image size by this relationship:

$$\text{True size} = \frac{\text{Image size} \times \text{Focus-structure distance}}{\text{Focus-film distance}}$$

Magnification is given by these relationships:

$$\text{Magnification} = \frac{\text{Focus-film distance}}{\text{Focus-structure distance}}$$

$$\text{Magnification} = \frac{\text{Image size}}{\text{True size}}$$

This inevitable enlargement in the image is the reason why pelvic measurements for obstetricians and bone measurements for orthopaedic surgeons cannot be made on the simple basis of putting a ruler against a conventional radiographic image of the parts concerned. Where measurements are necessary, some method of correction or some means of reducing enlargement must be used.

Long tube-film distances diminish the difference between the true size and the image size because they result in the tube-structure distance and the focus-film distance being more nearly the same. If in fact they could be the same, if no distances separated the structure from the film, then the relationship between them would be unity. The true size of the anatomical structure would then be exactly equivalent to the dimensions of its radiographic image.

It is to be noted that this magnification occurs even when projection is correct: that is, when the main planes of the structure are parallel to the film and the X-ray beam is aligned at right angles to them to pass through the area of diagnostic interest. It is to be distinguished from the elongation that can occur when projection is incorrect and from the opposite effect of incorrect projection which is foreshortening and can cause the image to be less than life-size. Elongation and foreshortening are both radiographic distortions and give a false impression not only of size but of shape and the relative proportions of the structure.

Magnification must also be distinguished from sharpness of outline in the shadow image. Although the factors of focus to structure and focus to film distances affect *both* the *size* and the *sharpness* of outlines in the image, these two features of the shadow are quite separate. Sometimes radiographers considering radiographic images seem confused between the two and even to believe that the two are the same entity. Yet confusion would disappear if they stopped thinking about radiographs and imagined instead the shadow cast by a hand placed between a light-source and a wall. It is at once obvious that the *size* of this shadow and the *sharpness* of its outline are two separate features. So are they for the radiographic shadow images that we daily assess.

An Appendix at the end of this book presents, in table form, factors in the radiographic image which we have discussed in this chapter.

Chapter 13
Management of the Quality of the Radiographic Image

In recent years many of those who are concerned with the work of diagnostic X-ray departments have investigated closely the quality of the radiographic image. They have considered the checking and the directing of the numerous elements in its production. In an earlier chapter (Chapter 12) we defined the quality of the radiographic image as its ability to reproduce in a visible pattern the varying transmission of X rays through the subject being radiographed. The image is of the higest quality if the reproduction is exact. This implies the least loss of diagnostic information in the complex conversion of the emergent radiation pattern from the subject to the visible pattern of photographic densities which is the image on the radiograph. This minimal loss of diagnostic information must be the aim of the X-ray department which is properly discharging its function as a producer of radiographs.

In this entirely technical context we might (if it is possible temporarily to overlook the patient) see the X-ray department as a small factory set up to manufacture radiographs. Management of the image seeks to control the quality of the end-product of that factory: that is, of the radiograph. What are the elements to be controlled in the manufacture of this product? It is plain that indeed there are many of them and the best starting point for clarification is to see all these components in the groups to which they belong. The groupings are as follows.

(i) Components relating to the processing procedures (development and subsequent stages of the cycle) to which the radiograph is submitted.

(ii) Components relating to the recording system which is used to form the visible image (in diagnostic radiography the system most often used is a combination of films and intensifying screens).

(iii) Components relating to the X-ray tube and the conditions of its use: this might be termed the technical system or the exposure unit.

(iv) Components relating to the subject of the diagnostic X-ray examination, to the determination of the required exposure and to the radiographer's assessment of the patient.

TABLE 13.1

Elements relating to the processing	Elements relating to the recording system	Elements relating to the X-ray tube and conditions of its use	Elements relating to the subject
(1) Constitution of developers	(1) Characteristics of film-materials	(1) Focal spot size	(1) Radiation-attenuating characteristics of tissues
(2) Replenishment of developers	(2) Characteristics of intensifying screens	(2) Tube rating	(2) Differentials in attenuation by different tissues
(3) Constitution of fixers	(3) Characteristics of cassettes	(3) Tube filtration	(3) Characteristics of organs and anatomical locations
(4) Replenishment of fixers	(4) Characteristics of film-stores	(4) Type of high tension generator	(4) Capability for movement of the part examined
(5) Temperatures used in processing		(5) Kilovoltage	(5) Focus-object and object-film distances
(6) Characteristics of processors		(6) Milliamperage	(6) Determination of required exposures
		(7) Exposure-time	(7) Radiographers' assessments
		(8) Beam collimation and centering	
		(9) Control of scattered radiation	
		(10) Focus-film distance	

Table 1 shows elements in the production of the radiograph arranged under these four headings. To practice management of the image is to seek to check and to direct towards an optimum result many of these components which are liable to test and to measurement. The meticulous exercise of such control costs time and costs money. So perhaps a question to be early considered is: what are the benefits of such practices?

THE BENEFITS OF CONTROL OF THE IMAGE

X-ray department is a very costly department of the hospital. The administering authority is required to spend large sums of money in the provision of equipment, material, services and staff so that the X-ray department may give efficient diagnostic aid for the clinicians of the hospital. Managers of any organization within which and upon which money must be laid out concern themselves with questioning how the money is spent.

is a jargon term to express this question: that is, cost-effectiveness. Cost-effectiveness means the ratio of the spending to the efficiency of production that follows in result. If the spending is high for relatively low efficiency, the cost-effectiveness is unfavourable. If the efficiency is high for high spending, then the cost-effectiveness could be accepted as satisfactory. If efficiency is high for low spending, then the cost-effectiveness is a sweet dream for any finance officer in any organization!

The benefits of close control in an X-ray department can be summarized by saying that the overall cost-effectiveness of the department is improved. In putting the case for spending time and money on such controls, there is no argument to submit to finance officers more compelling of consent than *that*. Here, however, we should perhaps enumerate some of the details which add up to improved cost-effectiveness. They are as follows.

(i) The number of repeated radiographs is reduced.

(ii) The rate of flow of patients through the department is improved.

(iii) The department's ability to meet the demands made upon its services (departmental capacity) is raised.

(iv) The quality of the radiographs produced is higher.

(v) Standardization of the radiographic results is achieved and is maintained.

(vi) The reliability and efficiency of automatic processors and of X-ray equipment are improved.

MANAGEMENT OF THE IMAGE

The rest of this chapter considers many of the items which are laid out in Table 1. We do not aim to discuss these comprehensively. Our plan is rather to describe various practices which help radiographers towards an improved management of the images (the radiographs) produced in their departments.

A useful way to begin a programme of improved management is to initiate an analysis of the department's rejected radiographs. This is done by placing these radiographs among four categories which indicate the reasons why each was rejected, as follows:

(i) overexposure or underexposure;

(ii) malpositioning of the patient, the central X-ray beam, the film;

(iii) motional blur;

(iv) processing faults;

(v) other reasons.

We put the exposure errors at the top of the list because these usually account for 50 per cent of the rejections and thus they cause much waste of money, material and time. We put the processing faults almost at the bottom of the list since these account for only a very small percentage of the rejected radiographs. Nevertheless if the processing system is not functioning correctly the image will be of impaired quality whatever is done to improve all other factors in its production.

We propose in the following pages to consider the management of the image in four main sections as indicated by the headings at the tops of the columns in Table 1. We begin with the processing because of its essential importance in the success of the whole production.

CHECKS FOR AUTOMATIC PROCESSORS.

When radiographically exposed film is taken to the darkroom it holds a latent photographic image: the first step has been accomplished in converting a radiation image which emerges from the patient (as a pattern of various transmitted X-ray intensities) to become a permanent visible image which can be viewed and interpreted. This visible and permanent image is a pattern of various photographic densities on the film and it is produced from the invisible and impermanent latent image by the procedures which make up the complete processing cycle.

The procedures of the processing cycle are today implemented through the functioning of automatic processors which are in widespread use. These processors are key units in the production of radiographs. In the radiographs from any department where diagnostic radiography is done a consistently high quality becomes possible only when systems of automatic processing function with a maintained uniformity. So it is important to have some relatively simple and quickly applied method of testing or monitoring the performance of these processors. In many departments it is not just a matter of making sure that one processor performs to a standard: it is often necessary to make sure that two or more processors are functioning to the the same level.

APPLYING SENSITOMETRY TO CHEMICAL RESPONSE

Sensitometric monitoring is a simple method of evaluating the performance of a processor in the development phase of its cycle: that is, checking its chemical response. Sensitometric monitoring is carried out by processing a number of film strips which have each been given a series of stepped exposures and then analysing the processed strips as we will explain later. So, for example, daily monitoring could be done by processing one such strip each day in each of the processors to be checked, the findings of the analysis being recorded. The records would reveal variations in the chemical response and show the need for adjustments to be made within the development phase of the processor. This is a monitoring routine which is easily applied and is within the competence of a radiographer.

Since the functioning of the processor is to produce radiographs with images made up by various densities, it is logical to check performance by processing a strip of film which will show various densities because it has received a series of stepped exposures. It is a direct method of testing the performance of a processor since measurements are made upon a film on which the processor has just acted, as it will on the radiographs which are developed by it in the course of the working day.

OBTAINING STEPPED EXPOSURES

The film strips which are processed in sensitometric monitoring must each show a number of densities to allow adequate measurements to be made. Twenty one steps of density are acceptable because they give 20 differences. The densities should include the range 0·25 to 2·0. The density steps are the results of stepped exposures which have a known step-to-step increment called the wedge constant. In any monitoring programme the series of stepped exposures must be reproducible exactly for all the control strips which are processed. The control films are better exposed and then immediately processed rather than exposed and then processed later: an aged latent image has been shown to be less sensitive than is a fresh one to variations in the performance of a processor. The phenomenon is known as latent image fade.

So the X-ray department which is to carry out a programme of sensitometric monitoring should have the means to produce a sustained series of control strips which have been exposed in exactly similar conditions precisely reproduced from day to day. There are two choices to be considered here as follows:

(i) stepped exposures to X rays using a conventional cassette with intensifying screens so that the exposures are to a combination of X rays and light from the screens (which is the commonest method of making radiographs);

(ii) controlled stepped exposures to light using for the purpose a special device called a sensitometer.

STEPPED X-RAY EXPOSURES

A radiographer might at first think that the control strips with which to monitor automatic processors could readily be produced without the aid of any special devices. We all know that we could give a film a series of exposures with a known step-to-step increment by working at a fixed kilovoltage and focus-film distance and varying the milliampereseconds by a given factor: for example, times two would give milliampereseconds values of 1, 2, 4, 8, 16, 32 and so on. Lead could be used to mask off those parts of the cassette which were not being used for exposure.

The difficulty in doing it this way is that it really would not be possible to guarantee that the separate exposures required for the serial steps of density would be exactly related to each other and exactly reproducible from day to day. Exactness in the conditons of exposure is extremely important since these film strips are to be used to monitor the performance of an automatic processor. Variations can be critical and can lead to misinterpretation of the result. There is, however, more latitude for variation when the series of exposures is to be used to establish relative film speeds.

The situation can be improved by making use of an aluminium step-wedge: each control film is then produced by making one X-ray exposure through the wedge. Twenty one steps of density would result if the wedge had twenty one steps. The wedge must be precisely (and expensively) constructed so that each step transmits to the film an exposure related to that which the preceding step transmits by a known factor which is called the wedge constant.

The modification to the first idea still fails to guarantee from day to day exact reproduction of the X-ray exposures. To achieve some degree of consistency the practical procedure should be standardized as much as possible. To that end, the following constituents of the test should always be the same:

(i) the X-ray set used;
(ii) the X-ray tube used;
(iii) the settings of kilovoltage, milliamperage and time;
(iv) the focus-film distance;
(v) the stepwedge;
(vi) the cassette to be used, loaded always with the same type and make of film.

If more than one processor is to be monitored, only one film should be exposed at the time of one test. It is then cut into as many strips as there are processors involved in the test. Each strip must hold all the steps of the wedge and is of course processed in a different processor.

USE OF A SENSITOMETER

A sensitometer is a device which is especially for the purpose of exposing photographic materials to light so that they receive exposures which can be carefully controlled as to the intensity and the quality of the light and the periods of exposure to it. Sensitometers thus provide a means whereby film strips to be used in X-ray departments for the monitoring of processors can be given exposures which are exactly related to each other and reproducible from day to day.

Commercially available sensitometers have the following features:

(i) a light source which may be a tungsten-filament lamp operating at specified voltage and amperage so that the intensity of the emitted light is always the same or may be an electroluminescent panel which emits light when excited by an electric current;

(ii) consistent control of the duration of the exposure which may be achieved by a timing device such as a shutter blade driven by a motor which has a constant speed or by means of an electronic timer;

(iii) temperature stabilization;

(iv) a means to attenuate the light through a scale of exposure steps with a known relationship. A device to provide such an exposure-scale is effectively a light-attenuating stepwedge with a wedge constant: it is known as a grey scale with related exposure steps. When a film is put into the sensitometer and is exposed to the light source, the light-attenuator is between the film and the light so that exposure is through the grey scale. On development the film shows a series of density steps which have a known exposure increment or wedge constant from each step to its darker neighbour. The twenty one exposure steps in an exposure attenuator which is to give 20 differences relate each to its adjacent step by a factor which is the wedge constant.

Such a sensitometer can be obtained specially adjusted for use in an X-ray department. The light source emits blue light and thus simulates for conventional screen-type X-ray film the exposure conditions which would apply in the usual radiographic practice of exposing the film to a combination of X rays and the light emitted from calcium tungstate intensifying screens.

USING THE FILM SAMPLES

The developed film strips used in processor-monitoring show a range of stepped densities resulting from stepped exposures. We have so far referred to twenty one stepped exposures related by a factor which is the wedge constant, the wedge being either an aluminium and copper stepwedge for radiographic exposure or a grey scale in a sensitometer. With twenty one steps, the wedge constant used is $\sqrt{2}$. This means that the factor relating exposures is 1·414 and the log exposure increment is 0·15 per step (0·1492 is the log of $\sqrt{2}$): there are thus 20 differences in small steps. Some wedges or grey scales have only 11 steps and a wedge constant of 2 has been considered suitable, the log exposure increment being 0·3 per step (0·3010 is the log of 2): this gives 10 differences in greater steps. The 21-step attenuator with a wedge constant of 1·41 provides more points of measurement and is a more exact tool. When the stepped exposures are made, there should be one shielded area of the film which receives no deliberate exposure and this area is to be used later to determine the density due to base plus fog.

The next stage of the test is to use the film strips so that information may be derived from them about the performance of an automatic processor in its development section.

The analysis of these films is based upon the measurement or the assessment of density. Records must be kept in order to reveal variation in performance. The densities may be objectively established as numerical values by being read on a densitometer. Simple visual comparisons without the aid of an instrument may be used if the X-ray department has no densitometer. Such assessment, as opposed to instrumental measurement, has a subjective element since it rests upon the judgement of a human observer. To some, this opportunity for error makes the method unacceptably inexact. Others will consider that since the radiograph emerging from the processor will be viewed by a human eye, there is no need to base a testing system on an instrument which is less susceptible to variation.

Deviations from the normal development conditions of the processor are revealed by (i) exposing; (ii) processing; (iii) evaluating these film samples every day. The aim is to check three important parameters. These are:

(i) speed;

(ii) contrast;

(iii) the density of base plus fog.

Of these three, speed is perhaps the most significant as an indication of a change in the development conditions. If the development section of the processor has so varied as to produce underdeveloped radiographs at the end of the cycle-time, there has been effectively a loss of speed since a given exposure elicits less density in the image as a response to development. Similarly if the change in performance has been in the direction of over-development there has been effectively a gain in speed since a given exposure elicits a response of greater density in the developed image. These changes in speed are noticeable indications in the radiograph that changes in the performance of the developer have happened.

It may be wished to keep the checks on a processor to a minimum so that they take up the least amount of time that is compatible with an adequate system. In that case, you should check the single parameter of speed and leave the other two untested. The change in speed is certainly the most sensitive indication that an automatic processor is failing to maintain standardized development.

MONITORING SPEED

After the control strips have been developed, consistency in speed is tested by measuring the density of a single step in the series of stepped densities which each strip shows. The step selected for the check must be the same one in all of the strips used for this daily monitoring programme. It should be one which develops to a density between 0·9 and 1·2 when the processor is working normally. Such a density falls towards the lower end of the straight-line region of the D log E curve (see Fig 13.1) and it

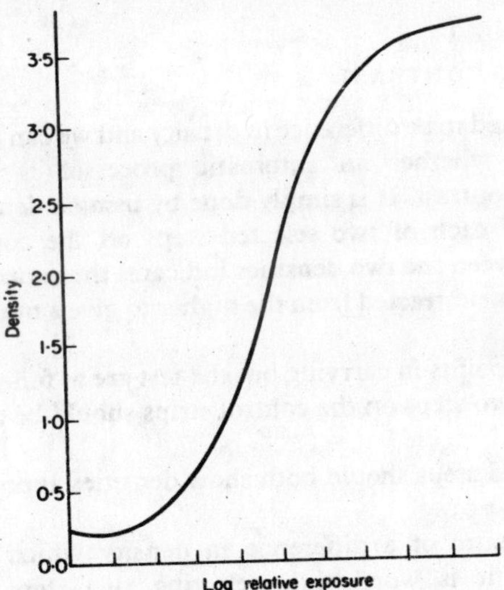

Fig. 13.1 D Log E Curve.

responds readily but without exaggeration to the changes in speed caused by aberrant development.

It takes only a very few minutes to make the measurement of density on just one step of each control strip and to graph the result as indicated in Fig. 13.2. Such a record shows whether speed is constant or variable as the days go by.

A question to be asked is: how much variation could be tolerated as an acceptably consistent result? The answer is that we could accept as

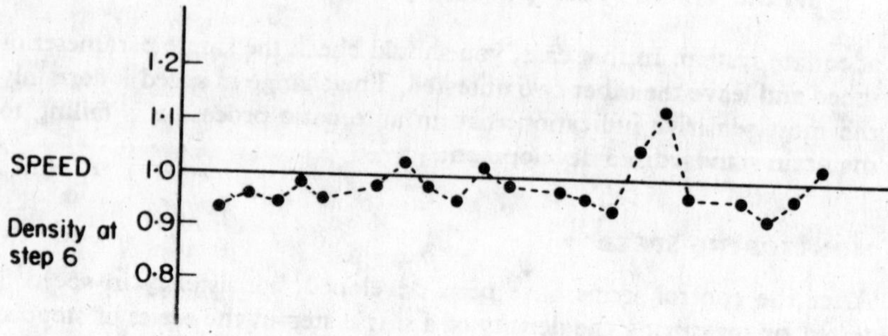

Fig. 13.2 Chart of speed test for processor.

tolerable density values which were 0·15 above or below the density measured on the selected step in the 0·9 to 1·2 range when the processor is operating normally. This is about plus/minus 15 to 20 per cent on average.

MONITORING CONTRAST

Contrast is stated to be difference in density and we can use this definition to determine whether an automatic processor is developing to a standardized contrast. It is simply done by using a densitometer to read the density of each of two selected steps on the control strips. The difference between the two densities indicates the contrast obtained: the lower density is subtracted from the higher to give a number which is the contrast.

Important points in carrying out the test are as follows:
(i) the same two steps on the control strips should be chosen for all the readings;
(ii) the selected steps should both show densities approximately within the range 0·25–2·0;
(iii) to make sure of a difference in density which is adequate for measurement, it is worthwhile selecting two steps which are not immediately adjacent but are separated by about seven steps. Fig. 13.3 shows the type of record which may be kept.

MONITORING THE DENSITY DUE TO BASE PLUS FOG

Increase in the density of base plus fog is not a sensitive indication of aberrations in the development section of an automatic processor. Deviations show themselves by changes in speed and in contrast at very early stages. Increase in gross fog is a much later effect.

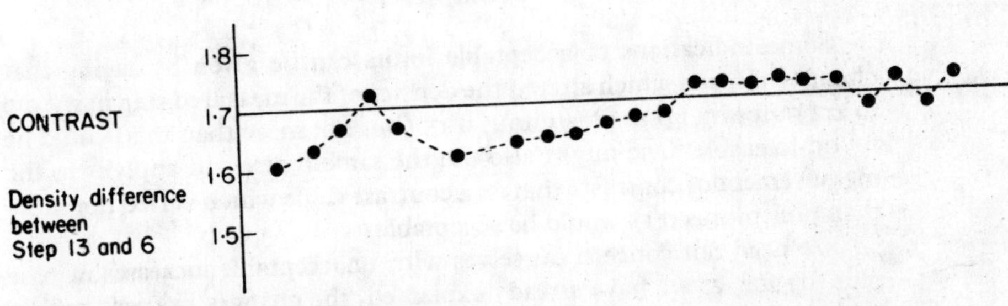

Fig. 13.3 Chart of contrast test for processor.

Gross fog is the density of the film base plus any density contributed by the development of unexposed silver halide. So gross fog is determined by the measurement of density in part of the film strip which was shielded from intentional exposure when the test strip was made. For what it may be worth, change in gross fog is thus easily checked. It can be understood that any change taking place must be towards an *increase* over the density obtained when the processor is working properly. Fig. 13.4 shows the type of record that may be kept.

CRITERIA OF ACCEPTANCE OF THE TESTS

Having taken the trouble to make tests as a check on the development section of an automatic processor and having established records of the type shown in Figs 13.2, 13.3 and 13.4, the next question for the tester is: how much variation in the graphs is considered tolerable? A general answer is to say that the acceptable variations may be in the 15 to 20 per cent range. Doubtless any diagnostic X-ray department may wish to set its own limits. What is certain are the following points: (i) a single value which shows itself as outside the level to be tolerated requires the action only of making a second test for there is little need to do anything else about it; (ii) *trends* of change *are* significant and will show themselves in the tests much before alterations in speed and contrast become unacceptably apparent in radiographs.

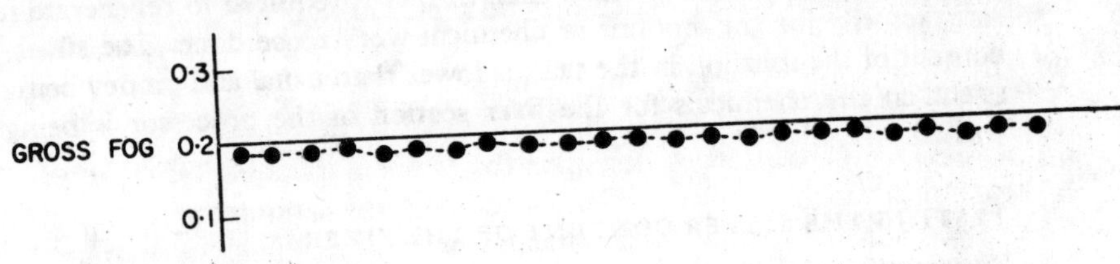

Fig. 13.4 Measurement of fog.

Some indications of acceptable limits can be given by saying that changes of speed which altered the density of the measured step in the 0·9 to 1·2 range by up to plus/minus 0·15 (but not more than this) could be found tolerable. One might also use the same figure and apply it to the measurement of contrast: that is, a contrast value which varied not more than plus/minus 0·15 would be acceptable.

We need not concern ourselves with unacceptable increases in base plus fog for, as we have already explained, the changes in speed and in contrast are early and significant pointers to deviation long before any revelations are made by the increased fog. An acceptable density due to base plus fog is around 0·20 to 0·23: if it is as great as 0·25 it is entering the useful density range in radiographs and from then on will deteriorate the contrast of the image.

TESTING THE ADEQUACY OF FIXER REPLENISHMENT

Following development of their images, radiographs in an automatic processor are next conveyed to the tank in which fixing is done. The basic action there is the conversion of unexposed, undeveloped silver halide to a soluble compound which is removed by water. As a result of this action, the fixer accumulates soluble silver complexes and a working fixer solution is bound to have a certain content of silver.

In an automatic processor the fixer is replenished for every film which is processed. If the rate of this replenishment is satisfactorily matched to the amount of chemical work to be done, the silver content of the fixer should not change very much. So checks on the silver content of the working fixer in an automatic processor indicate if the fixer replenishment system is achieving what it is intended to do: that is, to regenerate the fixer satisfactorily so that the radiographs will be fixed in the time allotted to this process.

If the fixer replenishment rate is inadequate the chemical work to be done exceeds the regeneration given and the quantity of silver in the fixer solution in the processor rises. If the replenishment rate is too high, more fixer is being added to the tank than in fact is required to regenerate it satisfactorily for the amount of chemical work to be done. The silver-content of the solution in the tank is lower than usual and money being spent on the chemicals for the fixer section of the processor is being wasted.

TESTING THE SILVER CONTENT OF THE FIXER

Silver-estimating kits are available commercially. They comprise booklets holding strips of special paper which has been impregnated with chemicals. When the paper strips are dipped into the silver-containing fixer, they become stained and the depth of the tone of a stain is related to the silver-content of the tested solution. The tone is darker as the silver-content in grams per litre of the fixer increases.

With the booklets of silver-estimating paper a chart is provided which shows the different tones of colour-change of the paper related to the content of silver. One such chart, for example, has eight steps of tone: the lightest one (being the original tone of the paper) is marked for 0 grams per litre and the darkest brown tone is given by 10 grams per litre: the figures in between are 1·0, 1·75, 2·5, 5·0 and 7·0 grams per litre.

The test is quickly performed. The silver-estimating paper is dipped into the fixing solution of the processor which is in the working tank and after a second or two the stain is established. The tint of the paper is then compared by eye with the tints on the chart and an assessment of the silver-content of the fixer solution is thus made. The test might suitably be carried out once a week and a record of the assessment should be kept so that it can be seen whether or not the quantity of silver present in the fixer is varying. The level should be between 5·0 and 7·0 grams per litre if the cycle of the processor occupies 90 seconds up to 3 minutes. Where processors have cycle-times longer than 3 minutes, amounts of silver up to 7 grams per litre are acceptable.

TESTING THE EFFICIENCY OF THE WASHING PROCESS

The purpose of the washing section in any processing unit is to reduce to acceptable levels the quantities of salts which are carried by the emulsion layers of films after they come out of the fixer solution. These salts deteriorate the image in time. They are all soluble and can be removed by water.

What the washing section aims to achieve is removal of these residual salts within the time that each radiograph remains in that part of the machine. Total removal cannot be accomplished and is in any case unnecessary. The requirement is to bring the level of the remaining salts low enough for the image not to deteriorate in the time for which it is to be kept. The level must be lower when the keeping-time is longer and in establishing acceptable levels a distinction is made between those films which are to be kept for archives and those which are to be kept for what might be termed ordinary usage. Radiographs kept as medical records in hospital fit into the group classified for ordinary usage.

Now clearly the test of time reveals the efficacy of the washing process in automatic processors and our successors need no special test for the efficacy of the washing given to our films in our X-ray departments today.

In the days after all our tomorrows, they have only to look at the radiographs which we processed years before to see whether there are stains upon them from the residual salts of fixing. But we are concerned *now* to control the radiographic images we produce and to assure ourselves that their quality is of the highest. An important part of this is their keeping properties. So how might we test that the automatic processor is washing efficiently enough?

There is a simple answer: apply chemical agents to the processed and washed radiographs to check the remaining salt-content of their emulsion layers. The necessary reagents are commercially available combined in a test-pack with a comparator-card. The card bears a set of tints which begins with a pale straw colour (corresponding to a low level of residual thiosulphate) and ends with a light tan (corresponding to a higher level of residual thiosulphate).

TESTING FOR RESIDUAL THIOSULPHATE

To carry out a test for residual thiosulphate, the supplied chemical reagent is spotted on a processed radiograph by means of a dropper. The area on the radiograph selected for the test must be a clear one and not carrying a developed density: the result of the test will be misleading if the reagent is applied to a region where there is developed silver. So an area where there is clear film base must be selected and one or two drops of the reagent are placed on it and left for two minutes. At the end of that time the reagent is blotted off and the brownish stain which is left on the tested area is then immediately studied. The stain will darken when exposed to light which is bright, especially if it is direct sunlight, so a long delay in assessing the depth of the colour will alter the result of the test. The depth of the colour of the stain indicates the amount of residual thiosulphate that the tested area contains, the colour being deeper for higher salt-content. So a colour which has been additionally deepened by 5 or 10 minutes exposure to light gives a finding from the test which is misleadingly high.

The colour of the stain is compared by eye as closely as possible with the set of tints on the comparator-chart. There may be only four tints as there are in the example shown in Fig. 13.5. If the comparison is done quickly in good, ordinary room-lighting, errors introduced by the stain's darkening as it is studied will be insignificant. Information on the comparator-chart relates the tones shown on it to amounts of thiosulphate and the levels of acceptability for keeping radiographs for normal use and for archival storage. For example, the chart shown in Fig. 13.5 brings

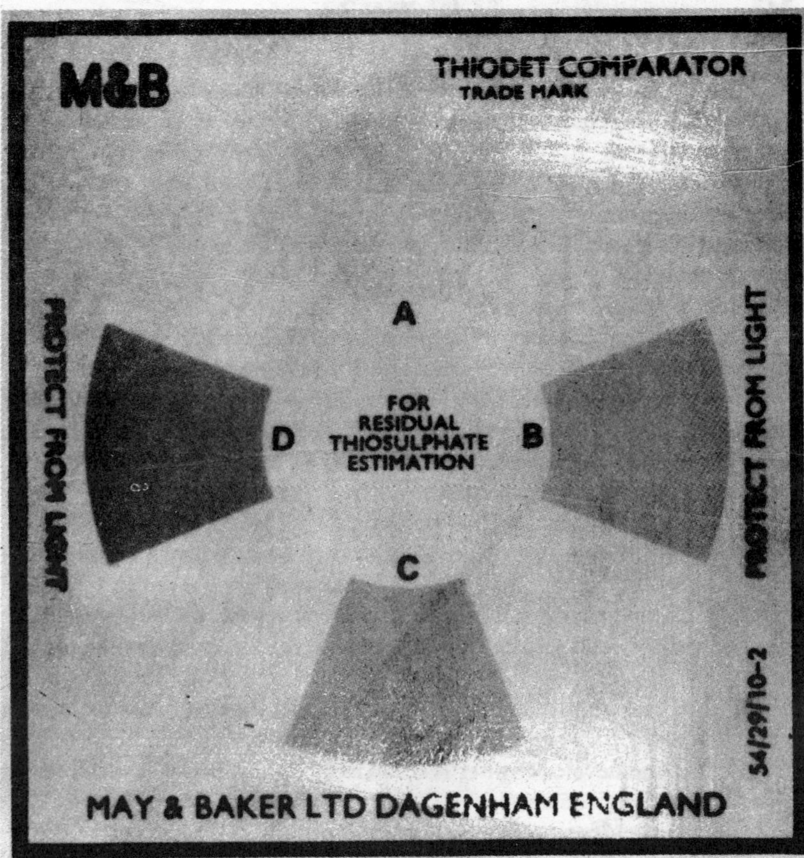

Fig. 13.5 Thiodet comparator chart.

with it the information that radiographs which have staining in the C–D range are acceptable for normal use and in the B–C range are satisfactory for archival storage.

SUMMARY OF PROCESSOR CHECKS

To conclude this section of the present chapter concerned with the management of the radiographic image, it has seemed to us worthwhile to bring together tests of the functioning of an automatic processor which should be systematically made if standardized results are to be achieved and maintained.

DAILY CHECKS ON DEVELOPMENT

(i) Prepare a sensitometric control strip for each processor to be monitored.

(ii) Process a strip in each processor about one hour after the unit has been switched on.

(iii) For each strip, assess those quantities which it is wished to monitor: speed, contrast, density of base plus fog. If only one of these is to be checked, it should be speed.

(iv) Record the findings. If there is little variation from those of the previous day the processor is satisfactorily developing radiographs.

(v) For a processor which has been performing satisfactorily, if a single test strip shows a result at variance with those preceding it, then a further test strip should be processed as a check on errors in the test.

(vi) If the variation is maintained, check the developer temperature. A rise in temperature leads to an increase in speed and a fall in temperature results in a loss of speed. The thermostat can be readjusted if necessary.

(vii) If the result of the test is a loss of speed and the developer temperature as it should be, then the following checks should be carried out:

  (a) that the replenishor and recirculating pumps are functioning satisfactorily to give recirculation of the developer;

  (b) that the developer filter is reasonably clean for if it is very dirty it will hinder recirculation;

  (c) that the developer-replenisher solution has been correctly prepared, for if too much water has been added to it the effect will be to reduce the speed of the developer.

(viii) If the result of the test is a gain in speed and the developer temperature is as it should be, then the next check to be made is on the preparation of the replenisher. If insufficient water has been added to it, the effect is to increase the speed of the developer.

(ix) If all the above sources of a change in the speed of the developer are investigated and are found not to be causing it, there remains the possibility that the replenishment-rate is ill-matched to the amount of chemical work to be done. If the replenishment-rate is too high for what is required, the developer is over-replenished and gains speed. If the replenishment rate is too low, the developer loses speed because it is under-replenished. If it is necessary to alter the replenishment-rate, the adjustment should be a small one (for example 5·0 millilitres). Time should be allowed for this to become effective before a further change is made.

WEEKLY CHECKS ON A PROCESSOR

Weekly checks on an automatic processor are best undertaken at the beginning of each working week after the machine has been switched on and has been running for a while so that conditions are stabilized. The tests to be carried out are as follows.

(i) Check and record the temperature of the developer.

(ii) Measure and record the replenishment rate of the developer.

(iii) Record the number of films processed during the week.

(iv) Record the number of developer packs used during the week.

(v) Check and record the temperature of the fixer: it should preferably be close to that of the developer.

(vi) Measure and record the replenishment rate of the fixer.

(vii) Record the number of fixer packs used during the week.

(viii) Measure and record the silver content of the fixer solution in the processor. Change in the silver concentration suggests that the replenishment of the fixer is not matched to the amount of fixing to be done. If the fixer is under-replenished, the amount of silver present rises. A fall in the quantity of silver shows that the fixer replenisher is being injected at a rate which is too high relative to the amount of fixing to be done.

(ix) Measure and record the temperature of the wash-water.

(x) Check the efficacy of the washing. If the result of the test shows the washing to be inefficient, the possible explanations are that:

(a) the water is flowing at too low a rate;

(b) if the water is tempered, its temperature is too low;

(c) the pump which circulates the washing water is faulty.

The flow-rate, the temperature and the functioning of the pump can be checked and appropriate action can be taken.

TESTS RELATING TO THE RECORDING SYSTEMS

In controlling the quality of the radiographs produced in diagnostic X-ray departments, radiographers find themselves concerned from time to time with checks relating to certain components of the record: these components are the films and the intensifying screens and the cassettes which hold the films and screens in combination for the radiographic exposure. Checks that the radiographer may make include the following:

(i) a determination of the relative speeds of two different films;

(ii) a determination of the relative speeds of different intensifying screens;

(iii) a check on a pair of screens in a cassette which appears to have an area where the contact between the screens is poor;

(iv) a check on a cassette which is suspected of letting in light when it is closed.

In the present section of this chapter we describe how such checks can be made.

COMPARING SPEEDS OF FILMS

In an earlier part of this book (Chapter 3) we considered the assessment of the speeds of X-ray films and comparisons which might be made between different materials. As a basis for comparison we used the D Log E curves of films which were to be compared and such curves certainly provide a means to obtain accurate results.

However, in the present chapter we are considering various tests that radiographers might undertake for the management of the radiographic image. Among these tests are those to be made in order to establish the relative speeds of films. It is unlikely that radiographers in busy X-ray departments would even consider tests of film-speeds which needed the making of D Log E curves and fortunately no such necessity exists.

An imprecise system of assessing relative speeds of films has been satisfactory to radiographers in the past. It has been often based on a practical comparison of the exposures required by different emulsions to produce radiographs which seem to the viewer to be comparable. This is simply a visual assessment made without reference to characteristic curves. It must vary between observers and for the same observer in different conditions of judgement. It is a subjective and not a mathematical evaluation.

However, an estimation of relative speeds made without the use of characteristic curves has less error if a densitometer is used in evaluating the results of a test and if the test is made by submitting the films to a controlled series of exposures. The procedure is as follows.

TIME-SCALE X-RAY EXPOSURES

(i) Under safelights, cut a long strip from each of the two films to be compared.

(ii) Put the two strips side by side into the same cassette and take the loaded cassette to the X-ray room.

(iii) Using the X-ray equipment and lead shielding for the cassette, give a series of stepped exposures, proceeding down the lengths of the film-strips and increasing the time-intervals of the exposures by a constant factor: say, times 2. One part of the film strips should remain lead-shielded so that no exposure is received there: this yields information as to which of the two films has a higher base-plus-fog density. The series of exposures might be as follows.

Steps on the film-strips	Exposures in milliampere-seconds
1	0
2	1
3	2
4	4
5	8
6	16
7	32
8	64
9	128
10	256

The time-interval of the exposure must be the only variable. The other conditions must remain constant: for example, 100 mA, 60 kVp, broad focus, 100 cm focus-film distance.

(iv) When the X-ray exposures are complete, process the film-strips together.

(v) Use the densitometer to compare the strips and locate the two steps (one in each strip) which match in density. Try to find a density which is in the middle part of the useful density range: say, somewhere between 1·0 and 1·5. Let us suppose that you have found the matched densities in the two shaded areas in Fig. 13.6. For the sake of clarity in the diagram we have left all the other areas on these imaginary film strips blank.

(vi) We can relate this density to the exposure required to produce it because the exposures were controlled for the test. So in Fig. 13.6 Film B required 16. milliamperseconds and Film A required 4 milliampere-seconds to give the same density. The ratio of these exposures is 16/4 = 4. So Film A is four times faster than Film B and requires only 25 per cent of the exposure necessary for Film B.

This test has the following sources of possible error.

(i) There might be no densities within the useful range which exactly matched between the two strips. It would then be necessary to select the two densities which showed the least difference.

(ii) There could be variations in the performance of the X-ray set within the series of exposures so that the exposure relationship between the steps was not precise.

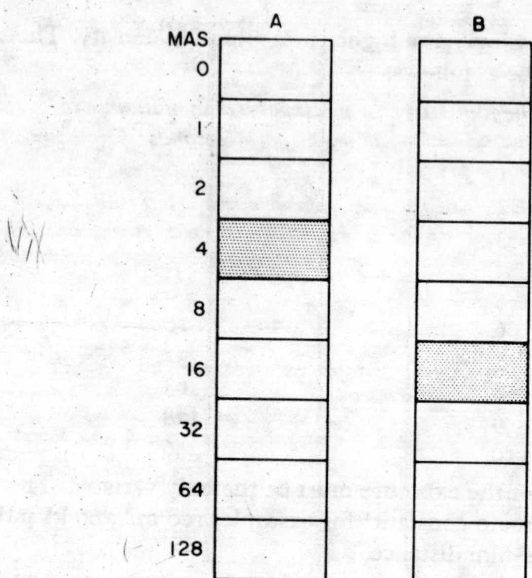

Fig. 13.6 Comparing film speeds: test strips.

INTENSITY SCALE X-RAY EXPOSURES

Errors arising from variations in the performance of the X-ray unit would be minimized if a single exposure through a large-area stepwedge were made, instead of the stepped series with varying milliampereseconds. The stepwedge should be placed on the cassette so that it covers both the film strips. The long dimension of the wedge must be in line with the long dimensions of the film strips so that both strips depict all the steps.

The stepwedge must be a calibrated one: that is, the exposure transmitted by each step must have a known relationship to the exposures transmitted through its neighbours in the wedge. If this is not so, when you try to interpret the results and find two steps in the strips which match in density, you cannot relate the exposures which produced that density for you do not know the relationship between the steps.

EVALUATING THE RESULTS

In the absence of a densitometer, the results of these tests could of course be judged subjectively. The matched densities in the two strips could be sought by eye and be selected on the basis of finding the two steps which looked most nearly the same density. It can certainly be argued that since radiographs are to be viewed by human observers then a visual judgement is good enough for the test strips.

COMPARING SPEEDS OF INTENSIFYING SCREENS

As well as the speed of the film which is used, the action of the intensifying screens between which it is held influences the radiographic density resultant from a given exposure. So radiographers may be concerned to discover the relative speeds of two sets of intensifying screens. Much of what we have said in the previous section on film-speeds is valid for the relative speeds of intensifying screens: so we here enumerate some points previously made.

(i) The tests may be a simple visual comparison of radiographs obtained with the two sets of screens, relating the exposures which were needed in each case to give similar results.

(ii) A more exact way is to produce two film-strips (one for each pair of screens) which show a series of density-steps resulting from a series of exposures stepped in a known relationship. The exposures could be time-scale X-ray exposures or could be intensity-scale exposures transmitted through a radiographic stepwedge as we have described for the testing of film-speeds. The tube voltage should be 70 kVp to ensure full activation of the back-screen.

(iii) As with the tests for the film-speeds in the previous section, the strips of film can be exactly evaluated by the use of a densitometer but to many will be acceptably assessed by a visual judgement.

A test to compare the speeds of intensifying screens can be undertaken as follows. Let us call one pair Screens F and the other pair Screens R.

1 Take a cassette which has no screens in it and place Screens F appropriately for use, leaving them loose and not fixed in place.

2 In safelighting conditions, take a film of suitable size for the cassette and screens and cut it in half along its longer dimension.

3 Load the prepared cassette with one half-strip and take care to place it correctly between the active surfaces of the screens which are loose in the cassette. Keep the other half-strip safe from radiation and light.

4 In the X-ray room, expose the cassette radiographically at 70 kVp using either a series of time-scale exposures or through a stepwedge to give intensity-scale exposures as earlier described.

5 Under safelighting, unload the cassette and put the film-strip in a place which is safe from radiation and light. Remove Screens F and replace them with Screens R, similarly left loose in the cassette. Reload the cassette carefully with the other half-strip of the divided film.

6   In the X-ray room repeat the technique of the exposure *exactly as before.*

7   In the darkroom, unload the cassette. Proceed to process both film-strips together, first making sure that you can identify each strip as to the screen-pair used for its exposure.

8   Compare the processed strips as we described before for the test of film-speeds and locate (with or without a densitometer) the two steps (one in each strip) which match in density.

9   Relate this density to the exposure between Screens F and to the exposure between Screens R required to produce it (as described on page 345 in the test for film-speeds).

10   Similarly determine the exposure ratio and thus ascertain the relative speeds of the two pairs of intensifying screens.

A NEW SYSTEM FOR EXPOSURE TECHNIQUES

For X-ray films a numerical expression of speed has not been used and X-ray films have been assessed as we have seen in terms of relative speed, one in comparison with another taken for its control. In the well-managed production of radiographic images it may be important to make statements on film speeds which are more exact than the previous practices imply.

A system intended to give a firm scientific basis to the selection and conversion of factors in an exposure technique has been developed by Dupont in the X-ray Technical Service of their Photoproducts Department. It is called a Bit System of Technique Conversion: in this context the word bit is an abbreviation of binary digit, one of the two digits (0 and 1) used in the binary notation (or the binary counting system) which is employed for computers. This new system involves the computerization of the many variables to be handled in the production of the image and it assigns bit values to them according to the effect on film density that each variable factor can achieve. Essentially what the Dupont Bit System does is to bring all the variables to a common currency in exposure units so that the variables can be readily manipulated to a predictable result when techniques are being changed.

The speeds of films and intensifying screens used are important variables in the production of the image and the Dupont system assigns bit values to them. In the tables which they publish we find, for example, that the Cronex Quanta III screens combined with Cronex 2 D C Film is a combination with a bit value of 18·2 and that the Cronex Par Speed screens combined with the same film have a bit value of 15·4. (See Fig. 13.7.) This Bit System is a useful and interesting approach to the

TABLE P
CRONEX® 2 FILM—SCREEN COMBINATIONS

Bit Speeds

Cronex® Screen	Cronex® Film				
	2 DC	4 & 6+	6	7	Lo-dose
Quanta III	18.2	17 8	17.9	16.9	
Quanta II	17.4	17.0	17.1	16.1	
Lightning Plus	16.8	16.4	16.5	15 5	
Hi Plus	16.4	16.0	16.1	15.1	
High Speed and SP	16.1	15.7	15.8	14.8	
Par Speed	15.4	15.0	15.1	14.1	
Fast Detail	14.5	14.1	14.2	13.2	
Lo-dose/2 (back only)	14.2	13.8	13.9	12.9	12.3*
Lo-dose (back only)	13.6	13.2	13.3	12.3	11.3*
Detail (Pair)	13.4	13.0	13.1	12.1	
Detail (back only)	12.7	12.3	12.4	11.4	

Extremity One	= 12.3
Extremity Two	= 13.3
Extremity Three	= 12.3

Combinations with speeds below 14.0 Bits are recommended for thin parts (extremities) only.

*These speeds do not apply at 30 kVp and with beam filtration typical of mammography.

Fig. 13.7 Bit System of Technique Conversion—Table P. Extract from *Bit System of Technique Conversion*, by courtesy of Du Pont (U.K.) Ltd.

problems that have previously existed because of the lack of absolute film speeds in diagnostic radiography.

There is more about the Dupont Bit System of Technique Conversion later in this chapter.

Today the radiographer's work is greater in scope than it used to be and we are concerned with more imaging systems than the traditional radiographic one which uses film/screen combinations to make the record In this extended world of what has been termed diagnostic imaging with many people investigating and evaluating factors which determine quality (or ability to yield diagnostic information) for imaging systems, perhaps the terms we have used and the comparisons we have made for film speeds must change.

TEST FOR SCREENS' CONTACT

A radiograph can easily be taken which will show whether there is uniformly good contact between the intensifying screens and the film in a cassette. The object radiographed is a sheet of zinc—or copper—which is 0·036 in. (0·91 mm) thick and is continuously perforated; the holes should have a diameter of 3/32 in. (2·4 mm) and a pitch of 7 to the inch (approximately 3 per cm).

The density recorded on the film during the test will be more easily measured if a hole is cut at or near the centre of the zinc sheet; the diameter of this hole should be at least half an inch (13 mm). The overall area of the zinc sheet should be great enough to cover completely the cassette which is to be tested and it must lie flat and in close contact with the cassette. If wished, the zinc can be tacked for protection to a wooden frame which will keep it rigid; the advantage of a copper sheet is that it is more durable.

To carry out the test the suspect cassette is loaded with its normal film and placed on the X-ray table with the zinc sheet in front of it, so that the surfaces of the cassette and the zinc sheet are closely in touch with each other. An X-ray exposure is made at an anode-film distance of not less than 59 in. (1·5 m) using an X-ray tube with a focal spot of 1·0 mm–1·5 mm: this should be centered upon the centre of the cassette. The filtration of the X-ray tube should be not more than 2 mm Al equivalent and the recommended kilovoltage is 50 kVp. The exposure should be sufficient to produce on the central unobstructed area of the film a density (see Chapter 3) of 2–4 on full standard development; for example perhaps an exposure of 4 or 5 milliampereseconds in the case of a film/screen combination of medium speed. The film is then processed and viewed.

intensifying screens dark areas appear on the radiograph (see Figs. 13.8 and 13.9). These areas will be readily visible when the radiograph is viewed in the normal way on an illuminator fitted with the usual fluorescent tubes, provided that the density of the image is high enough. The aim should be to obtain a really 'black' radiograph of the 'holes'; that is, a density in the perforated areas of 4.

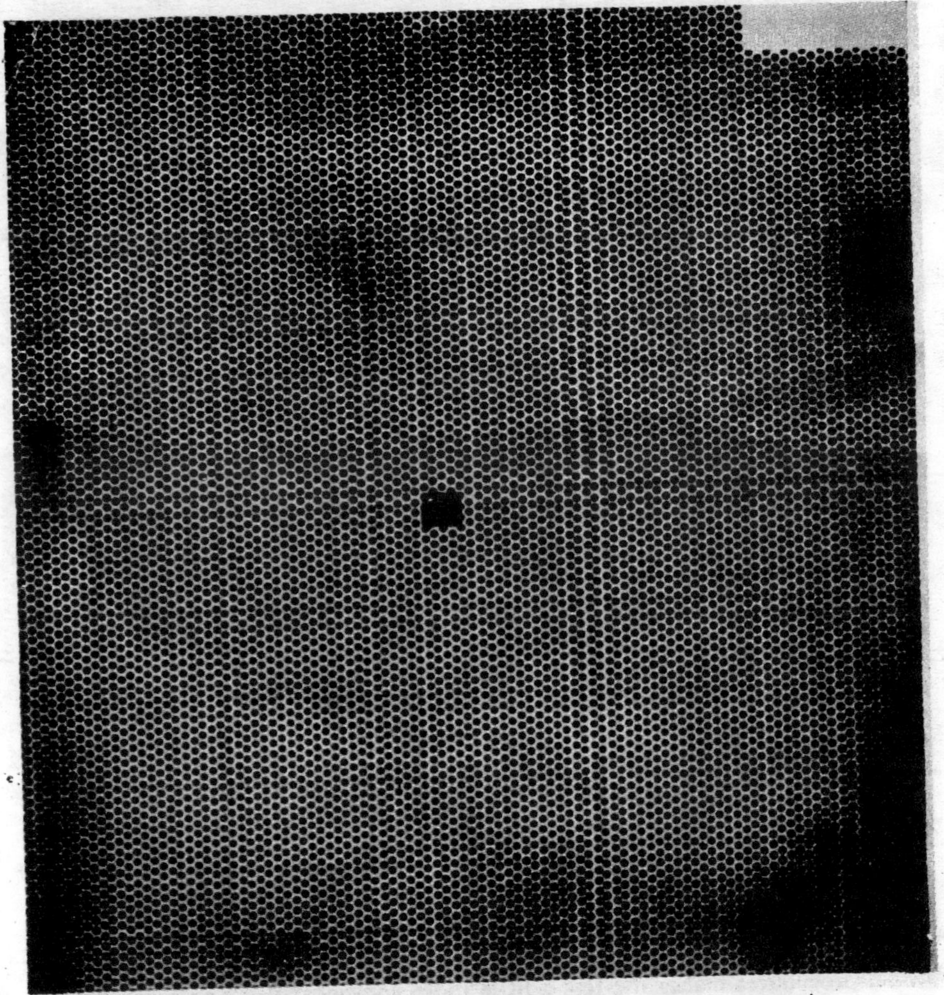

Fig. 13.8 The test radiograph of a perforated metal sheet obtained from a cassette in which screen contact is good. The central cut-out area facilitates the measurement of density. *By courtesy of G. M. Ardran.*

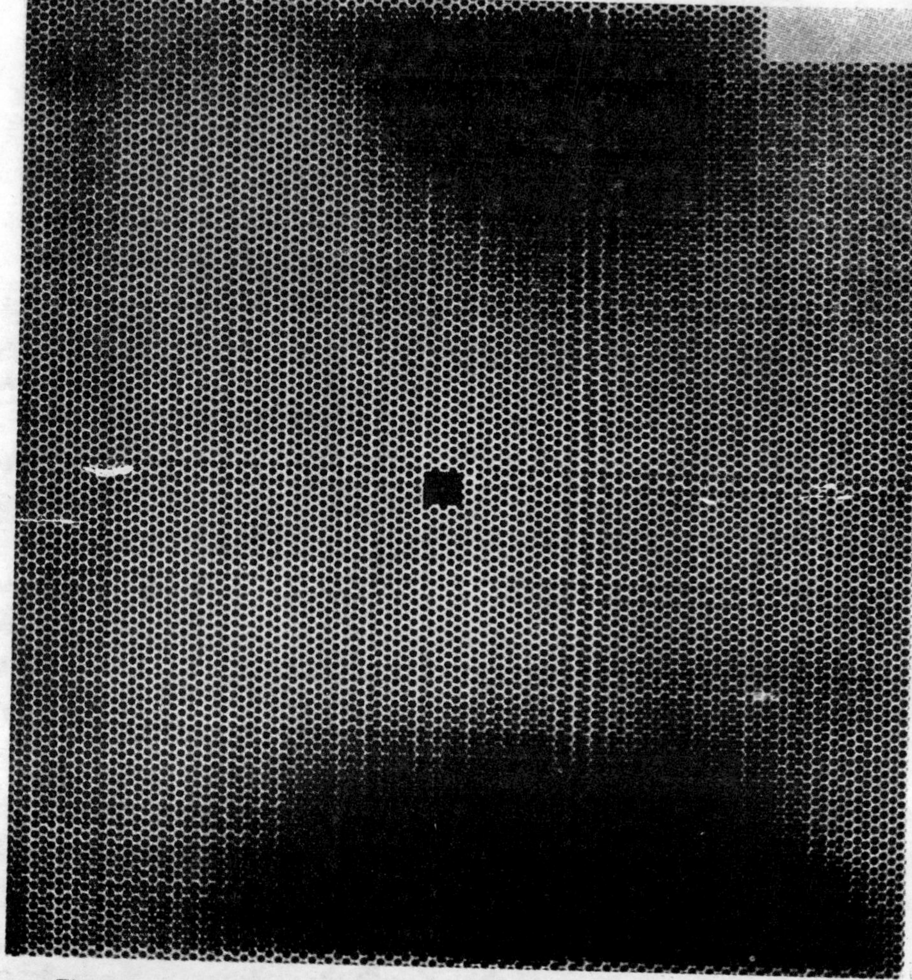

Fig. 13.9 The test radiograph obtained from a cassette in which screen contact is poor. *By courtesy of G. M. Ardran.*

At lower densities the effect is less readily apparent. It is not visible at densities of about 1·2 or less. At densities between about 2 and 3 it can be seen if the film is studied from a distance of 12 ft. (4 m) or more; or alternatively if it is viewed through a reducing lens which gives an image equivalent to looking at the film from this distance. Either of these procedures makes the test a little more complicated for radiographers than it need be and as few X-ray departments possess densitometers as standard equipment, the practical advantages of using enough exposure to obtain maximum density of the film are evident.

The results of a screen-contact test performed in this way are much easier to assess than if merely a flash exposure of a perforated metal sheet—or wire mesh—is given and the radiograph examined for evidence of unsharpness at the edges of the holes or wires. Detail unsharpness must occur whenever there is poor contact between a film and intensifying screens but blurring is likely to be less immediately apparent to the eye—especially if it is only slight in degree—than is a simple area of blackness on the radiograph. The dark patches result from scattering of the light of the screens over areas of the film which should not have been exposed as they underlie the metal of the test object. This procedure readily indicates areas where only slight loss of screen-film contact is present.

There is not much of lasting effect that can be done for a cassette which is failing to maintain contact between the intensifying screens. It is best to take a long term view of economy and discard it.

TEST FOR LIGHT LEAKAGE

Following a number of fogged films physical inspection of a cassette usually makes evident the admission of extraneous light and the points at which it has entered. Broken fastenings or hinges, buckled corners or loose fronts are the likely culprits.

However if the condition is suspected rather than self-evident a test for light leakage can be made very simply by exposing a loaded cassette to an intense light. The exposure should be for 6 successive periods of 15 minutes each. Each side and each edge of the cassette in turn should face a 100 watt pearl tungsten lamp (operating at its rated voltage) which is at a distance of 4 ft. (1·22 m) from the cassette. (British Standard 4304: 1968). Processing the film will reveal on it patches of fog if leakage is present, the area of their situation being unequivocal evidence of where the light is entering. An edge darkening of not more than $\frac{1}{8}$ in. (3·2 mm) is insignificant.

CHECKS RELATING TO THE X-RAY TUBE AND ITS OUTPUT

FOCAL SPOT TEST

It is possible to make radiographic tests of the focal spot of an X-ray tube by using the 'pinhole camera' principle. This is done by covering the portal of the X-ray tube with a sheet of radiopaque metal which has a pinhole in its centre: the chosen metal is usually lead. Through the pinhole a radiographic exposure is made on a film in a cassette which is placed at right angles to the X-ray beam emerging from the pinhole. The result is a 'pinhole picture' of the effective focus of the X-ray tube as shown in Fig. 13.10.

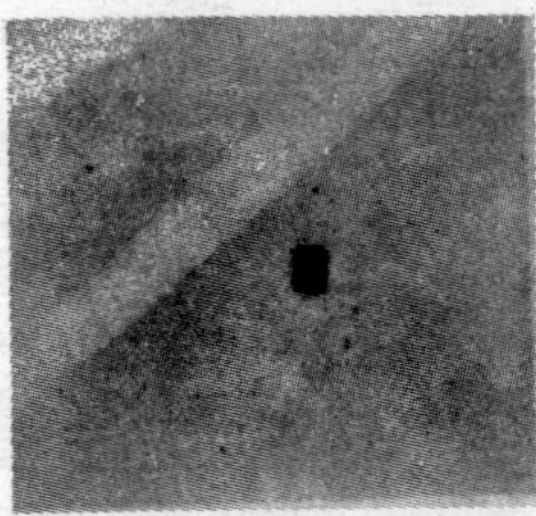

Fig. 13.10 Pinhole of focal spot

If this test is to give accurate information on the size and shape of the focal spot, it must be carried out in exacting conditions. Stringent requirements are specified for the shape and dimensions of the pinhole; for the location of the pinhole directly beneath the focal spot of the X-ray tube; for the distances separating the focal spot from the pinhole and the pinhole from the film; for the type of film used; for the exposure given and the density of the resultant image; for the viewing conditions in which the result is assessed. It is therefore not a test which can be readily done by a radiographer in an X-ray department as one of several procedures established in a system for quality control. It is a test among others which might be carried out by a medical physics department associated with a radiological service.

For tests that radiographers can apply in the setting of the X-ray department there is a series of available test tools. One of these sets of tools is known as the Wisconsin Radiologic Test Tools. They have been developed by individuals in the Medical Physics and Engineering Center of the University of Wisconsin Department of Radiology. Among these tools is one for testing the focal spot of an X-ray tube.

THE WISCONSIN FOCAL-SPOT TEST TOOL

The focal-spot test tool in the Wisconsin range has a pattern in heavy metal mounted in a frame (see Fig. 13.11). The test is made by making a radiograph of this pattern and Fig. 13.12 shows such a radiograph. The pattern is produced by means of slots in the metal and in the radiograph

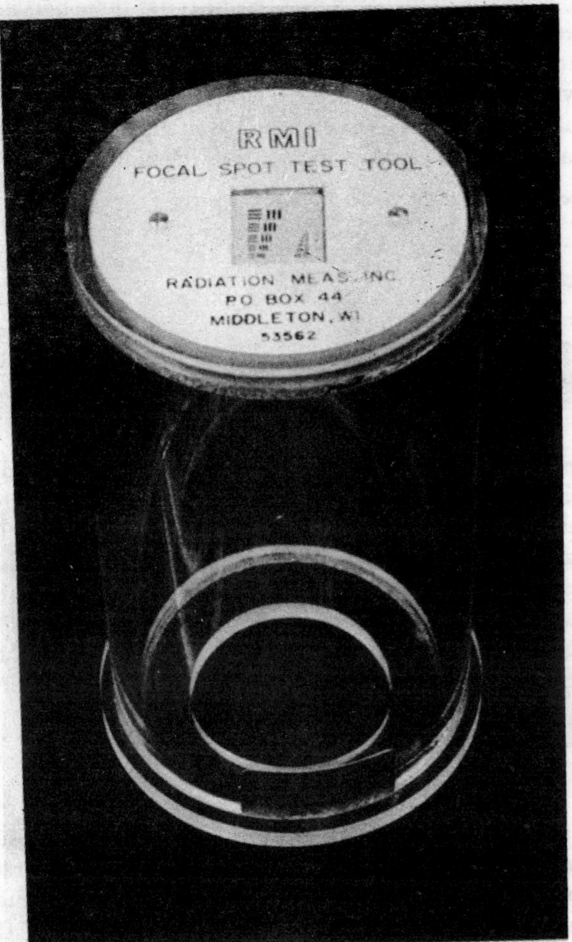

Fig. 13.11 Wisconsin Test Tool for size of focal spot

these slots appear as 'black bars' of density where the radiation has passed through the slots, alternating with the 'white strips' where the radiation has been attenuated by the heavy metal.

As can be seen from the radiograph, the bar pattern consists of 11 groups of bars which diminish in breadth and in length as the serial number of the group rises, there being 6 black bars in a group. Thus the spacing of the slots for the group numbered 1 is 0·6 line pairs (that is, a black bar and a white strip) per millimetre and for the group numbered 11 the spacing of the slots is 3·35 line pairs per millimetre.

As the radiograph in Fig. 13.12 shows, the numbered groups of bars consist of paired sets of identical bars; each set has three bars arranged to lie in a direction which is at right angles to the three bars of the paired set in the group The radiograph is made on X-ray film which is for direct exposure without intensifying screens (for example, dental X-ray film of the occlusal size). The focal-spot of the X-ray tube is 18 inches from the test pattern and the pattern is 6 inches from the film.

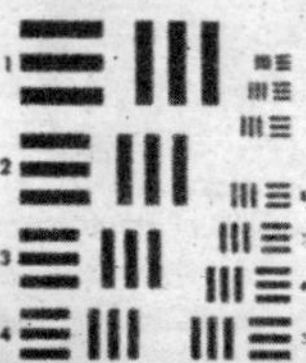

Fig. 13.12 Radiograph for size of focal spot

Assessment is made by looking at the numbered groups and trying to judge which is the group of smallest bars in which *all six bars* (that is, two sets of three bars at 90° to each other) can be clearly seen by the eye as separate black bars in the image. Then a chart is consulted to discover the size of the effective focal spot which is capable of resolving that group of bars. For example, if the group of smallest bars which is clearly resolved is number 4, then the nominal size of the focus is 2·0 mm; if the smallest bars resolved are those of group numbered 8, the nominal size of the focus is 1·0 mm.

TESTS FOR TIMERS

A traditional method of testing the accuracy of an X-ray exposure-timer is to carry out a 'spinning-top test'. This involves the use of a radiopaque disc (the spinning-top) with a hole in it. A radiograph as in Fig. 13.13 is made of the top while it is spinning and the pulsations of the X-ray generator are registered on the film as a series of 'black spots'. These black spots are produced because the hole is moving and is over a different part of the film for each pulse of current through and voltage across the X-ray tube in the alternating cycle of the a.c. mains supply. The number of the spots is counted and this gives the duration of the exposure. Thus, for example, a single-phase generator with full-wave rectification puts a pulse of current through the X-ray tube for every half-cycle of mains alternation. If the mains frequency is 50 cycles per second (50 hertz) then in one second there are 100 pulses of current and voltage. If the X-ray exposure lasts for 0·1 second there will be 10 spots to be counted in the test

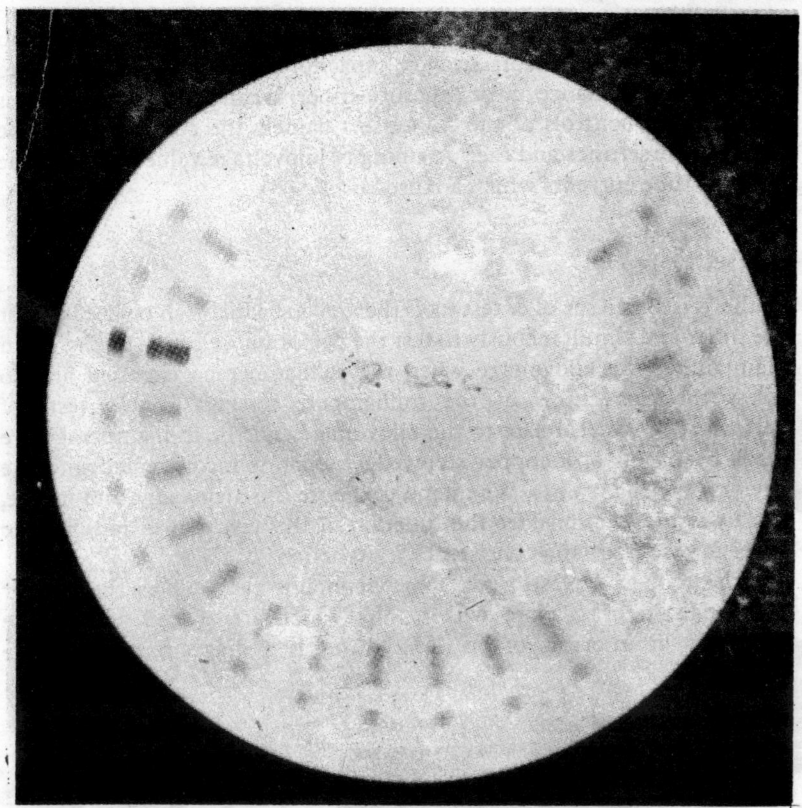

Fig. 13.13 Spinning top test

radiograph and if the exposure time is o·c
spot represents o·o1 second for such a gen
such a frequency.

...are three-phase generators o...
slight ripple as opposed to discrete pul...
discharge units with maintained continuous voltage outp
these types supplies for the X-ray tube a voltage characterise...
pulses which give well separated images of black spots when a sp...
top test is made. So the accuracy of exposure-timers on such units cannot
be checked by means of the old spinning-top and another device must be

used. Below we describe a test tool that can be used on single-phase and on three-phase generators and on capacitor discharge X-ray units to check the performance of the exposure-timer. It can also be used to assess certain other controls of the X-ray set: namely the consistency of the milliampere settings and the sustaining of kilovoltage values through the range of tube currents which are used.

A TIMING TEST

In the Wisconsin series of test tools there is one which can be used to test the timer and simultaneously to test the performance of the X-ray set in maintaining the kilovoltage when the milliamperage is raised and to assess the correctness of the milliampere settings. These tests of performance which relate to the kilovoltage and the milliamperage are made by means of a copper stepwedge which is incorporated into the device. (See Fig. 13.14). We intend to ignore this stepwedge and its use. Let us at present consider the function of this test tool in judging the timer for accuracy and consistency in its action.

The tool is a plastic box which contains (as well as the copper stepwedge) a brass plate with 4 slits which are spaced around the periphery at intervals of 90°. Fig. 13.15 is a diagram to show the

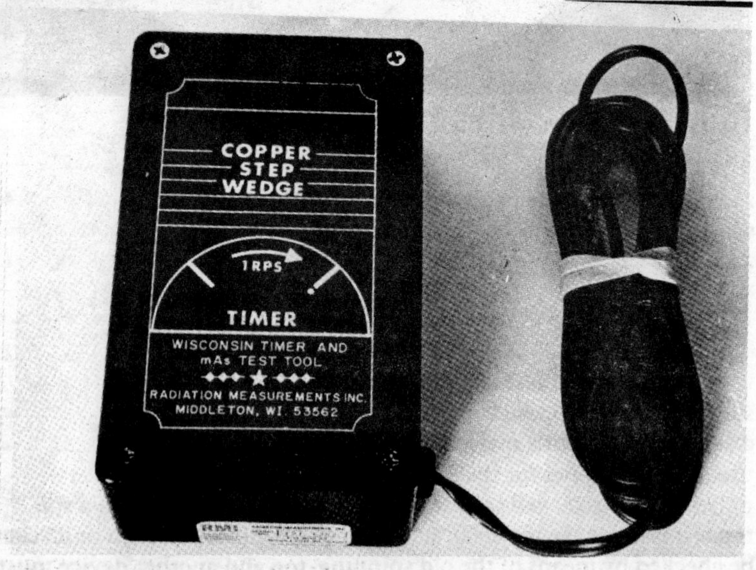

Fig. 13.14 Timer test tool

arrangement. The presence of a hole close to one of the slots allows this disc to be used as a conventional spinning-top with the counting of 'black spots' or impulses if the X-ray generator is of the single-phase full-wave rectified type. For other generators, as will be seen, the test is made by using the wedge-shaped region of density which is produced by exposure through the moving slits.

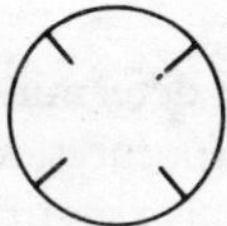

Fig. 13.15 Timer test tool

The brass plate is rotated by a motor which revolves it at a speed of one complete revolution per second: that is, in one second a point on the periphery of the disc moves from a starting position through 360°. A suggested technique is to make four separate exposures, placing the exposures in each quarter of a film of 24 cm by 30 cm size. The loaded cassette is put on the X-ray table and the timing tool is placed on the quarter which is for use, lead being used to screen the other three quarters of the cassette. The X-ray tube is centered directly above the tool and the collimator is adjusted so that the beam covers only the area which is to be used for the test tool. When the exposures are being made, the motor in the tool is running and the brass plate is rotating.

The exposure settings might be as follows: focus-film distance 100 cm (or 40 inches), 60–80 kVp (Wisconsin's suggestion is for 80 kVp on single-phase generators and 70 kVp for three-phase generators); 10 milliampereseconds. The four separate exposures differ from each other only in the settings of time and milliamperes: so they are given as (i) 25 mA for 0·4 second; (ii) 50 mA for 0·2 second; (iii) 100 mA for 0·1 second; (iv) 500 mA for 0.02 second. If the generator were of the three-phase type then higher milliamperages and shorter times would be available. If it were wished to test these, further exposures could be made using a second film.

It is to be noted that in the series given the milliampereseconds are maintained at a value which is constant for the four exposures. If the test is *solely* for the performance on the timer, this constancy of milliampereseconds is most important and the main requirement is to achieve a series of wedge-shaped densities which look more or less alike or not widely different and are easily perceptible. A further important point is that for any given X-ray set absolute accuracy of the timer is not essential:

for example, if a timer set for 0·02 second actually gives an exposure-time of 0·025 second it does not matter very much so long as the timer maintains that inaccuracy of 0·005 second on every occasion that the 0·02 setting is used. In trying to achieve a standard radiographic result from any X-ray set, consistency of performance by the timer is much more important than absolute accuracy. On each setting, the timer is not stringently required to perform without error: it *is* required to perform without variation.

So any test of the timer must determine its consistency of action. This is done by means of a series of exposures of the test tool as described, with each time-setting used for several exposures. Thus for example, the series given on the previous page might be repeated four times. The first film used could have four exposures with 25 mA for 0·4 second: the next film would carry four exposures with 50 mA for 0·2 second: the third and the fourth films would be similarly used for the settings at 100 mA for 0·1 second and 500 mA for 0·02 second. So could the consistency of the timer be tested.

Figs. 13.16 to 13.19 show the radiographic results of a test carried out by means of this tool. At the top the copper step-wedge shows as a series of densities but we are ignoring these.

It is the dark arcs of density which appear in the radiographs of the rotating disc with which we are presently concerned. The measurement of these arcs indicates whether the exposure-timer is or is not functioning correctly.

The slit on the disc moves through 360° in one second since the disc is rotating at a rate of one revolution per second and the slit describes a complete circle in that time. So in, for example, 0·2 second the arc produced should be 72°; 0·1 second should give an arc of 36°; 0·05 second draws an arc of 18°; and 0·02 second should show an arc of 7·20°. The darkened arcs can be measured by means of a specially designed protractor which gives the corresponding exposure-time to be checked against the time-setting on the control console.

Slight variations can be considered acceptable but the shorter the time-setting is then the slighter is the permissible variation, for the obvious reason that a small variation can be a very large proportion of a very short exposure time. As examples of what can be tolerated we submit the following: for an exposure of 0·2 second, acceptable angles are 68° to 76°; for an exposure of 0·1 second, 34° to 38°; 0·05 second, 15° to 20°; and for 0·02 second, within 5° to 9°.

To take the arcs shown in Figs. 13.16 to 13.19:

(i) 0·4 second should show an arc of 144° but here the arc is 120°. (Fig. 13.16).

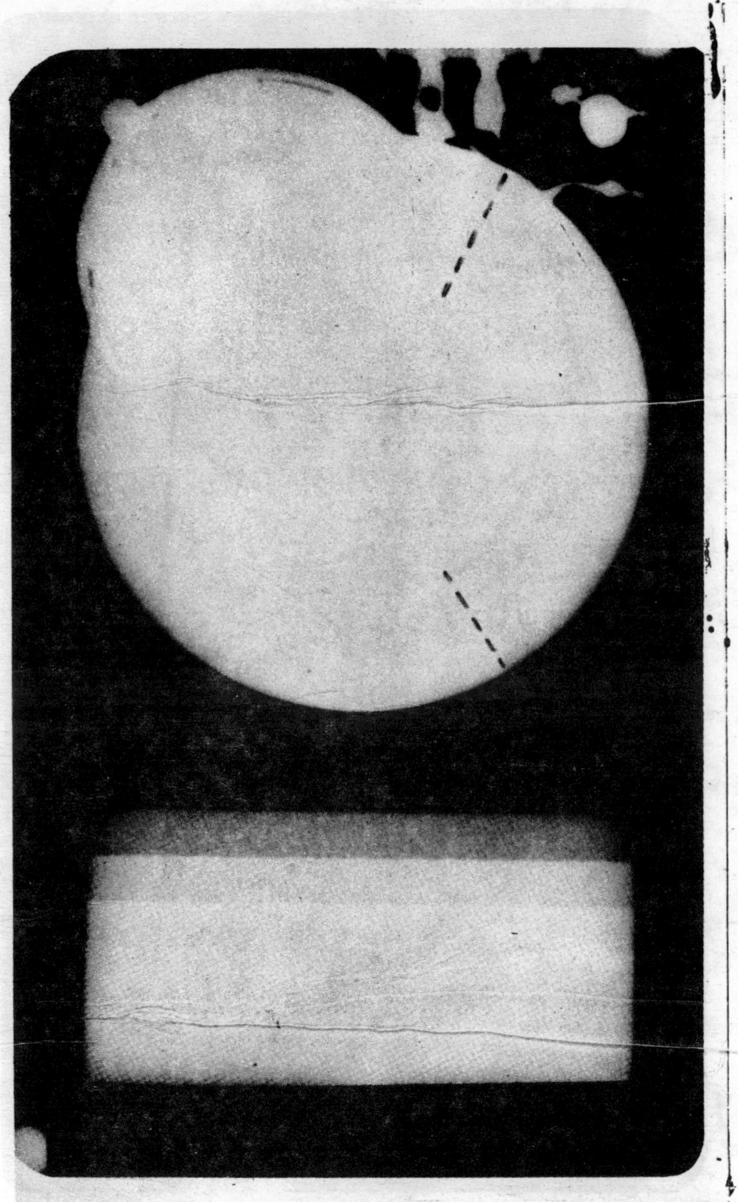

Fig. 13.16 Timer test

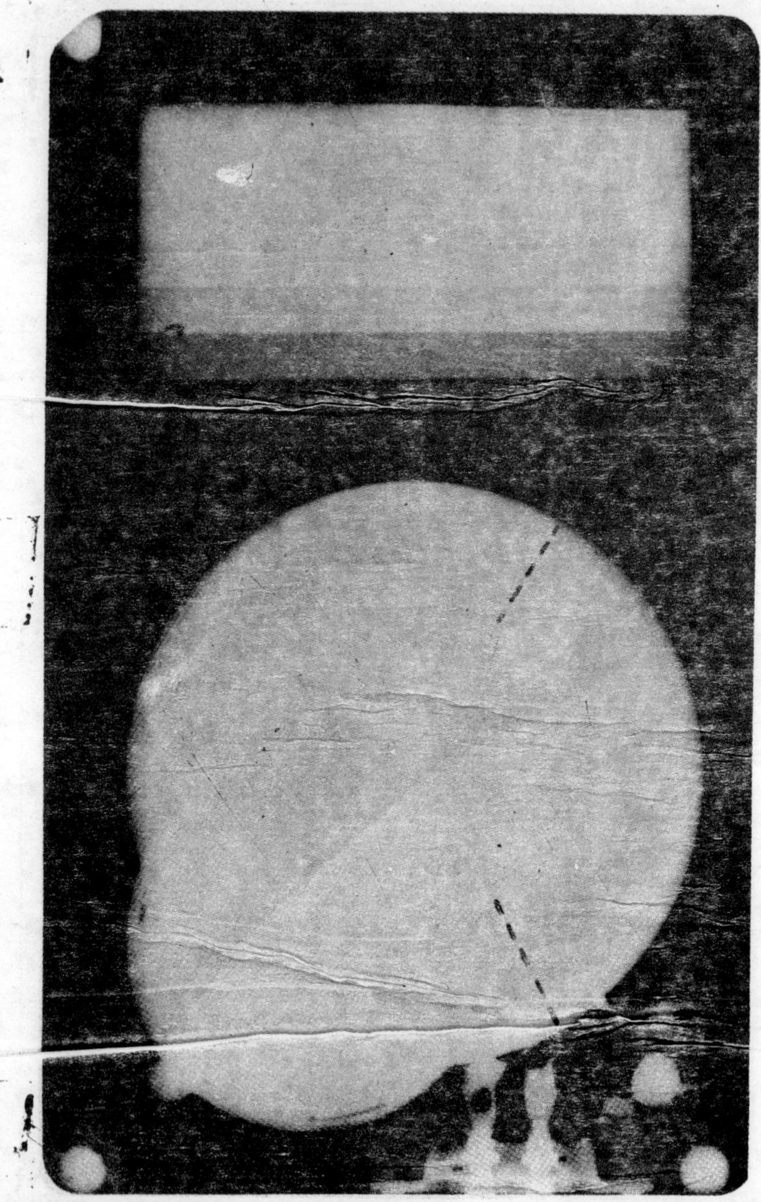

Fig. 13.17 Timer test

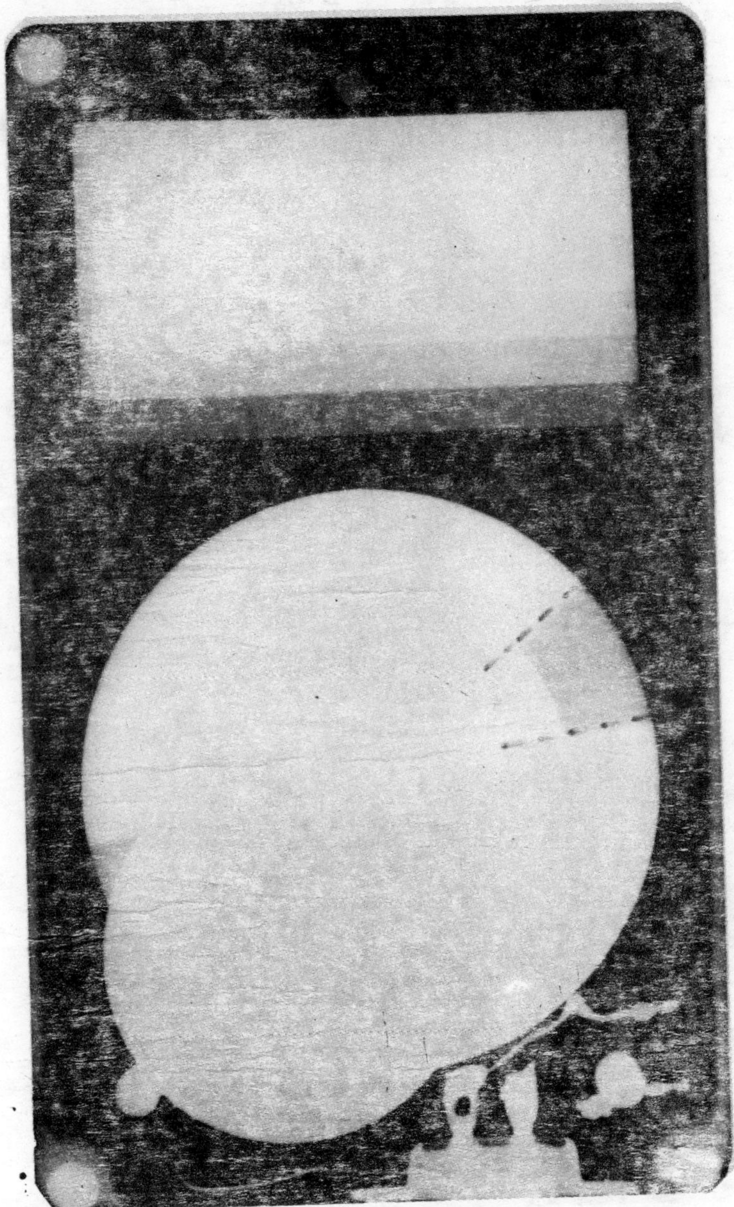

Fig. 13.18 Timer test

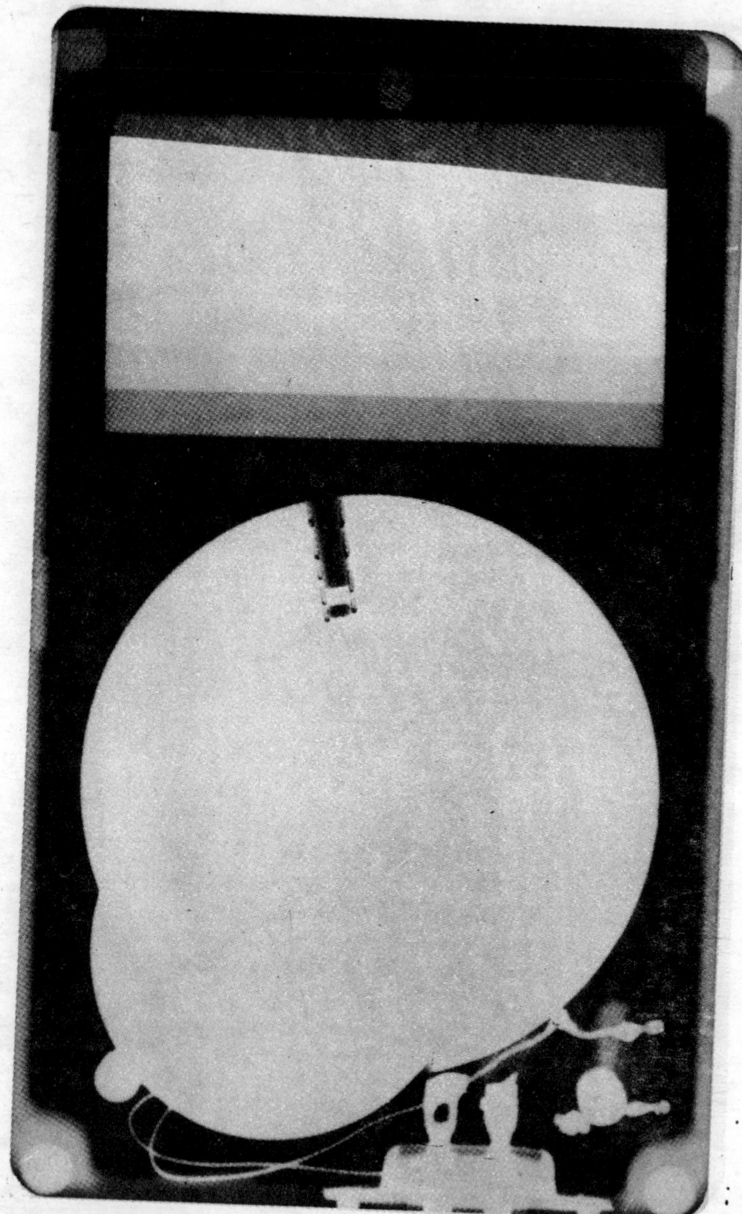

Fig. 13.19 Timer test

(ii) 0·2 second should show an arc of 72° but here the arc is 60° (Fig. 13.17).

(iii) 0·1 second should show an arc of 36° but here the arc is 32°. (Fig. 13.18).

(iv) 0·02 second should show an arc of 7·2° but here the arc is 5°. (Fig. 13.19).

TESTING THE MILLIAMPERE SETTINGS

The Wisconsin test tool which we have described here has a function to test the milliampere-settings of an X-ray set. It does not give information on actual milliampere values but it does allow some assessment as to whether the milliampere-settings used in the test give a radiographic result that matches the one expected.

If the exposures earlier described for the timer-tests are made as given at the same milliampereseconds for the whole of the series, then the test also yields information on the consistency of the milliampere-settings.

If the various milliampere settings which are used (in this case 50 mA, 100 mA, 200 mA, 500 mA) are consistently related to each other, then the dark arcs produced by the exposure (in this case 10 mAs) through the moving slit will all be of equal density. This statement is true provided that the following conditions are met:

(i) that the timer is accurate;

(ii) that the lack of reciprocity (see page 386) is insignificant;

(iii) that the kilovoltage was maintained at a given value (60 kVp here) despite the rise in milliamperes (of which there is more on page 367);

(iv) that the processing conditions were the same for all four images.

If these conditions are met the density of the arcs will be the same over the milliamperes used so long as the milliamperes values are consistently related to each other and are approximately those stated on the settings of the selector. From a setting which provides an irregular milliamperage the arc has a density which is less than that of the others or greater than that of the others, according to whether the actual milliamperage is lower or higher than the expected value.

More satisfactory for the measurement of density for the purposes of this test is to use an aluminium stepwedge rather than this Wisconsin tool. Fig. 13.20 shows a radiograph which has on it a range of densities produced by exposures through a stepwedge: five seperate exposures have been made and there are five images of a stepwedge which has eleven steps. What has been said in general about the density of the exposed arcs in the Wisconsin tool is also true of the densities in the images of the stepwedge: they should match step for step. It is best to select a step with

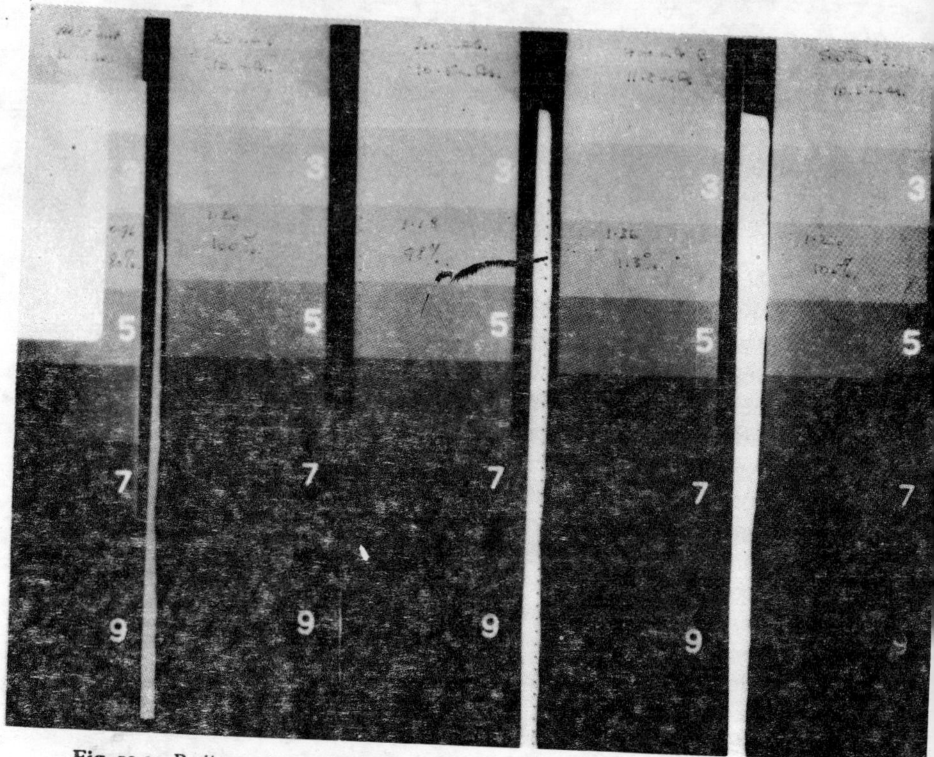

Fig. 13.20 Radiographs of stepwedge

a density of about 1·0 for the purposes of comparison and then check whether the same step has the same density in all the images.

For the radiograph in Fig. 13.20 all the five separate exposures were made at 60 kV. The cassette was on the table-top with a focus film distance of 40 inches and the central X-ray beam was centered to the wedge for each exposure. All the exposures were at 10 mAs (or as near 10 mAs as the controls would allow) and the milliampere settings were as follows: 100 mA, 200 mA, 300 mA, 400 mA, 500 mA. Lead was used to screen those parts of the cassette which were not serving as the exposure area.

On the processed radiograph, the tester first selected a step of the wedge with a density close to 1·0: in Fig. 13.20 this is step 4. The range of densities shown in the original radiograph of the illustration is from 0·96 on the 100 mA setting to 1·36 on the 400 mA setting. In order to express helpfully the changes of density produced by the irregular milliamperages, the different densities of step 4 are expressed as a percentage on one of the others selected as the 100 per cent standard. As can be seen, for Fig. 13.20 the density taken as the standard 100 per cent is 1·20 on step 4 at the 200 mA setting and 10 mAs. The other densities expressed as a percentage of that are as can be seen: 80 per cent on 100 mA setting, 98 per cent on 300 mA setting, 113 per cent on 400 mA setting and 105 per cent on 500 mA setting.

A density-difference which is as small as or less than 15 per cent will not be perceptible in the radiograph by the human observer. So in the case of the X-ray set which was tested in Fig. 13.20 there is no need to consider any re-adjustment of the settings by an engineer except perhaps in the case of 100 mA which shows a 20 per cent difference in density. However, it must be admitted that visually all these stepwedge strips acceptably match step for step.

A test for the consistency of the milliampere-settings can be made in an entirely different way by ionization dosimetry. This is a method which uses ionization chambers to measure the instantaneous dose at a point. If all other conditions of operation of an X-ray tube stay the same, then dose is proportional to milliamperage. Irregularity in the milliampere-settings is revealed by irregularity in the expected linear relationship of dose to milliamperes.

It will be realized that ionization dosimetry uses an ionization chamber and not a film as the 'detector' of the radiation leaving the X-ray tube. It is arguable that the method of ionization dosimetry is preferable to one based on the use of films since there are fewer variables to be taken into account.

TESTING FOR MAINTENANCE OF KILOVOLTAGE

A stepwedge test as described for Fig. 13.20 can be used to check whether a given kilovoltage maintains itself over a range of milliamperages. A test with this stepwedge *does not* answer the question: what is the actual kilovoltage across the tube? *It does* answer the question: is the kilovoltage available from a particular setting of the selector maintained when the milliamperage is raised?

Perhaps the student is asking: why should the kilovoltage not be maintained since milliamperage and kilovoltage are separately controlled? The actual kilovoltage available from any given setting of the selector is modified by the voltage drop that occurs in the high-tension transformer when the exposure is made and the load current (tube milliamperage) flows. The magnitude of this voltage drop is proportional to the load current and so it becomes greater as the load current increases: that is, as the tube milliamperage is raised. So any given setting of the kilovoltage selector actually provides for the X-ray tube a kilovoltage which becomes lower in value for each increase in milliamperage. In the circuitry of the X-ray set, compensation can be arranged for this effect, there being provided for the generator an additional voltage which is intended to match the voltage drop that occurs when the load current flows. This compensation is variously called the *kilovoltage compensation*, the *milliamperage calibration* or simply the *calibration* of the generator.

If the compensating voltages in fact match the voltage drops that occur, then the kilovoltage available from any given setting of the selector is maintained over the whole range of milliamperages used. If the compensating voltage does not match the voltage drop that occurs at any given selected milliamperage, then the kilovoltage will be lower (under-compensation) or higher (over-compensation) than it should be. A kilovoltage that is correctly maintained through all milliamperages is essential in assuring the quality of the radiographic result. The most important control of contrast in the image which can be varied by the radiographer is the selection of appropriate kilovoltage.

A series of exposures made with a step-wedge as described on page 365, for Fig. 13.20 allows the stepwedge to be used to test the kilovoltage compensation of the high-tension generator. It is essential in this test that the milliampereseconds used remain the same throughout the test and that a kilovoltage-setting which is about the middle of the available range should be selected and be unchanged throughout the test. The only variables in the series of exposures constituting the test are the milliampere-settings and the time-intervals.

Fig. 13.21 shows the results in one such series of test exposures made at the settings indicated. The kilovoltage was 60 kVp on the selector. If the kilovoltage actually available is correctly compensated at the five different milliamperages used, then the penetrating ability of the beam remains the same and the five images of the stepwedge should appear to be alike: that is, all five should show penetration of the same steps of the wedge.

The reader should realize that the five images of the stepwedge are not bound to match in density step for step. Densities match step for step only if the following requirements are met:

(i) that the timer is accurate;

(ii) that the lack of reciprocity is insignificant;

(iii) that the kilovoltage was in fact sustained through the changes in milliamperage;

(iv) that the processing conditions were identical for all five images.

A viewer looking at the original radiograph against a bright light can

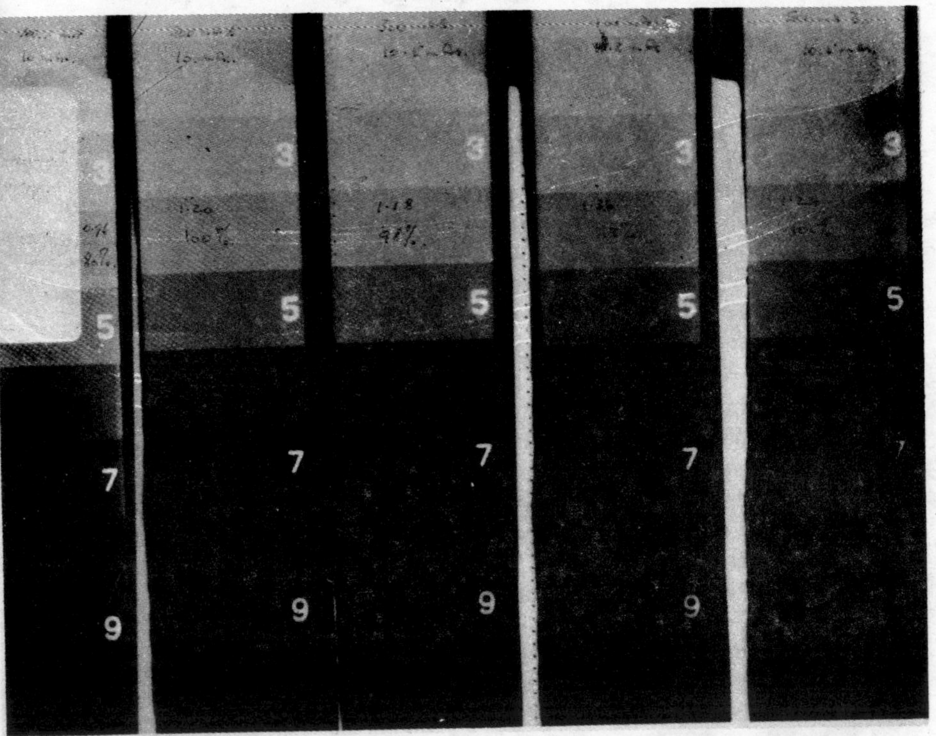

Fig. 13.21 Radiographs of stepwedge

ın fact differentiate in all five strips the eleven steps of the wedge which are recorded on the film. This indicates that there was no significant change in kilovoltage over the five different milliamperages which were used.

In the previous paragraphs we have described how exposures through a stepwedge may be used to check that kilovoltage is maintained over a range of milliamperages. Such a test does not measure the kilovoltage actually applied to the X-ray tube. If the means are available to make such a measurement, it is of course unnecessary to use a stepwedge for checking whether the kilovoltage varies with the milliamperage used. The kilovoltage available from a particular setting of the control can be measured over a range of milliamperages. This test gives a more precise result than does the use of stepwedges in the way described.

MEASURING TUBE-KILOVOLTAGE

Careful selection of the kilovoltage across the X-ray tube is a most important factor altered by the radiographer to determine contrast in the resultant image. Variations in the effective penetrating power of the X-ray beam change significantly the differential absorptions by the tissues to be traversed. Yet direct knowledge of the kilovoltage applied for any given setting of the selector is not available to radiographers through conventional control consoles.

It may be considered to be unimportant that kilovoltage settings should provide exactly the value which is stated. In choosing kilovoltage, the radiographer makes a subjective judgement which is empirically based, although modified by knowledge of the principles which are involved. More important perhaps than the accuracy of the settings is their consistency: any given setting should provide a value of kilovoltage which is repeatable and for that setting remains the same whenever the setting is used.

In assuring the quality of the radiographic result it is necessary to check the kilovoltage applied from the control-settings of the X-ray sets which are in use. If all the X-ray sets consistently provide kilovoltages close to the stated values, the radiographers are much more likely to achieve a high standard of work that is reproducible and is maintained. It may be possible for one radiographer working with one X-ray unit to make adjustments through familiarity with the inexactness of the settings (so long as the settings are consistent in their erroneousness) and so to achieve a satisfactory radiographic result on every film which is exposed. But in a department with several X-ray sets and many radiographers if the kilovoltages actually available differ widely from the values stated by the settings, then these variations are a plentiful source of repeated radiographs. With so much present emphasis on the conservation of materials and energy and on limits to expenditure, such repeats are intolerably wasteful.

Several methods are available for estimating the kilovoltage applied to the X-ray tube. Some of them are not such as would be used readily by a radiographer making a check on the X-ray sets of the department: so there seems little point in describing them here. Instead we concern ourselves with a technique that can be applied easily and quickly by radiographers. This technique uses an X-ray film to detect the radiation emerging from the tube and it is based upon the use of a special cassette.

THE WISCONSIN TEST CASSETTE

The Wisconsin test cassette is a special cassette which can be used to determine by a radiographic method the effective kilovoltage across the X-ray tube when the test was made. The accuracy of the result is assessed as generally within plus/minus 2 per cent and certainly within plus/minus 5 per cent. At 100 kV, 2 per cent is a 2 kV variation and 5 per cent is a 5 kV variation. While some people might say that a 5 kV change makes to the radiograph a difference which is perceptible to the viewer's eye, most would doubtless agree that in the general run of radiographs a 2 kV change does not appreciably alter the image.

The cassette (see Fig. 13.22) allows the kilovoltage to be assessed in four regions: 60 kVp region; 80 kVp region; 100 kVp region; 120 kVp region. It is said to be most accurate in the first two regions and least accurate in the highest one. It has higher accuracy when it is used on three-phase generators as compared with single-phase ones.

The cassette further enables its user to estimate the half-value thickness (half-value layer) of the X-ray beam which comes out of the

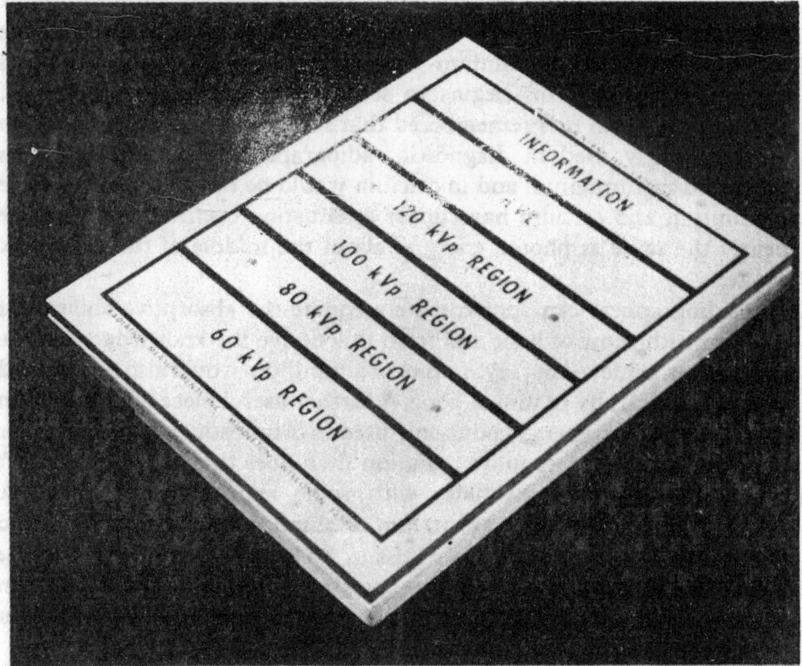

Fig. 13.22 Wisconsin test cassette

tube when it is energized at the 60 kVp setting. Students may recall from their study of physics that the half-value thickness of an X-ray beam is a statement about its penetrating power. The half-value thickness is defined as being the thickness of a stated material which is required to reduce the intensity of an X-ray beam to half its original value: the Wisconsin cassette gives an expression of the half-value thickness (half-value layer) in equivalent millimetres of aluminium.

As an indication of the penetrating power of an X-ray beam, the peak kilovoltage at which it is generated makes an incomplete statement. To know the peak kilovoltage is to know of a heterogeneous beam only its minimum wavelength and the related maximum energy for a photon. Radiographers could well question the usefulness of knowing only *that* when they must concern themselves with the ability of a beam to penetrate the tissue of the human body and to have an effect on a film and produce a radiograph. At least the half-value layer gives an indication of the effective penetrating power of a heterogeneous beam since to specify the half-value layer is to indicate the beam's attenuation by the material which is used to state the half-value layer.

When the Wisconsin test cassette is used to determine the half-value layer of the beam produced at 60 kVp, the radiographer gains knowledge of what thickness of aluminium will reduce this beam to one half of its original intensity. This begins to seem a potentially useful piece of information when it is remembered that for the photon energies which are commonly used in diagnostic radiography the half-value layers expressed in aluminium and in calcium would be nearly the same, since aluminium and calcium have linear attenuation coefficients which are nearly the same at photon energies about the middle of the diagnostic range.

Radiographers can approximately equate the absorptive abilities of calcium with those of bone and from this derive the knowledge that the attenuation achieved by, say, 10 mm of aluminium would also be achieved (nearly enough) by 10 mm of bone. A further useful piece of information is that at a photon energy commonly used in diagnostic radiography bone removes about 5 times more radiation than does the same mass of soft tissue. So we could estimate, with some approximation, that the attenuation achieved by, say, 10 mm of aluminium and of bone would also be achieved by 50 mm of soft tissue. So knowledge of the half-value layer of a beam of X rays when it is expressed in millimetres of aluminium is a piece of information which can be of some use to the radiographer who is selecting exposure factors.

A further important point is that a beam generated at 60 kVp which has a very low half-value layer (say less than 1·5 mm of aluminium in contrast to around 1·8 to 2·0 mm of aluminium) must be a beam with a long range of photon energies. This suggests that there is insufficient equivalent aluminium filtration in the tube to remove the low photon energies which will be absorbed in the patient's skin: so this X-ray tube is giving the patient a dose of needless radiation which is not contributing to the radiographic result at all.

On the other hand, if a beam of X rays generated at 60 kVp shows a half-value layer which is thicker than the expected figure of around 1·8 to 2·0 mm of aluminium, then the implication is that the effective filtration in this X-ray tube has *increased*. Such could be the case in a long-used X-ray tube, subjected to heavy loading, where there has been considerable deposition of hot tungsten on the glass envelope of the tube. The layer of metal over the window through which the X rays emerge from the glass insert acts as a filter if it is thick enough and removes some of the photons in the beam which have lower energies. Thus the beam becomes effectively more penetrating and the half-value layer increases in thickness. So this finding may give warning of the state of an ageing X-ray tube and predict its failure.

THE CONSTRUCTION OF THE WISCONSIN CASSETTE

Fig. 13.22 shows the external appearance of the Wisconsin test cassette. The four regions of kilovoltage from 60 kVp to 120 kVp are seen marked on the outside of the cassette, as are the panels for half-value layer and what is described as *Information*: this last one is intended to bear lead legends or other markers which may identify the particular X-ray set which is being tested and the date of the test.

Fig. 13.23 shows an exploded view of the Wisconsin test cassette so that the different constituent parts can be seen. Working inwards from the front of the cassette the various elements are as follows.

1 A sheet of copper which is $\frac{1}{16}$ inch thick and is large enough to cover the four regions where the kilovoltages are to be assessed but does not extend over the region where the half-value layer is to be measured. This sheet of copper is intended to act as a filter and remove some longer wavelengths from the heterogeneous beam which comes out of the X-ray tube. With the photons of lower energy thus removed, the energy-range of the remainder in the beam is narrower and the attenuation by the copper wedges which are the next elements in the cassette becomes almost a linear function of photon-energy.

2 Underneath the copper sheet are four copper stepwedges, one for each of the four kilovoltage regions: 60 kVp, 80 kVp, 100 kVp and 120 kVp. They each have a different range of thickness as appropriate to

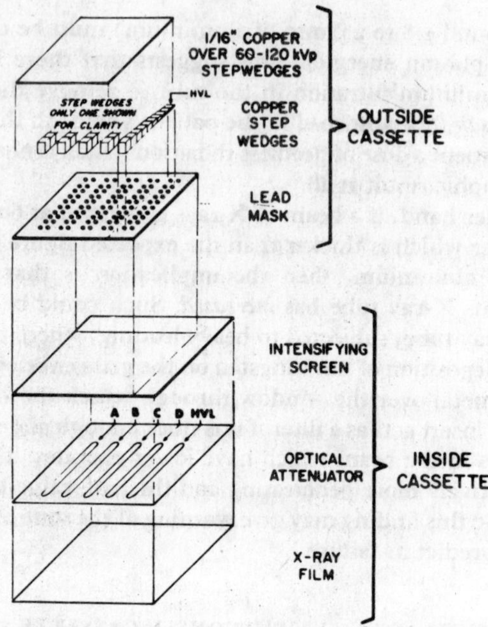

Fig. 13.23 Wisconsin test casssette

the kilovoltage to be measured. Thus, for example, the copper stepwedge for the 60 kVp measurement has a different thickness-range from its thin to its thick end than does the wedge for the determination of tube-voltage in the 120 kVp region. These stepwedges are used in the measurement of kilovoltage as will be seen. Alongside these stepwedges is a fifth copper stepwedge which is used for the measurement of half-value layer: it is *not* covered by the copper sheet as are the other four for that does not extend into the half-value layer region of the cassette. The important point is that the measurement of kilovoltage is to be done *after* the beam has had the photons of low energy removed from it: that is, a filtered beam is used. The measurement of half-value layer uses an unfiltered beam because the half-value layer depends upon the range of energies in the primary beam which emerges from the X-ray tube.

3   Underneath the copper stepwedges is a lead sheet with holes in it. There are ten columns of holes with ten holes to a column. The columns are grouped as five pairs, there being one pair of columns in each of the five regions of the cassette: 60 kVp, 80 kVp, 100 kVp, 120 kVp and lastly the half-value layer region. In each pair of columns, the left-hand column of holes is positioned so that each hole is beneath a copper stepwedge in

an arrangement of one step of the wedge for each hole: thus each hole is covered by a different thickness of copper. The right-hand column of holes in each pair of columns is *not* beneath a copper stepwedge. The use of the lead sheet improves the contrast of the radiographic result (seen in Fig. 13.24) by absorbing scattered radiation.

4   Beneath the lead sheet with the holes is an intensifying screen which extends through all the 5 regions of the cassette. It is a single screen, there being no other in this cassette. The use of a single screen instead of a pair eliminates the effects of possible changes in the relative speeds of different screens.

5   Beneath the intensifying screen is an optical filter which is designed to filter the light which the intensifying screen emits when it is energized by X rays. This optical filter or attenuator is arranged in bars so that it filters the light emitted from the parts of the screen which are beneath the right-hand column of holes in each pair of columns in the lead sheet. This action of the bars of the optical filter is effectively to reduce the speed of the intensifying screen in those areas which are covered by the filtering bars.

6   The last essential in this test cassette is the film which is the detector of the radiation.

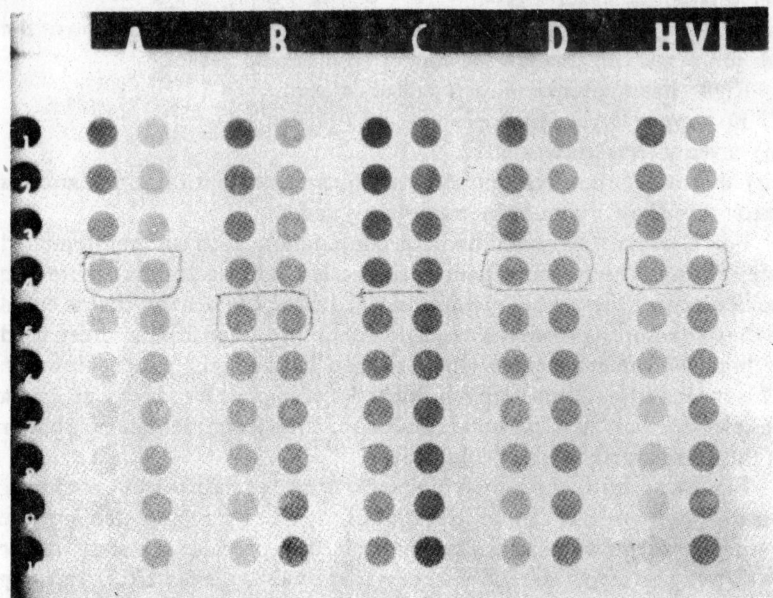

Fig. 13.24 Radiograph of test cassette

PRINCIPLE OF OPERATION OF THE WISCONSIN TEST CASSETTE

We have described as a component of the test cassette a lead mask with columns of holes arranged in pairs. It will by now be realized that in each pair of columns:

(i) the right-hand column of holes has the optical attenuator beneath it but no absorbing copper stepwedge above it and the circular densities which are produced as images of the holes (see Fig. 13.24) result from a combination of an unattenuated X-ray beam and an attenuated light from the screen: the attenuation of light does not vary down the column of holes for the optical filter achieves a fixed degree of attenuation.

(ii) the left-hand column of holes has a different thickness of copper absorber above each hole but no optical attenuator under any of the holes and the circular densities in the radiograph (see Fig. 13.24) are the result of an X-ray beam which is variously attenuated by the copper stepwedges and an unattenuated light from the screen: the copper stepwedges increase in thickness down the columns.

So for the circles of density shown in Fig. 13.24 the situation is as below.

Left-hand column of each pair of columns:

(i) copper X-ray absorbers;

(ii) unattenuated screen;

(iii) circles show a density-gradient, density diminishing down the column as the thickness of the copper absorbers increases.

Right-hand column of each pair of columns:

(i) no copper X-ray absorbers;

(ii) attenuated screen;

(iii) density of the circles is nearly uniform as the optical attenuation is fixed: this density should be between 0·5 and 2·0.

For a copper absorber used in conjunction with an unattenuated intensifying screen (the situation in the left-hand columns) there is a particular thickness which results in a radiographic density that is equal to the one resulting from the use of an attenuated intensifying screen used without a copper absorber (the situation in the right-hand columns). This means that there is a given thickness of copper stepwedge at which a circle of density in a left-hand column matches its immediate neighbour in the adjacent right-hand column.

Fig. 13.24 shows three matching pairs of circles indicated by enclosing hand-drawn lines. It can be seen that in the 60 kVp region step 4 of the copper absorber was the thickness required to produce a match: in the 80 kVp region step 5 was the thickness that produced a match: at 120 kVp step 4 was the thickness of copper absorber needed to achieve a match.

If the attenuation of the intensifying screen is fixed (as we have seen it is in this cassette) the thickness of copper required for a match in density increases with rising kilovoltage. Furthermore, it is almost a linear function of kilovoltage when the X-ray beam has had its spectral distribution narrowed by the use of the copper sheet described on page 373. So 'match thickness' can be used to measure kilovoltage and also (as it is here) to estimate the half-value layer for a beam generated at a given kilovoltage (in this case 60 kVp). Fig. 13.24 shows the two columns of circular densities in the half-value layer region of the cassette with a matching pair enclosed in a hand-drawn line.

For the determination of half-value layer, the energy-distribution of the beam emerging from the X-ray tube must be left unchanged and the spectrum is not narrowed by passing the beam through the copper sheet. It is for this reason that as described on page 373 the copper sheet does not extend over the region of the cassette where the half-value layer is to be measured.

Wisconsin test cassettes are each calibrated individually by the manufacturers (Radiation Measurements Inc.) against a master standard cassette. They come to the user accompanied by calibration data which allow 'match thicknesses' or step numbers to be related to kilovoltage-values and to half-value layers.

METHOD OF USE OF THE WISCONSIN TEST CASSETTE

When the Wisconsin test cassette is used to check a particular X-ray set for the exactness of its kilovoltage-settings, comparing actual kilovoltage-values with those indicated on the control panel, and for the estimation of half-value layer at 60 kVp, five exposures must be made: one exposure on each of the four kilovoltage regions of the cassette and one on the half-value layer region. For each exposure, the areas of the cassette which are not being used must be masked with lead and it is most important that this lead shield is adequate. At least 2 mm of lead (*not* a lead-rubber sheet) must be used.

The cassette is loaded with any type of X-ray film and is put on the X-ray table, placed as is any conventional cassette with its front aspect towards the X-ray tube. The long sides of the cassette should be parallel to the long anode-cathode axis of the X-ray tube. This is so that the columns of holes and the copper stepwedge absorbers lie along lines at right-angles to the anode-cathode axis of the X-ray tube: such a placing will prevent the anode heel-effect from significantly modifying the findings of the test. The X-ray tube should be centered to the long central axis of the cassette-front and will be directly over each of the five measuring regions of the cassette in its turn as the area to receive exposure.

Exposures are made in series over each region separately with the other regions masked with lead and with the beam-collimator so adjusted that the whole of a region is irradiated to its complete length and width. When the half-value layer region is being exposed, the area next to it which is marked Identification should be included within the field: lead letters or other markers for radiographic identification placed in this panel before exposure can record data relevant to the test.

Before the exposures are made, the line voltage compensator of the generator should be set as precisely as possible if it is a manual control and the kilovoltage-settings each in their turn should be accurately made. If the generator of the X-ray set which is being tested does not provide the higher kilovoltages which are marked on the cassette, then those regions are not used and no exposures are made for them.

The 60 kVp setting on the generator must be checked as correctly providing 60 kVp before testing the half-value layer. This means that you must re-load the cassette with a second film and make the half-value layer test separately, for you cannot know the result of the test of the 60 kVp setting until you have processed the film on which it was made. Fig. 13.25 shows a radiograph taken to test the half-value layer.

Exposure factors for the Wisconsin test cassette which are suggested are set out below.

Region of the cassette	Focus-film distance	kV setting	mA	Time in seconds
A 60 kVp	50 cm (20 inches)	60	100	1·0
B 80 kVp	100 cm (40 inches)	80	100	0·5
C 100 kVp	100 cm (40 inches)	100	100	0·12
D 120 kVp	100 cm (40 inches)	120	100	0·04
HVL	100 cm (40 inches)	60	100	0·03

There are some points about these exposure factors to be noted as follows.

(i) The milliamperage and the times should be set to give values of milliampereseconds which are as close as possible to those in the table.

(ii) In the resultant radiograph (see Fig. 13.24) the density of the circles in the right-hand column of each pair (which is considered as a reference column) should be between 0·5 and 2·0. If the density is outside this

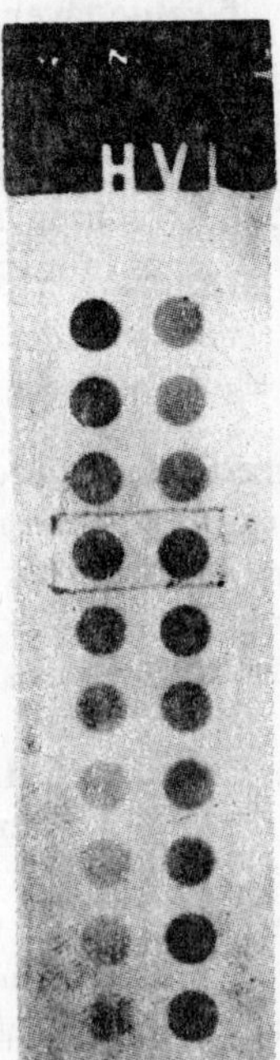

Fig. 13.25 Radiograph of test cassette

range, then the cassette should be re-loaded and the test should be repeated with an increase in the milliamperseconds-values if the density is less than 0·5 and a decrease in the milliamperseconds-values if the density is more than 2·0.

(iii) The milliamperseconds-values which are to be used for three-phase generators should be half those which are used with single-phase units because a three-phase generator gives a higher radiographic output for every kilovolt and milliampere used. This is a result of the rippling voltage waveform which is applied to the X-ray tube and enables it to produce useful X rays throughout the cycle of the alternating mains supply. Such a condition of operation is to be contrasted with the pulsating voltage waveform from a single phase generator in which the voltage falls from the peak kilovoltage and reaches zero on three occasions in the period of one full cycle of mains alternation.

(iv) The milliamperseconds-value for the half-value layer test which is undertaken at 60 kVp is much lower than that given for the test of the 60 kVp setting itself. The explanation for this lies in the copper sheet which covers the 60 kVp to 120 kVp stepwedge absorbers but does not cover the stepwedge in the half-value layer region of the cassette. The beam of radiation reaching the film in the half-value layer region has not had the range of energies of its photons narrowed by the removal of those photons which have low energy. There are therefore more photons (that is, greater intensity of radiation) reaching the film in that area of the cassette than in the other four regions of measurement.

INTERPRETING THE RESULTS OF THE TEST

When the film has been processed, it is viewed to determine the results of the test. As can be seen in Fig. 13.24 the radiograph shows a series of circles of density arranged in columns. Across the top the letters A (60 kVp region), B (80 kVp region), C (100 kVp region), D (120 kVp region) and HVL indicate the five regions of the cassette which are available for the tests.

It can be seen that the circles are arranged, as would be expected from a description of the cassette, in paired columns, one pair in each region of the cassette. The right-hand column of each pair shows circles with no change of density and is considered to be the reference column: the circles of density are produced through the optical attenuator which modifies the light from the single intensifying screen in the cassette. The left-hand column in each pair shows circles of density produced through the copper stepwedges which attenuate the X-ray beam and these show a range of diminishing densities down each column. In the original of Fig. 13.24 all the circles which head the five left-hand columns had densities in the range 1·0 to 1·5; all the circles which are at the lower ends of the five left-hand columns had densities in the range 0·25 to 0·75. Another feature of the radiograph shown in Fig. 13.24 at the viewer's left hand is a column of circular densities labelled 1 to 10 downwards. The figures indicate the ten steps of each of the five copper stepwedge absorbers which are in the cassette over the the left-hand columns in the A, B, C, D and HVL regions. It is obvious from the radiograph that step 1 is the thin end and step 10 is the thick end of each copper stepwedge.

To interpret the radiograph you should take each of the five pairs of columns in turn. With the aid of a densitometer, measure densities and locate in the paired columns the step where a circle in the left-hand column has a density to match that of the adjacent circle in the righ-hand column. This has been done for sections A, B and D in Fig. 13.24.

It can be seen that in section A step 4 produced the matched density, in section B step 5 gave the match and in section D step 4 is the level of the circles which match. If there is no densitometer, the circles must be matched by eye and this clearly introduces subjective variables which must affect the accuracy of the result. The manufacturers of the Wisconsin test cassette say that the visual assessment is approximate at plus minus 3 kVp: good viewing conditions and visual acuity in the assessor must be presumed.

If in any of the paired columns there is no density match, you should note the two steps between which the match may be assumed to occur as indicated by the arrow in Fig. 13.24. If there is a match, note the step at which it occurs.

Each Wisconsin test cassette is calibrated by the manufacturers against their master cassette and comes to the user with calibration data. This information relates the step-numbers at which matches occur to the actual kilovoltages across the X-ray tube at each of the four settings indicated on the cassette and in the fifth section to the half-value layer at 60 kVp in equivalent millimetres of aluminium.

The manufacturers of the Wisconsin test cassette suggest that acceptable variations in kilovoltage from the selected values are less than 5 kVp at the 60 kVp and 80 kVp settings and less than 8 kVp at the 100 kVp and 120 kVp settings. A half-value layer finding that is low (say, about 1.0 mm Al) suggests that the added aluminium filtration which is required for the protection of patients is no longer in place. A half-value layer finding which is high (say, 6.0 mm Al) suggests that an ageing X-ray tube is near the end of its useful life.

MANIPULATION OF EXPOSURE FACTORS

Whether a radiographic image is produced by the action of X rays directly, or by a combination of X rays and fluorescent light from intensifying screens, the result is obtained because the photographic emulsion has absorbed some energy. There are many variables which influence this absorption of energy. These variables are assessed by the radiographer in selection of radiographic techniques, and they form a complex which now will be examined in more detail.

The variables involved can be seen to come under two main headings. They are (i) variables which constitute the exposure factors; these amount to statements concerning the conditions of operation of the X-ray tube: and (ii) variables which modify the selection of exposure factors if a correctly exposed radiograph is to result; this group embraces certain factors in the use of the X-ray tube and accessory equipment as well as variations connected with the subject of the radiographic examination.

THE EXPOSURE FACTORS

Statements on the operating conditions for the X-ray tube which we call the exposure factors comprise the following;
(i) the X-ray tube voltage, expressed in kilovolts;
(ii) the X-ray tube current, expressed in milliamperes;
(iii) the tube-film distance, expressed in inches or centimetres;
(iv) the time-interval of the exposure, expressed in seconds.

In the absence of a patient the intensity of the X-ray beam can be considered as more or less constant over the whole surface of the film. This statement can be made because in practice there is little noticeable difference; in actual fact there is less intensity of radiation at a point of measurement beneath the anode end of the X-ray tube than at a point of measurement beneath the cathode end. The effect is demonstrable on film if very short tube-film distances are used, but in most radiographic examinations it is ignored.

It can be said that the photographic effect (or the amount of silver deposited, or the blackening of the film) depends upon the intensity of the X-ray beam producing the reaction. If the intensity of the X-ray beam is increased the photographic effect is increased, and similarly the two decrease together. The current through the X-ray tube, the voltage across it, and the distance separating it from the film alter the intensity of the X-ray beam reaching the film. The time-interval of the exposure is in effect the length of time during which energy is given to the film, and so the total amount of energy received by the film depends (if all other factors are equal) on the exposure-time. Thus all these factors influence the photographic effect in their several ways as discussed in the following sections.

THE X-RAY TUBE VOLTAGE

Altering the tube voltage alters two characteristics of the X-ray beam— its penetrating power and its intensity. These are two distinct features, as the colour and the brightness are separate characteristics of a beam of visible light.

The effect of a change in ability to penetrate by the X rays, and consequent alteration in the contrast of the radiographic image, has already been discussed in Chapter 12. In this section we are now concerned with the change in *intensity* that follows alteration in tube voltage, and the consequent change in photographic effect.

The change in intensity that occurs when kilovoltage is altered cannot be considered as an entirely simple matter. The basic statement which *is* simple is that when kilovoltage is raised the intensity of radiation leaving the X-ray tube also is increased. Difficulties arise when we wish to know the relationship more precisely, and we ask by what factor is the intensity increased.

It has been said that the intensity of the X-ray beam increases approximately as the square of the tube voltage in kilovolts peak, and that X-ray intensity is proportional to kVp^2 or kVp^3 depending on filtration. These have been used as acceptable statements and student radiographers have been given the exercise of calculations involving the assumption that they are true, though approximate in character. The X-ray intensity reaching the film holder after passing through the patient increases by a higher power, and is proportional to kVp^4 or kVp^5 according to the part being radiographed. This relationship is further modified by the nature of the beam being considered, that is whether it is being produced by a high tube kilovoltage or a relatively low one and the proportion of long wavelengths to short wavelengths that it contains.

The practising radiographer finds slight application for this knowledge, and is little interested in the intensity of the X-ray beam as it comes off the anode of the X-ray tube or even as it emerges from the tube housing. Radiographers *use* X-ray beams, and are therefore concerned most with the results on the film of these physical phenomena. What a radiographer needs is the answer to this question: *Since intensity increases with increase in tube voltage, if I raise the tube voltage, by how much should I decrease the time-interval of the exposure to achieve a radiographic result in which film blackening looks more or less the same?*

Here again there is no simple answer which is not an approximation. If intensifying screens are used, there is alteration in the intensification factor with tube voltage which theoretically affects the result. An increase of 10 kVp from, say, 50 kVp to 60 kVp does not have the same effect on the film as an increase of 10 kVp from 90 kVp to 100 kVp. This can be appreciated if some numerical examples are worked out on the basis of the fact that the amount of energy reaching the film is proportional to kV^4. For example, a change from 50 kV to 60 kV would require the time interval of the exposure to be reduced by a factor

$$\left(\frac{50}{60}\right)^4 = 0{\cdot}48$$

A change from 90 kV to 100 kV would require the time to be reduced by a factor

$$\left(\frac{90}{100}\right)^4 = 0{\cdot}66$$

So the change in time required for a change in kilovoltage depends on the ratio of the kilovoltages concerned. Differences in waveform between X-ray sets, and perhaps also differences in performance in one X-ray set when its loading is low or sufficiently high to be near its limit, are other factors which add to the complexity of the situation.

There is some help obtainable towards simplifying this complexity. It comes from the Bit System developed by Dupont to which we referred in an earlier section of this chapter (page 348). This system establishes a common currency for the variables of the exposure by assigning Bit values to them in accordance with their effects on density in the radiograph. Thus, to take examples from the tables published by Dupont (see Fig. 13.26), 50 kVp has a Bit value of 4·6, 60 kVp has a Bit value of 6·0 and 110 kVp has a Bit value of 9·8: obviously Bit values must rise with kilovoltage since the intensity of the beam and hence resultant density in the radiograph increase with raised tube voltages.

On the basis of the Bit System and the Dupont tables it is simple to find out what change in milliampereseconds must be made to compensate for any change in kilovoltage and give a radiograph of similar density (but of course different in contrast). For example, it can be done from the tables by adding up Bit values as follows. Suppose that you have a technique which uses 64 kVp and 0·4 second and that it is wished to modify this to 85 kVp and a shorter time. The question then to be answered is: what is the new shorter time of exposure that is required?

$$64 \text{ kVp} = 6·4 \text{ Bits}$$
$$0·4 \text{ second} = 11·0 \text{ Bits (see Fig. 13.27)}$$

The sum of these is 17·4, so that is the total Bit value of the original exposure factors.
The new kilovoltage is:

$$85 \text{ kVp} = 8·4 \text{ Bits}$$

This value is deducted from the original total and gives:

$$17·4 - 8·4 = 9·0 \text{ Bits}$$

This means that the new time of exposure which is being sought must have a value of 9·0 bits. For the tables:

$$0·1 \text{ second} = 9·0 \text{ Bits}$$

So 0·1 second is the new exposure-time required to give at 85 kVp the same result as 0·4 second at 64 kVp.

The radiographer selects kilovoltage for a radiographic examination

TABLE H

kVp	=	Bits
153	=	11.4
147	=	11.2
141	=	11.0
135	=	10.8
130	=	10.6
125	=	10.4
120	=	10.2
115	=	10.0
110	=	9.8
106	=	9.6
102	=	9.4
98	=	9.2
94	=	9.0
91	=	8.8
88	=	8.6
85	=	8.4
82	=	8.2
80	=	8.0
78	=	7.8
76	=	7.6
74	=	7.4
72	=	7.2
70	=	7.0
68	=	6.8
66	=	6.6
64	=	6.4
62	=	6.2
60	=	6.0
58	=	5.8
56	=	5.6
55	=	5.4
54	=	5.2
53	=	5.0
51	=	4.8
50	=	4.6
49	=	4.4
47	=	4.2
46	=	4.0
45	=	3.8
44	=	3.6
43	=	3.4
42	=	3.2
41	=	3.0
39	=	2.8
38	=	2.6
37	=	2.4
35	=	2.2
34	=	2.0
33	=	1.8
31	=	1.6
30	=	1.4
29	=	1.2
28	=	1.0
27	=	.8
26	=	.6
25	=	.4

Fig. 13.26 Table H Bit values

TABLE K

Fraction Seconds	=	Bits	=	Decimal Seconds
6	=	15.0	=	6.32
		14.8	=	5.50
5	=	14.6	=	5.00
		14.4	=	4.20
4	=	14.2	=	3.70
		14.0	=	3.20
3	=	13.8	=	2.80
2-1/2	=	13.6	=	2.50
		13.4	=	2.10
2	=	13.2	=	1.83
		13.0	=	1.60
1-1/2	=	12.8	=	1.40
1-1/5	=	12.6	=	1.20
		12.4	=	1.05
1	=	12.2	=	.920
		12.0	=	.800
3/4	=	11.8	=	.700
3/5	=	11.6	=	.600
		11.4	=	.525
1/2	=	11.2	=	.455
2/5	=	11.0	=	.400
		10.8	=	.350
3/10	=	10.6	=	.300
		10.4	=	.265
1/4	=	10.2	=	.230
1/5	=	10.0	=	.200
		9.8	=	.175
3/20	=	9.6	=	.151
2/15	=	9.4	=	.132
		9.2	=	.115
1/10	=	9.0	=	.100
		8.8	=	.087
1/12	=	8.6	=	.075
1/15	=	8.4	=	.066
		8.2	=	.057
1/20	=	8.0	=	.050
		7.8	=	.044
1/24	=	7.6	=	.038
1/30	=	7.4	=	.033
		7.2	=	.029
1/40	=	7.0	=	.025
		6.8	=	.022
1/50	=	6.6	=	.019
1/60	=	6.4	=	.0166
1/72	=	6.2	=	.0143
1/80	=	6.0	=	.0125
1/90	=	5.8	=	.0110
1/105	=	5.6	=	.0095
1/120	=	5.4	=	.0083
1/140	=	5.2	=	.0072
1/160	=	5.0	=	.0063
1/180	=	4.8	=	.0053
1/215	=	4.6	=	.0046
1/250	=	4.4	=	.0040
1/280	=	4.2	=	.0035
1/333	=	4.0	=	.0030
1/360	=	3.8	=	.0026
1/430	=	3.6	=	.0023
1/500	=	3.4	=	.0020
1/560	=	3.2	=	.0017
1/666	=	3.0	=	.0015
1/780	=	2.8	=	.0013
1/860	=	2.6	=	.0012
1/1000	=	2.4	=	.0010

Fig. 13.27 Table K Bit values

usually on the basis of previous experience. The following considerations will affect the choice.

(i) Knowledge of what has been used before, of the performance of the X-ray set in use, and of the practice of the department.

(ii) The need for adequate penetration of the subject.

(iii) Recognition of the fact that higher kilovoltage reduces radiation contrasts in the subject, and allows a wider range of tissue differences to be recorded together.

(iv) Knowledge that when higher kilovoltages are used intensity increases and times of exposure can be decreased; this is very marked when 'high kilovoltage techniques' (100 kVp to 140 kVp range) are used.

THE X-RAY TUBE CURRENT

The intensity of the radiation emerging from the X-ray tube can be considered to be proportional to the X-ray tube current as it is indicated by the controls and recorded on the milliampere meter of the X-ray set. This is a direct proportion; for example doubling the tube current increases the intensity by the same factor.

The radiographer is again concerned less with the intensity of the X-ray beam emerging from the X-ray tube than with the effect upon the film; that is to say less with the emitted intensity than with the quantity of radiation that the film receives. This is proportional to the product of the tube current (mA) and the time for which it flows (S), the result being milliampereseconds (mAs).

When the film is exposed directly to X rays without the use of intensifying screens, a milliampereseconds value of (say) 20 mAs produces the same effect whether it is delivered as a tube current of 20 mA passing for 1 second, of 200 mA pasing for 0·1 second, or of 400 mA passing for 0·05 second. Provided that the product of tube current and time remains the same, the photographic effect is unchanged, irrespective of the separate values of milliamperage and time. This interchanging of intensity and time follows the law which is called the Law of Reciprocity. This is valid for X radiation acting on photographic materials.

When intensifying screens are in use the effect on the film is produced mainly by visible light emitted by the screens in response to X radiation. In this case there is reciprocity failure: this means that high intensities of light acting for short times and low intensities of light acting for long times do not produce the same photographic effect with the product Intensity × Time staying constant; at both extremes the effect is to produce less density than a reciprocal relationship leads one to expect.

High tube currents passed for a short time and low tube currents passed for a long time may not produce the same result in comparison with each other, and indeed may not compare in effect with intermediate values of tube current and time, even though the milliampereseconds are the same in all these cases.

In practice radiographers regard reciprocity failure as having no practical significance, and assume that milliamperes and time are interchangeable whether intensifying screens are used or not. If 50 mAs has given a reasonable result in a certain examination and it is wished to shorten the time because the patient cannot keep still, then the new time-interval is derived by multiplying the tube current and dividing the time by the same factor; for example it might have been 50 mA for 1 second, and it could become 200 mA for 0·25 second. Here again the justification for such disregard of scientific fact is that the assumption works, perhaps because in any given examination radiographers are not likely to change milliamperage over a very wide range.

As with other factors of exposure, the radiographer selects milli-ampereseconds on the basis of previous experience. The following considerations will affect the choice.

(i) Knowledge of what has been used before, of the performance of the X-ray set in use, and of the practice of the department.

(ii) The need for adequate film density.

(iii) Assessment of the likelihood of subject-movement, taking into consideration the state of the patient, the nature of the examination, and the body-part involved.

(iv) The assumption that milliamperage and time are in effect interchangeable.

THE TUBE-FILM DISTANCE

Since the X-ray beam is divergent from its source, it covers an area which increases in size with distance from the source. The energy of the beam is therefore spread over a large area and the intensity (which may be defined as the energy reaching unit area in unit time) is thus diminished. The intensity varies inversely with the square of the distance from the source.

The student is surely familiar with this law known as the Inverse Square Law, and doubtless has been taught the conditions in which the law breaks down—namely when the source is not a point and when scattering or absorption occurs in the intervening medium. It will be realized from the discussion on geometric unsharpness earlier in Chapter 12 (if from no other head of knowledge) that the source of radiation in an

X-ray tube is *not* a point. When radiographers are concerned with X-ray beams there is generally a patient of appreciable if varying size occupying *some* of the distance through which the beam travels to reach the film; in this patient's tissue scattering and absorption occur.

It is now easy to reach the conclusion that in diagnostic radiography the law strictly is not valid. Yet radiographers assume that in the conditions of their work the Law of Inverse Squares is sound and applicable. In practice it proves to be a reasonable assumption, once again justified by the fact that it seems to work. When it is realized that the usual tube-film distance is great in comparison with the size of the source, and that the larger proportion of this distance is occupied by air and not the subject's tissue, the apparent validity of the law may be explained.

Radiographers therefore use the Law of Inverse Squares when computing alterations in exposure required by distance changes. Since intensity decreases with increase of distance, exposure must be increased to compensate for this; and at shorter distances must similarly be decreased. The exposure must be altered by a factor related to the *squares* of the distances involved.

This factor is found simply by the ratio

$$\frac{(\text{New distance})^2}{(\text{Old distance})^2} \text{ or } \frac{(\text{Old distance})^2}{(\text{New distance})^2}$$

It is easier to use this ratio if the *greater* of the two distances is placed 'on top' in the relationship. The student should take care *always* to do this and keep firmly in mind that (i) increase in distance requires increase in exposure, decrease in distance requires decrease in exposure, and (ii) multiplication by figures greater than unity increases quantities, division by figures greater than unity decreases quantities. Then problems involving the law of inverse squares can be tackled without dismay and with success. If the new milliampereseconds value is required to be greater than the previous one, then simply multiply the old milliampereseconds by the distance ratio; if the new milliampereseconds value is required to be less than the previous one, then simply divide the old milliampereseconds by the distance ratio.

For example: *If 16 mAs give a reasonable radiograph of a chest at a focus-film distance of 4 feet, what milliampereseconds must be used if the distance is increased to 6 feet?*

The new distance is the larger of the two figures so it is put 'on top' and the distance ratio is:

$$\frac{(\text{New distance})^2}{(\text{Old distance})^2} = \frac{6^2}{4^2} = \frac{36}{16}$$

The new milliampereseconds must be more than 16 mAs (since the distance has been increased), so the new value is:

$$16 \times \frac{36}{16} \text{ mAs}$$

If 10 mAs give a good radiograph of the knee at a focus-film distance of 40 inches and the examination must be made in conditions which impose a distance of 30 inches, what milliampereseconds must be used?

The old distance is the larger of the two figures so it is put 'on top' and the distance ratio is:

$$\frac{(\text{Old distance})^2}{(\text{New distance})^2} = \frac{40^2}{30^2} = \frac{1600}{900}$$

The new milliampereseconds must be less than 10 (since the distance has been decreased), so the new value is:

$$\frac{10}{1600/900} \text{ mAs} = 5 \cdot 6 \text{ mAs approximately}$$

It may be of help to give some correction factors for certain changes of distance and we give a few below. The arithmetic has been done to yield approximate answers, which may be easier to remember and are adequate in use. Exposure selection is often an imprecise procedure.

Changing distance:		Multiple mAs by:
From 30 ins. to 36 ins.		1·5
36 ins.	40 ins.	1·25
30 ins.	40 ins.	1·75
48 ins.	60 ins.	1·5
60 ins.	72 ins.	1·5
48 ins.	72 ins.	2·25

		Divide mAs by:
From 36 ins. to 30 ins.		1·5
40 ins.	36 ins.	1·25
40 ins.	30 ins.	1·75
60 ins.	48 ins.	1·5
72 ins.	60 ins.	1·5
72 ins.	48 ins.	2·25

We have given the above guide in the hope that we may help radiographers who, faced with the need to work out a new technique adapted to a changed tube–film distance, can manage to recall these figures. Our experience tells us that in practice the radiographer is a rarity who in the course of a busy day will pause to calculate a new milliampereseconds-value on the basis of the inverse square law, even with the ready availability of electronic calculators to come up quickly with an accurate result. The tendency is to guess at the adjustment needed and to get a radiograph which is underexposed or overexposed. The radiographer had forgotten that the *square* of the distance is the operating figure and this means that what seem relatively small changes in tube–film distance require larger changes in milliampereseconds if the density of the radiograph is to remain unchanged. So if tube–film distance is changed by a factor of two (for example 2 metres is reduced to 1 metre) the milliampereseconds must change by a factor of four (for example 20 mAs would be reduced to 5 mAs).

The Dupont Bit System to which we have previously referred can certainly help with adjustments to be made in milliampereseconds when tube–film distances are to be changed, just as it can with other variables in the exposure technique. Suppose, for example, that 20 mAs has resulted in a satisfactory radiograph for which a tube–film distance of 72 inches (183 cm) has been used. Let us further suppose that the radiographer then is required to use a distance of 44 inches (112 cm) and wants to know what new milliampereseconds-value must be set in order to get the same result.

Consulting the Dupont Bit System tables, we find that for tube–film distances:

72 inches = 5·0 bits and 44 inches = 6·4 bits (see Fig. 13.28)

So the change in Bit values which is considered here is:

$$5·0–6·4 = -1·4$$

The appropriate column in the tables shows that a bit change which is minus 1·4 as it is here (the distance is shorter and the milliampereseconds are to be decreased) carries with it a milliampereseconds-factor which is 0·38 (see Fig. 13.29).

To calculate the new milliampereseconds-value we use this relationship:

New milliampereseconds = previous milliampereseconds
                                × the milliampereseconds-factor.

So in this case the milliampereseconds required are:

$$20 \times 0·38 = 7·6$$

The experienced radiographer selects the tube-film distan for an X-ray examination with the following points in mind:

TABLE F FOCAL-FILM DISTANCE		
Inches =	Bits =	Centimeters
6.7	12.0	17
7.3	11.8	18.5
7.7	11.6	19.5
8.3	11.4	21
9.0	11.2	22.5
9.5	11.0	24
10.0	10.8	25.5
10.6	10.6	27
11.4	10.4	29
12.2	10.2	31
13	10.0	33
14	9.8	35
15	9.6	38
16	9.4	40
17	9.2	43
18	9.0	46
19	8.8	48
21	8.6	53
22	8.4	56
24	8.2	61
25	8.0	64
27	7.8	69
29	7.6	74
31	7.4	79
33	7.2	84
36	7.0	91
39	6.8	99
41	6.6	104
44	6.4	112
48	6.2	122
51	6.0	130
55	5.8	140
58	5.6	147
63	5.4	160
67	5.2	170
72	5.0	183
77	4.8	196
83	4.6	211
88	4.4	224
95	4.2	241
102	4.0	259
109	3.8	277
116	3.6	295
125	3.4	318
136	3.2	345
144	3.0	366
154	2.8	391
165	2.6	419
176	2.4	447
180	2.2	457
203	2.0	516
218	1.8	554

Fig. 13.28 Table F Bit values

(i) Knowledge of what has been used before and of the practice in the department.

(ii) Long tube-film distance reduces geometric unsharpness and enlargement in the image.

PERCENTAGES

TABLE T

Bit Change	% Increase (+) % Decrease (—)	Dosage or mAs Factor*	Relative mAs or Arithmetic Speed
+ 5.0	+ 3100%	32.00X	3200
+ 4.8	+ 2720%	28.20X	2820
+ 4.6	+ 2360%	24.60X	2460
+ 4.4	+ 2040%	21.40X	2140
+ 4.2	+ 1760%	18.60X	1860
+ 4.0	+ 1500%	16.00X	1600
+ 3.8	+ 1310%	14.10X	1410
+ 3.6	+ 1130%	12.30X	1230
+ 3.4	+ 970%	10.70X	1070
+ 3.2	+ 812%	9.12X	912
+ 3.0	+ 700%	8.00X	800
+ 2.8	+ 592%	6.92X	692
+ 2.6	+ 503%	6.03X	603
+ 2.4	+ 425%	5.25X	525
+ 2.2	+ 357%	4.57X	457
+ 2.0	+ 300%	4.00X	400
+ 1.8	+ 247%	3.47X	347
+ 1.6	+ 200%	3.00X	300
+ 1.4	+ 163%	2.63X	263
+ 1.2	+ 130%	2.30X	230
+ 1.0	+ 100%	2.00X	200
+ .8	+ 74%	1.74X	174
+ .6	+ 51%	1.51X	151
+ .4	+ 32%	1.32X	132
+ .2	+ 15%	1.15X	115
0	0	1.00X	100
— .2	— 13%	.87X	87
— .4	— 24%	.76X	76
— .6	— 34%	.66X	66
— .8	— 42%	.58X	58
—1.0	— 50%	.50X	50
—1.2	— 56%	.44X	44
—1.4	— 62%	.38X	38
—1.6	— 67%	.33X	33
—1.8	— 71%	.29X	29
—2.0	— 75%	.25X	25
—2.2	— 78%	.22X	22
—2.4	— 81%	.19X	19
—2.6	— 83%	.17X	17
—2.8	— 86%	.14X	14
—3.0	— 87%	.13X	13
—3.2	— 89%	.11X	11
—3.4	— 91%	.09X	9
—3.6	— 92%	.08X	8
—3.8	— 93%	.07X	7
—4.0	— 94%	.06X	6
—4.2	— 95%	.05X	5
—4.4	— 95.5%	.045	4.5
—4.6	— 96%	.04X	4
—4.8	— 96.5%	.035	3.5
—5.0	— 97%	.03X	3

*New mAs   Old mAs X mAs Factor

Fig. 13.29 Table T Bit values

**(iii) Long tube-film distance requires greater radiation intensity from
the X-ray tube to obtain adequate film density. This needs greater
electrical power input which may impose the use of larger focal spots;**

these increase geometric unsharpness. Or it may be necessary to use longer exposure times; these increase the chance of unsharpness due to movement.

(iv) Short tube–film distance increases geometric unsharpness. Structures remote from the film are recorded less sharply than those close to the film and if a short tube–film distance is used the differential is increased. This can be useful. For example in an anteroposterior projection of the sternoclavicular joints a short tube-film distance will 'blur out' the shadows of the upper dorsal vertebrae, in an occipitomental view of the nasal sinuses a short tube–film distance will aid dispersion of the shadows of structures in the middle and posterior fossae of the skull.

(v) Very short tube–film distances imply short tube–skin distances. Where these are less then 6 inches, repeated exposures carry risk to the patient of damage to the skin.

(vi) Where subject–film distances are very short, the tube-film distance can be decreased without the geometric unsharpness becoming objectionable.

As a general rule tube–film distances are standardized for particular examinations in a given X-ray department. For example, chests may be examined at 2 m, nasal sinuses and extremities at 75 cm, abdominal viscera at 100 cm. This standardization is essential if satisfactory and repeatable results are to be obtained.

THE EXPOSURE TIME

The total amount of energy received by the film depends on the intensity of radiation reaching the film and the time for which it does so.

From a practical point of view the exposure-time is considered to be the period of time during which the X-ray tube is energized, and the period during which radiation reaches the film is taken as being the same.

From what has been said in the foregoing sections, the relationship between exposure-time and the other factors of exposure can be appreciated. It can be summed-up as follows.

Exposure time can be decreased when : kilovoltage is raised, milliamperage is raised, tube-film distance is shortened.

Exposure time must be increased when : kilovoltage is lowered, milliamperage is lowered, tube-film distance is increased.

In selecting an exposure-time for an X-ray examination, the radiographer's choice is affected by the following considerations.

(i) Knowledge of what has been used before, of the performance of the X-ray set in use, and of the practice of the department.

(ii) The need for adequate film density.

(iii) Assessment of the likelihood of subject movement, taking into consideration the state of the patient and the nature of the examination and the body-part involved.

(iv) The assumption that milliamperage and time are in effect inter-changeable.

(v) Knowledge of the way in which alteration in kilovoltage, milli-amperage and tube-film distance modifies exposure-time.

THE SELECTION OF EXPOSURE FACTORS

The foregoing sections have been a discussion of the way in which the exposure factors modify each other. It is clear that certain features of technique and of the subject alter their selection. The choice of exposure factors will now be considered further.

The student doubtless has realized that the selection of exposure factors in radiography is not a precise process limited by exact definitions. Certain general rules are used for guidance and certain features can be standardized in practice—for example tube-film distances, films, inten-sifying screens, and processing procedures. Modern methods of automa-tion both in processing and in exposure techniques are an advance in standardization which cannot fail to aid the radiographer by making procedures more exact. The variables that must be considered, and the several quantities that must be assessed by the radiographer on an empirical basis may make it almost surprising that in practice a reproducible standard of results has long been obtained.

The following factors modify exposure selection.

(i) Type of unit.

(ii) Use of filters.

(iii) Size of field.

(iv) Use of a secondary radiation grid.

(v) Use of intensifying screens.

(vi) Speed of film.

(vii) Developer and development technique.

(viii) Absorption in structures radiographed.

COMPARABILITY OF UNITS

It might be expected that if the controls of two X-ray units are set to give the same factors of milliamperage, kilovoltage, and time they would yield comparable results if the subject and other conditions of operation also are standardized. This is not necessarily so, and in practice it is not possible in transferring factors between X-ray sets to secure precisely similar results in every case. There are various explanations for this.

A distinction has been made between the performance of four-rectifier full-wave sets and sets in which the X-ray tube is supplied with constant potential. The radiation output for every kilovolt and milliamp in the tube factors is improved when the X-ray tube is energized by a voltage which is steady or rippling and is not varying in a cyclical manner from maximum to zero values. Truly constant potential should give better output than potential with a ripple, and both should be better than voltage with the waveform of conventional full-wave and half-wave sets.

So for the same values of kilovoltage and milliamperage and the same exposure-time, a constant potential unit should produce greater image density. It may be noticeable that radiographs produced by such units are somewhat flatter in contrast than those given by units in which the voltage is pulsating. The long wavelengths produced by the low tube voltages of the cycle are eliminated from the beam, and this results in a beam of which the *average* wavelength is shorter for the same tube voltage. The beam is therefore effectively more penetrating; this levels out absorption differences in the subject resulting in lower image contrast.

Now that we have considered the case of constant potential units and four-rectifier units and the differences between their radiographic outputs for a given setting of the controls, the reader may be wondering if there is any difference between four-rectifier units (giving full-wave rectification) and self-rectified units. A four-rectifier generator with its full-wave rectification provides two pulses of current and voltage for the X-ray tube for every one cycle of mains alternation (hence it is called two-pulse equipment). In the same period of time, a self-rectified unit gives one pulse of current through the X-ray tube (hence its description as a one-pulse generator).

There is a fallacious argument which proceeds along these lines. *If the controls for both these sorts of unit are set for the same time of exposure, the same milliamperage and the same kilovoltage, because the self-rectified set is passing current for only half the time that the other does* (one pulse in comparison with two pulses for every complete cycle of mains alternation) *the radiographs exposed on the one-pulse set must have less density than those exposed with the other.* **The italicised statement is in fact erroneous and the radiographs (other factors being equal) could be expected to look similar in density; the radiation output of the two sets in these conditions could be expected to be effectively the same.**

The explanation of the last statements in bold type is as follows. In these X-ray units our knowledge of the milliamperage has been traditionally based upon the reading on a moving-coil milliampere meter. Being energized by a pulsating milliamperage which varies cyclically with the mains alternations, the meter reads the average of many different instantaneous values. It is this average value which radiographers know and discuss as one among what we call 'the exposure factors'.

Now in the case of the self-rectified unit, the peak value reached in the cycle of change is considerably above this average, being about three times greater. In the case of the two-pulse equipment, the peak is much closer to the average, being only about 1·5 times greater. It is this difference in relationship between the average and the peak values that accounts for the similarity in radiographic outputs of the two sorts of X-ray sets when their controls are placed for the same settings. The self-rectified set is passing current for only half the time that the other is but the peak value which the current reaches in its cycle of change is twice as great.

Having said all that, we must admit as an anticlimax that it is all somewhat academic. In practice, which radiographer needs to compare the performances of one-pulse and two-pulse X-ray sets, needs to use the same exposure factors on both or wishes to transfer factors between them?

Where two X-ray sets seem to be comparable (for example both may be conventional full-wave sets) there can still be differences in radiation output, although the controls are set to give the same milliamperage and kilovoltage for the X-ray tube. Control and measurement of tube voltage and tube current are not direct procedures. There are also complexities of voltage stabilization, kilovoltage compensation at different tube currents, space charge compensation to be arranged. It is very likely that two X-ray sets with the same settings on their controls and meters do not operate with precisely identical values in milliamperage and kilovoltage and precisely identical waveforms.

AVAILABILITY OF SELECTIONS

The traditional radiographer had three selections to make: kilovoltage, milliamperage and exposure time (seconds). This independent selection of the three factors is today known as three-component technique.

To modern radiographers other possibilities are available, for some controls offer a two-component technique. One selector is for the kilovoltage and the other is for milliampereseconds: this quantity is the product of the tube current and the exposure time. Such two-component techniques provide a given milliampereseconds as the highest possible current and the shortest possible time, taking into account the rating of the X-ray tube with which the generator is being used.

The third type of selection available removes from the radiographer the need to select exposure factors. It is called programmed automatic exposure control and one pushbutton on the control panel activates the setting of kilovoltage, milliamperage and time. A series of such pushbuttons is marked with anatomical parts and types of examinations and when the radiographer presses a particular button appropriate factors are preselected. To put some flexibility in the system so that it may adjust to patients who are not 'average', there are plus and minus settings which allow 'more exposure' and 'less exposure' to be given. So it is only within this limited range of decision that the radiographer acts.

Any readers who are using only such equipment perhaps need not concern themselves with much of the content of this chapter. They have little need to spend time on the inspired guesswork on which many selections of exposure factors depend.

USE OF FILTERS

A modern X-ray tube is constructed as a glass insert in a ray-proof metal housing. The insert is smaller than its housing, the space between them being filled with oil both for insulation and for cooling. The X-ray beam coming from the focal spot of the tube therefore penetrates the glass envelope of the insert, the oil surround, and the port of the housing. These materials act as a filter on the beam, removing some of the components of longer wavelength. The total effect is described as the inherent filtration of the X-ray tube.

Current codes of practice may require the permanent total filtration of an X-ray tube to be increased above the inherent value. An additional aluminium filter to the X-ray tube is inserted so that the combined effect of this filter plus the filtering action of the tube materials is equivalent to the required level.

The reason for this requirement is that such filtration removes from the X-ray beam the long wavelengths which will be absorbed by the patient's superficial tissues. They do not contribute to the radiographic image of the parts examined, for they are insufficiently penetrating to reach the film, and their sole achievement is to provide the patient with a dose of unnecessary radiation.

Since the radiation being removed from the beam could not reach the film through the patient, the use of such filtration requires no alteration in exposure factors and may be disregarded in selecting them. In some cases, however, there is an appreciable difference to be detected in the *appearance* of radiographs taken with such filtered beams; this is noticeable particularly in the case of extremities radiographed on direct-exposure film. The contrast of the image appears to be less and the radiograph seems much 'flatter'. This may be due less to any reduction in contrast within the image itself as to the fact that the background to the image is greyer in tone. If the soft radiation which the filter removes is left in the beam it can reach those parts of the film not covered by the patient. Being absorbed by the emulsion it serves to enhance the blackness of the surround.

Additional filters, or filters of materials such as copper or iron, may sometimes be added to diagnostic tubes as a special practice. When such filters appreciably reduce the radiation output of the tube to the film they must be taken into account in selecting exposure factors. The increase required will depend on the characteristics of a particular filter and its attenuating action on the beam.

Special filters are sometimes used to solve the problem of subjects which show a wide range of capacities to absorb X rays—for example the dorsal spine in an anteroposterior projection, and the pregnant abdomen in a lateral projection. In these cases a filter might be used which is wedge-shaped, being thin over those parts of the subject which are most absorptive and thick over those parts of the subject which are least absorptive. Inserted at the tube head or placed between the patient and the film, the filter *plus* the subject ensure a more even absorption of the beam. Exposure factors are then selected with the most absorptive parts of the subject in mind.

SIZE OF FIELD

Modern X-ray units are invariably equipped with beam-limiting devices in the form of multi-plane or double-leaf diaphragms. Also provided are radiopaque cones which can be fitted additionally to the tube-head, giving another means of limiting the beam. The use of these is to define the area of irradiated tissue, thus reducing both dose to the patient and the production of scattered radiation.

This reduction in scatter improves the contrast of the image but at the same time lessens its density since less radiation is reaching the film. When a very small field of irradiation is used it is necessary to increase the milliampereseconds factor in the exposure by some amount. The amount required will depend on the restriction of the field and must be determined empirically for the size of diaphragm or cone in use for a particular examination. It may vary from an increase of 25–30 per cent to some much higher value.

USE OF A GRID

The functions of a secondary radiation grid are to transmit primary radiation which forms the image on the film, and to absorb scattered radiation which impairs the distinctness of the image. The efficiency with which a grid performs the first function is known as its transmission efficiency, and its degree of achievement in regard to the second is known as its screening efficiency. The two functions show incompatibility, and a grid with high screening efficiency has less transmission efficiency. When a grid is used exposure factors must be increased, since a result is less radiation reaching the film.

The exact increase required depends on the characteristics of the grid being used, the amount of both primary and secondary radiation which it removes, and the kilovoltage range being employed. It is therefore impossible to give precise figures for adapting exposure techniques to the use of grids. In practice radiographers work by somewhat general rules, without making use of detailed information on the characteristics of the grids in their departments.

As a practical procedure, exposures would be increased by a factor of approximately 3 for a stationary grid; and by factors of approximately 3 to 4 for a moving grid of 6–1 or 8–1 ratio. The change in the exposure factors can be made by increasing the milliampereseconds, or by increasing the kilovoltage, or by a smaller increase in both. Very high ratio grids with high screening but reduced transmission efficiency require a greater increase in exposure. High ratio grids are used only with high kilovoltage techniques which involve special selection of factors and make the use of a grid essential in most cases. In these techniques it is unlikely that radiographers will be required to make comparisons between exposures with and without grids.

The Dupont Bit System to which we have earlier referred can remove at least some of the guesswork to be done if a technique is to be modified by the use of a grid when previously one was not used or by a change to another grid of different characteristics. In the Dupont tables there is a section relating to grid-transmission of the primary beam at 80 kVp. The use of no grid carries a Bit-value of 10. Ranged below 10 in the column are Bit-values assigned to various sorts of grid: these range from 9 Bits for a 60 line grid of 4:1 ratio down to 7 Bits for an 8:1 cross-hatched grid.

Suppose that a technique has been used which is 20 mAs at 80 kVp with the use of a grid which has the characteristics of 60 lines and 6:1 ratio. This has produced a radiograph which is satisfactory in density but is lacking in contrast because of the effects of scattered radiation. So it is decided to improve the technique by using a grid which has the characteristics of 103 lines and 10 : 1 ratio. The question then to be decided is : what increase in milliampereseconds is necessary to compensate for the decreased transmission by the grid which has higher ratio and more lines to the inch?

Looking in the Dupont tables (see Fig. 13.30), we find that for the two grids the Bit-values are :

  60 lines 6 : 1 ratio   8·4 Bits
  103 lines 10 : 1 ratio 8·0 Bits

The difference is :

$$8\cdot4 - 8\cdot0 = 0\cdot4 \text{ Bits}$$

So there is 0·4 Bits to be made up by increasing the milliampereseconds. For a change of 0·4 Bits, the tables show a milliampereseconds-factor which is 1·32 (Fig. 13.29).

So the new milliampereseconds required are :

$$20 \times 1\cdot32 = 26\cdot4$$

TABLE N
GRID TRANSMISSION
(80 kVp)

Ratio	= Bits
None	10.0
4 : 1 60L	9.0
5 : 1 80L. 6 : 1 60L	8.4
8 : 1 80L. 10 : 1 103L	8.0
12 : 1 103L	7.6
5 : 1 Cross Hatched	7.4
16 : 1 80L	7.2
8 : 1 Cross Hatched	7.0

Fig. 13.30 Table N Bit values

It is perhaps worth pointing out to the student that any factor by which the exposure must be increased (sometimes called the grid-factor) when the grid is used is determined by the transmission characteristics of the grid and by the kilovoltage used. The kilovoltage varies the penetrating ability of the radiation emerging from the X-ray tube and this must affect the amount of radiation that the grid transmits. So any firm statement which assigns a value to a grid-factor can strictly be true only for a stated kilovoltage and certainly would not apply for all the kilovoltages used. This is why the Dupont Bit-values which apply to transmission by a grid have a stated kilovoltage (80 kVp) to accompany them.

USE OF INTENSIFYING SCREENS

Intensifying screens and the difficulties in expressing a factor of intensification as a single absolute value have already been discussed in Chapter 5. In practice radiographers are most often concerned with comparing the relative performances of different screens in use in their departments. In doing this they may not undertake any very exact tests, and rely mainly on a simple visual comparison of radiographic results, together with some information from the manufacturer. The radiographs under inspection may be test films made with a stepwedge, or they may be clinical radiographs in examination of a patient. In any case the conclusion reached on the necessary modifications to exposure are neither exact nor inflexible. Some such statement as this might be made: *The new screens are probably about twice as fast as the old, so we can divide the milliampereseconds by 2.* With other conditions of exposure the same, the use of faster screens reduces the milliampereseconds required.

A modern approach to the management of the radiographic image requires stricter evaluation of the speeds of intensifying screens than the above description permits. The use of stepped exposures and a densitometer makes it possible to determine the relative speeds of intensifying screens with sufficient exactness. We refer our readers to tests described in an earlier section of this chapter (see page 347).

SPEED OF FILM

It is doubtless clear to the student by now that the speed of the film used must alter the selection of exposure factors. Faster materials require less exposure to produce the same film density. The advantages in using them are that shorter exposure-times can be employed, better radiographic results can be obtained with X-ray sets of low output, and a smaller dose is given to the patient. As explained in Chapter 3, the speed of X-ray films has not been stated as an absolute value, and in the selection of exposure factors the speed of the film does not appear as a precise quantity.

When using a new X-ray film, the radiographer, aided by information from the manufacturer, compares it with another film the performance of which is already known. For example, it may be said that the new film is twice as fast as the old one; or perhaps that the exposures can be reduced by one-third for the new film. The radiographer then understands that in the first case the milliampereseconds value may be reduced to one-half of that used for a comparable examination with the old film; and in the second case that the milliampereseconds required are two-thirds of the value previously used.

Comparison in performance between the two films may be made by exposures with a stepwedge or based on clinical radiographs. In either case these are usually visual assessments without exact measurements and the required modifications to exposure factors are judged in this way.

Films which differ in speed often differ also in contrast, so that it may be impossible to secure with material of two different speeds results which are exactly comparable. The object of the radiographer's assessment is therefore not so much to decide whether two radiographs are identical, but to determine whether the one made on new film with the new exposure is approximately comparable with the old, and is acceptable in the quality of its image.

In an earlier section of this chapter and also in Chapter 3 we have described how comparisons may be made between the characteristics of different film-materials and how relative film-speeds may be tested.

DEVELOPMENT TECHNIQUE

The effective speed of a film material (as well as its contrast) can be altered by the composition of a developing solution and by the technique of development in use. The effect of development time on the characteristic curve of an emulsion was mentioned in Chapter 3, processing factors in the contrast of the image were discussed in Chapter 12 and developers and their use were considered more fully in Chapter 6. Here it may be sufficient to sum up the situation with general statements, and say simply that important factors are: the constitution of the developer and the activity of the developing agents in it, the degree of exhaustion of the solution, the temperature of the solution, the development time, and the amount of agitation given to the films during immersion in the developer.

Since there are so many variables here which alter both speed and contrast, the radiographer would find it quite impossible to select exposure factors in relation to them if they were not standardized as far as possible. In departmental practice features such as the constitution of the developer, its replenishment against exhaustion, the temperature of the solution, and the development time are standardized in the use of automatic processors.

In manual processing the amount of agitation cannot be standardized and is usually inadequate. The benefits of automation include complete standardization in agitation, temperature, time, and replenishment.

The Dupont Bit System to which we have previously referred has a section in the related tables which is concerned with optimum development. This section assigns Bit-values to the development time (that is, the time of immersion of the film in the developer), to the temperature of the developer and its activity (see Fig. 13.31).

TABLE Q
OPTIMUM DEVELOPMENT
Is Obtained When

Time Bits + Temp. Bits + Developer Activity Bits = 15.0

Developing Time* (Sec.) = Bits	TEMPERATURE (°F) = Bits = (°C)		Developer = Activity Bits
220 = 7.0	106 = 7.4	= 41.0	Cronex® XMD[1] = 5.0
190 = 6.8	104 = 7.2	= 40.0	Cronex® XLD[2] = 4.8
160 = 6.6	102 = 7.0	= 39.0	Cronex® MCD[3] = 4.7
136 = 6.4	100 = 6.8	= 38.0	Cronex® XAD[4] = 4.4
117 = 6.2	98 = 6.6	= 37.0	
98 = 6.0	96 = 6.4	= 36.0	**USES**
86 = 5.8	94 = 6.2	= 34.5	
72 = 5.6	92 = 6.0	= 33.5	1. High contrast 90 sec. & 3½ min.
61 = 5.4	90 = 5.8	= 32.0	
52 = 5.2	88 = 5.6	= 31.0	2. Cine & hand tank.
43 = 5.0	86 = 5.4	= 30.0	3. Medium contrast
38 = 4.8	84 = 5.2	= 29.0	90 sec. & 3½ min.
33 = 4.6	82 = 5.0	= 28.0	
28 = 4.4	80 = 4.8	= 26.5	4. 3½ min. with high
23 = 4.2	78 = 4.6	= 25.5	water temperature
20 = 4.0	76 = 4.4	= 24.5	
17 = 3.8	74 = 4.2	= 23.5	
15 = 3.6	72 = 4.0	= 22.5	
13 = 3.4	70 = 3.8	= 21.0	
11 = 3.2	68 = 3.6	= 20.0	

*Immersion Time; no crossovers

Fig. 13.31 Table Q Bit values

The statement is made that optimum development is obtained when:

$$\text{Time Bits} + \text{Temperature Bits} + \text{Activity Bits} = 15 \cdot 0$$

We find, for example, that immersion in Cronex[R] XMD (5·0 Bits) for 20 seconds (4·0 Bits) at a temperature of 33·5°C (6·0 Bits) sums at 15·0 Bits and should give optimum development.

ABSORPTION IN STRUCTURES

Exposure factors are selected to obtain a good radiographic record of structures under examination. The choice of factors must clearly be modified by the structures themselves, and also by the presence of extraneous materials such as splints and dressings of varying radiopacity; these may range from plaster of Paris which is moderately radiopaque to aluminium or wood or inflated plastic sheaths which are virtually radioparent.

No attempt will be made here to suggest specific exposure factors for given examinations. This is never an entirely satisfactory process. In any case the student obtains knowledge and practice in the selection of factors through experience in the X-ray department; this is more useful than anything written here.

It is already clear that a considerable number of variables modify exposure selection, and by no means the least of these are variations within the subject. Human tissues absorb an X-ray beam to different extents, matter which has high atomic number absorbing it most heavily. The absorption that takes place depends not only upon the nature of the tissue which is traversed but also upon the energy of the X-ray beam, beams of high energy being absorbed less heavily than those of low energy.

In human subjects bone, muscle, fat, and air are all found, and show descending degree of radiopacity, normal bone absorbing radiation to a marked extent, and air showing virtually no absorption. Different structures therefore need different exposure factors (that is different radiation dose) if a radiograph of adequate density, penetration, and contrast is to be obtained.

Where body parts are of the same composition, thick parts absorb more radiation than thin ones and require more exposure (more milliamsvendances and/or kilovoltage). Assessment of thickness alone, however, is not an entirely reliable guide; for example two patients whose trunks appear to be relatively similar in thickness may indeed be very different in radiopacity. One man may have several inches of fat on his torso, and another man several inches of well-developed muscle, the muscular subject requiring greater penetration. Two people of the same weight can be very different subjects radiographically—one may be a healthily developed child, the other a frail old woman in whom age has atrophied muscle and decalcified bone so that little penetration is needed. Even the same subject at different times can show variation. When John Smith is brought into the accident department with a fractured tibia which he has just acquired on the sports field, the structures of his leg absorb radiation much more heavily than they do some weeks later when disuse has atrophied muscle and made the bone osteoporotic. In choosing exposure factors the radiographer applies knowledge of the nature of bodily structures and of disease processes, as well as an understanding of the radiation physics concerned with the absorption of X-ray beams.

It must be understood, however, that a dilemma exists because in selecting exposure-factors the radiographer is choosing conditions of operation for the X-ray tube: that is, the current, the voltage, the time-interval of energization and a tube-film distance. But what counts in the production of the radiographic image is the energy that reaches the film: that is, the exposure-dose which the film receives. *That* is not at all the same as the dose delivered towards the film from the X-ray tube for it is modified by the absorption-pattern which the subject presents; and also by such factors as the size of field, the tube–film distance and the use of a grid as we have mentioned in the preceding pages.

What the radiographer aims to do is to make an informed guess as to the dose that reaches the film from the use of a given set of exposure-factors in a given set of circumstances. With experience the radiographer has a fair chance of obtaining a satisfactory result since in practice the latitude for the guesswork is wide: an error of up to 200 per cent may still give an acceptable radiograph.

Yet clearly a close control of the quality of the image requires that the guesswork should be minimized, for you cannot standardize the skill of human guessers and even with only one guesser you cannot absolutely ensure a consistently reproducible result whatever the exactness of the guesses.

The Dupont Bit System of technique conversion which we have been describing in some of the previous pages minimizes guesswork in the selection and manipulation of technical factors. The tables published by Dupont display Bit-values for all the variables that radiographers must handle, including Bits assigned to the changes required in a radiographic technique because of the presence of pathology: for example, the condition in a bone of healed osteomyelitis requires an addition of 4 Bits while a bone necrosis requires the subtraction of 5 Bits.

This system as has been explained brings all the variables to a common currency and it is based on considerations which relate to the exposure-dose which is required by and is received by the film in a given set of circumstances. Dupont include some suggested Bit-totals as guides: for example, the Bit-total suggested for a lateral view of the lumbar spine is 63·6 Bits. It is claimed that correct exposure exists when:

Kilovoltage-Bits + Milliampereseconds-Bits + Film/Screen-Bits + Grid-Bits + Tube/Film-Bits + Anatomical Thickness-Bits = Guide Bit-total.

The careful formulation of techniques along these lines must help towards ensuring a well-managed, standardized and reproducible result.

Chapter 14

The Presentation of the Radiograph

Correct presentation of the radiograph is an important part of the radiographer's responsibilities, though this is not always apparent to the new student. In the more immediate issues of obtaining correct radiographic positioning and determining acceptable exposure factors we should not lose sight of certain features which can affect the ultimate value of the radiograph to those who use it. What are these features? What is required in a radiograph in addition to an adequate demonstration of the part examined?

Very simply the answer is *identification*. Any radiograph whatsoever should have included on it, preferably in indelible form, the following information.

1   The subject's name and/or record number. If the name alone is used, the surname is insufficient; initials or a first name should also appear.

2   The date on which the radiograph was taken.

3   A correct sign of the right or left side of the subject.

4   If the film is one of a sequence, proper indication of its position in the series; for example, 'control exposure', 'post-micturition', '10-min. after injection' and so on.

To this it is sometimes thought desirable to add:

5   the patient's date of birth.

The provision of this information is properly a charge on the radiographer, for clearly the person who exposes the film is best able to relate it accurately to the part examined, the time or interval of the examination and the identity of the subject. Consequently errors are unlikely to occur if the radiographer in practice and at the time of the film's exposure can record on it its correct identification.

This is not always possible depending on the marking system in use. Nonetheless, the theoretical responsibility remains and the radiographer who will not in fact actually mark the films as they are taken has an indisputable duty to ensure that whoever does mark them has accurate legible data from which to work. One scribbled label accompanying 3 or

4 cassettes into a darkroom is not an adequate discharge of this responsibility. It constitutes an open invitation to error, particularly when another group of cassettes similarly treated arrives simultaneously on the darkroom bench.

To facilitate the proper identification of films a number of systems and devices are generally available.

OPAQUE LETTERS AND LEGENDS

Opaque letters and legends permit the radiograph to be marked by means of the X-ray exposure itself. The letters or numerals may be themselves radiopaque; that is they may be separate lead characters and used to make up any appropriate signal, or they may be painted in lead on Perspex plaques available either individually or already composed into useful legends; for example 'erect', 'supine'. Alternatively the letters or figures may be radioparent on an opaque base, that is, they are incised on a metal square or strip and thus provide dark characters on a clear ground. Some examples of these varieties are shown in Fig. 14.1.

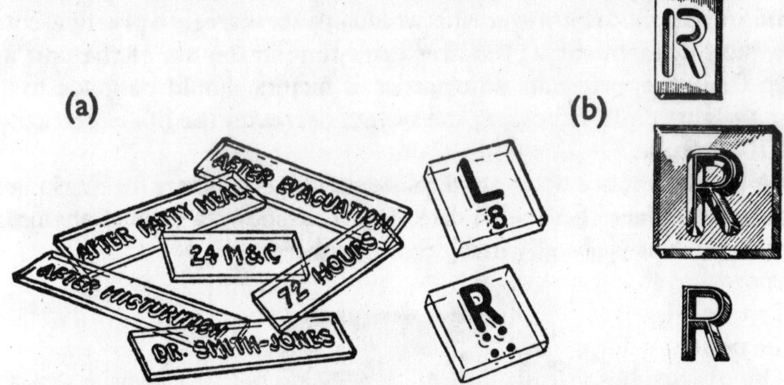

Fig. 14.1. (a) Radiopaque legends and letters for use in marking radiographs. These are engraved on a Perspex base and filled with a radiopaque material. The small character seen under the L and the group of dots under the R are to identify the radiographer. *By courtesy of Cuthbert Andrews.*

 (b) Markers for radiographs.
   Upper: The letter is incised in a thin piece of metal.
   Centre: The letter is lead, mounted in a Perspex plaque.
   Lower: Single lead character.
By courtesy of Picker International Ltd.

In the case of individual characters it is usual to provide two or three small metal frames in which the letters or numerals can be contained. These frames or holders may be suitable for clipping to the edge of a cassette held vertically and for lying flat on the surface of a cassette or direct-exposure film.

Prepared legends of the kind described and the letters R and L for anatomical recognition are useful when correctly employed. They should be fastened to the cassette with adhesive tape before making the X-ray exposure, attention being given to the following points.

1 The character or legend should not be placed in a position where it may obscure a feature of diagnostic importance.

2 If the irradiated field is limited by a cone or collimator to an area appreciably smaller than the dimensions of the cassette, it is useless to place a radiographic marker close to the borders of the latter as it will receive no X-ray exposure and will consequently fail to appear on the film.

It is appreciated that these two considerations tend to be mutually opposed. In order to avoid the possibility of obscuring some significant area of the radiograph it is sensible to place these markers at one edge of the cassette. As a general rule this is correct procedure.

In order to avoid the circumstances described in (2) above, it is theoretically possible to give the area of the cassette which contains the marker a separate X-ray exposure if cover is first provided for the original radiographic field. However, this would appear scarcely a practical course in a busy department. It requires extra time in the use of the unit and, even though appropriate adjustment of factors should be made to give just a slight 'flash' exposure, the system decreases the life expectancy of the X-ray tube.

A better practice no doubt is to use smaller characters for marking the film and to place these with care. Fig. 14.2 shows a typical anatomical marker such as is used by many radiographers.

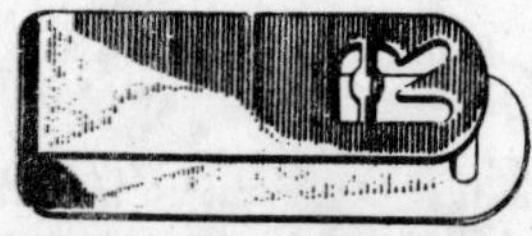

Fig. 14.2 Anatomical marker suitable for placing over the edge of a cassette to record on the film either the R or the L. It can be used in either vertical or horizontal positions. *By courtesy of Picker International Ltd.*

The clip form is generally convenient, particularly when films are taken with the cassette vertically placed. The letters are approximately 12 mm × 9 mm and the dimensions of the clip such that on most cassettes the R or L appears within 5 cm of the film's edge.

However, for say an occipitomental view of the nasal sinuses taken with a localizing cone on an 18 cm × 24 cm cassette, this type of marker is unreliable. It is sometimes visible, for example if the film is badly centred in relation to the patient or from the effects of secondary radiation, but in many cases the letter is not easy to read or is not apparent. Fig. 14.3 shows how a smaller single character may be used to

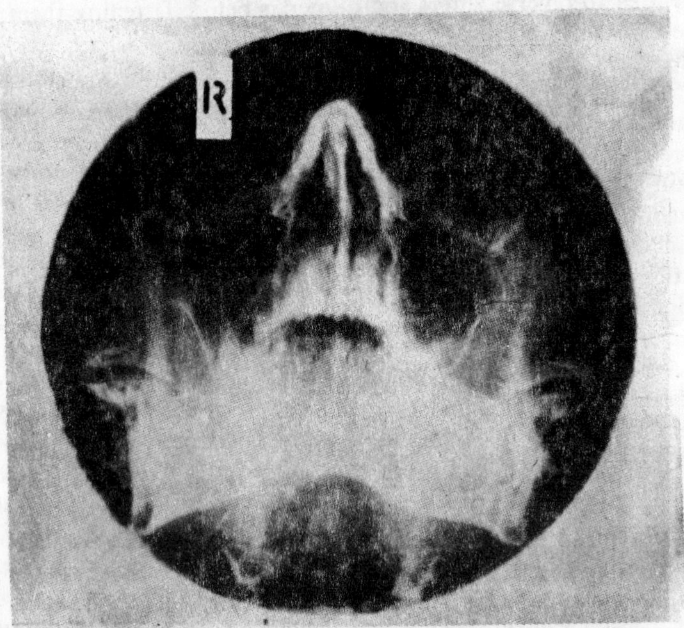

Fig. 14.3. Occipitomental projection, with anatomical identification.

better advantage in these circumstances. Its dimensions are 0·8 in. by 10 mm. Thought must be given to its position in order to avoid overshadowing of important structures; indeed it is true that any marking system needs to be used intelligently.

ANTERIOR PROJECTIONS

The marking of any radiograph for which the anterior aspect of the patient faced the cassette may require special attention. It is usual to present radiographs for report in the correct anatomical position; that is, the subject's left is on the observer's right, and conversely. This means that in the case of posteroanterior or anterior oblique projections the observer must read the film from the aspect which faced *away* from the

X-ray tube during the exposure. If opaque legends of the type described are positioned on the cassette so that they are legible to the radiographer from the tube aspect—and this after all is the natural tendency—then they will not be readable by whoever must report on the appearances, unless the film is first removed from the illuminator and the legend examined from the other side. To avoid this the radiographer should remember to reverse letters and numerals before fastening them to the cassette for any anterior projection.

Markers of the kind shown in Fig. 14.2 are generally available as A.P. or P.A. in type. In the latter the R and L are cut out as a mirror image and are intended to be used for anterior projections in order to avoid the difficulty described above. However, it is well to remember that there are certain disadvantages in having both types in circulation in the department.

So long as only one kind is available there can never be any doubt of the tube aspect of a film and sometimes certainty on this point is needed and indeed of crucial importance. As shown in Fig. 14.2, the tube aspect is bound to be that one from which the R and L is normally readable. It may be believed that certainty of this kind outweighs the slight disadvantage of viewing the letter as a mirror image on anterior projections. The minor difficulty in vision is certainly not of a nature to create confusion between the right and left sides. It must be admitted that in any case the availability of both types of marker does not necessarily ensure their correct use and so entirely preclude the necessity of reading the letter in reverse from time to time. A radiographer in a hurry may fail to observe the type of marker employed, or having second thoughts of the plan of technique—perhaps in the case of a patient who has multiple injuries—may easily forget to alter the marker to match it. In these circumstances the observer might be in doubt over the correct film aspect and the determination of the right and left sides.

PERFORATING DEVICES

Films, and indeed other records, may be perforated with letters or figures as a means of identification. Machines for doing this are available. A simple pliers type may be used for 1 to 3 letters. More elaborate presses cover a larger range of letters and may be suitable for including the date and the hospital's name.

Compared with other marking systems this method appears not very useful. Obviously most applicable when a large number of radiographs has to be marked with the same legend (such as the date or the hospital's identity), the necessity to change letters frequently makes these perforating devices quite unsuitable for names, even in a department which might not be considered very busy.

Rather more handy and reliable is a machine which perforates a lead strip which can be taped by the radiographer to the cassette before exposure. Letters are selected by turning a handle to the required character and pressing it down. The machine will cut the strip on completing the desired word. In this way not only the patient's name or number can be composed but other useful data, such as 'left', 'right', 'prone'. Strips of the latter kind can be used many times before they are discarded.

ACTINIC MARKERS

The use of individual, opaque or other characters to build the patient's name and possibly the date as well and thus record these on his radiograph is a procedure often too time-consuming in many radiodiagnostic departments. In some specialized examinations it may be an applicable method.

For example, such an arrangement might be placed in the exposure area of a rapid film or cassette changer and the information would then be automatically recorded on all films in that patient's series. In this type of case the time required to compose the name and position it suitably on the apparatus is very small in relation to the demands of the whole procedure and the ratio makes the system worthwhile.

However, it is usual for a rapid film changer to include a built-in identification system which prints on the radiographs information typed on a special card, when this is inserted appropriately in the equipment: this marker is able at the same time to record the position of each radiograph in the series exposed.

In general, actinic markers work either like direct printing boxes or like simple cameras and the radiation employed to affect the film is light. Their use in radiodiagnostic departments is almost universal.

An actinic marker, properly employed, has several attractive characteristics, because it:

1 provides permanent identification;
2 is economical of time;
3 shows information neatly and uniformly;
4 reduces the likelihood of error.

Actinic markers require some part of the film, usually a rectangular stip along one edge, to be protected from X rays during the normal radiographic exposure. This is in order to have in an established position on every film an area of unchanged silver halide suitable for receiving the exposure from the marker. Methods of accomplishing this will be considered in a later section.

DIRECT PRINTERS

A typical example of a direct printer is shown in Fig. 14.4 and is similar in principle to a photographer's printing box. If desired it can be sunk in the top of the darkroom bench so that the top of the marker is at a continuous level with the working surface.

The details to be recorded, that is the patient's name and number, the date and other significant information, are first written or preferably typed on a thin sheet of paper, small enough to occupy the window of the box (about 63 mm × 20 mm) and thin enough to be translucent to light. The model shown in Fig. 14.4 has a magnetic bar which holds the titling paper in position over the window and the window itself is illuminated by a safelamp within. These are clearly useful refinements which give the operator greater certainty and thus save time on the procedure.

The undeveloped radiograph is placed on the marker between the

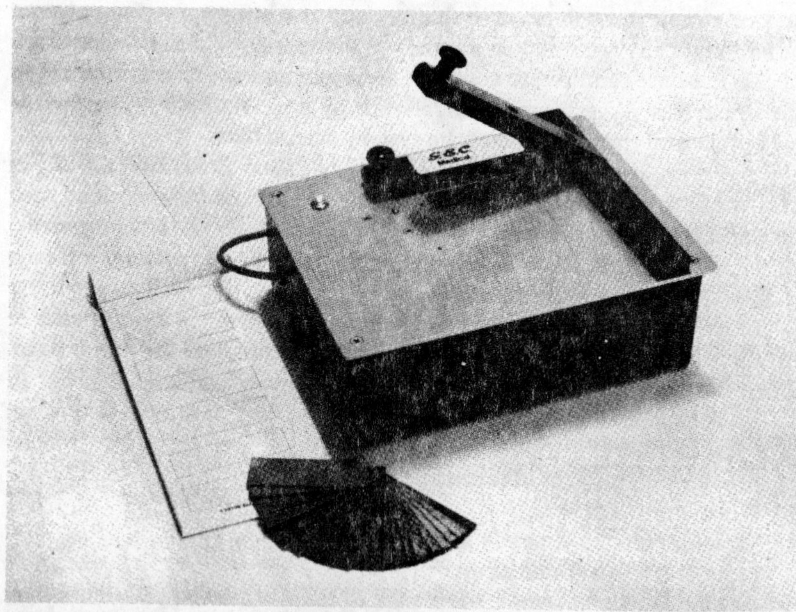

Fig. 14.4. An actinic marker of a printing-box type. Also shown are a pad of titling papers, which can be printed with a hospital's name, and a number of lead blockers for fitting to cassettes. *By courtesy of Picker International Ltd.*

guides so that the protected area of the emulsion lies over the window. The spring pressure pad is them pressed down and this automatically illuminates suitable lamps within the box. The light from these reaches the film through the slip of translucent paper, thus recording on the emulsion any information it contains; the legend will appear white on a dark ground.

In principle the device is admirably simple. In practice certain other features are desirable if the marker is to be fully efficient. These are concerned with the production of a consistent density of background in order to obtain on every radiograph a level of contrast which permits the legend to be easily read by the transmitted light of a standard X-ray illuminator. Variation of this background density obviously will occur with—

(a) variation of the light intensity due to fluctuations in the electrical supply;

(b) variations in emulsion speed of the film to be marked;

(c) variations in processing.

These effects may be such as to make the legend virtually unreadable because the ground is either too faint or too dark.

In order to eliminate the possibility of variations occurring under (a) above, good photographic markers of this simple type should operate from the discharge of a capacitor, which itself is fed from a stabilized supply provided by a neon valve within the unit. A few seconds are required to charge the capacitor prior to every operation but this interval normally occurs in the usual procedure of unloading cassettes and is not noticed by the technician.

Most photographic markers incorporate a control which is adjustable to meet any alteration in film speed. Direct exposure emulsions require exposure to an increased intensity of light and usually there is a specific setting on the marker for these. Equally the trial introduction in any given department of a screen-type film faster than that habitually employed could create difficulties if the marker had no means of reducing the light intensity, nor indeed would it be suitable for supply to a wide range of users. In some cases the potentiometer which provides this flexibility is freely available to the operator. In others it is intended for adjustment by the manufacturer's technician or engineer, either at the time of installation or on any subsequent request.

Variations in processing are not the responsibility of those who manufacture actinic film markers and of course do not normally occur in those departments where automatic systems are employed. However, one type of marker includes in the legend what is called a density reference. This is a small rectangle which will not alter in tone so long as processing is consistent. Its function is detective rather than prophylactic; it does not prevent the occurrence of these density variations but may reveal their source when they are noticed to be present.

The legibility of the information depends both on the background density and the difference between this and the lettering. Ideally, then, the latter should be recorded on the film as an area of no density at all. To this end it is important that the original writing or typing should be adequately black. The use of a ball-point pen is preferable to pencil. An ordinary sheet of carbon paper placed so that its active surface is in contact with the *back* of the titling paper can be used to enhance the opacity of the characters to transmitted light. A black fibre tip pen is helpful, too.

In another printing marker of this kind the required information is written on a special carbon stencil with an empty ball-point pen, preferably upon a hard surface. On the radiograph the legend then appears black on a white ground, since the carbon is opaque to light except where its surface is incised by the style. It is a matter of opinion which form is easier to read.

PHOTOGRAPHIC MARKERS

Actinic markers which photograph the information to be put on the radiograph (in distinction to photographically printing it) are rather more elaborate instruments. Like a camera, an actinic marker of this type has a lens which receives and converges light (in this case from the patient's card), focusing it upon a film (in this case the radiograph).

An opaque card is used instead of a thin sheet of paper and this is placed against a guide, face downwards, on the window of the marker, with the undeveloped radiograph not on top of it but beside it. The card is illuminated from below, as opposed to transilluminated, and its image projected through 180° on to the film. This is done, as shown in Fig. 14.5 by means of two aluminized mirrors each of which reflects the light through 90°. Between the two mirrors is a lens and a diaphragm.

Perhaps an advantage of this principle is that the photographed image may be smaller than the original card. This allows the original to be written more boldly or to have greater content relative to a direct printing device producing a legend of equivalent size.

Like the first one, this marker copies the data in white characters on a black ground. It may have an exposure control for different speeds of emulsion. This control—and we may note again its analogy with the mechanisms of a camera (Chapter 15)—takes the form of variation of the

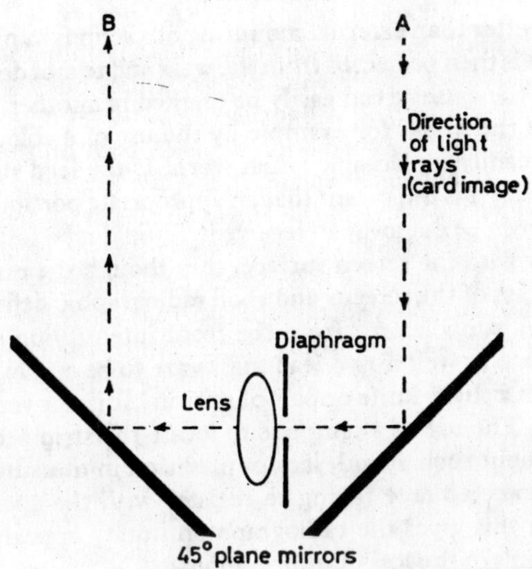

Fig. 14.5. Sketch to illustrate the operation of a photographic marker. The image from a card situated at A is transferred to a radiograph placed alongside the card at B. Control of exposure is obtained by varying the aperture of the diaphragm; this varies the amount of light passing through the lens.

diaphragm aperture and not directly of the exposure's duration which is fixed.

MASKING THE IDENTIFICATION AREA

The employment of any kind of actinic marker necessitates the provision on every film of a clear area which does not receive radiation during the radiographic exposure. This is achieved by the use of a thin lead mask which is mounted in relation to the front intensifying screen in the same position on every cassette. It corresponds in size to the window of the actinic marker and is situated where it is unlikely to obscure any radiographic detail of value, often for example in the lower left or upper right corner.

It is commonly advised that the film be protected from any fluorescence of the back screen as well, by means of either a twin lead strip or opaque adhesive tape. However, the practice is certainly not essential.

It is feasible to mount the principal lead strip on the front of the cassette. This gives clear indication to the user of its position; necessary information if the identification is to appear always in the same position on the radiograph and not reversed top to bottom so that the lettering appears upside down to the observer.

However, better than external mounting of a strip is to place it within the cassette as it is then protected from the wear and tear of daily handling. The outside of the cassette can easily be marked in another way to show the situation of the mask, for example by the use of a coloured label or tape which is readily replaceable when worn. If the lead strip is placed within the cassette it is important that an appropriate portion of the front intensifying screen be cut away to receive it. Should it be fastened simply *on* and not *flush* with the screen surface, thin though the mask is, it will impair the contact of the screens and spoil radiographic definition.

Excision of a suitable area from the front intensifying screen—and from the back one as well if two lead masks are to be employed—can be undertaken with a sharp knife or pair of scissors. It is not very easy work and needs care. The use of a template to locate the strip accurately is a great help. Without such an aid, lack of precision in measurements may result in the protected area failing to register with the aperture of the marker. At best this gives the radiograph an untidy appearance and at worst it may result in the loss of information.

The statement is sometimes made that the use of a lead mask is unnecessary. The rationale of this is that in the exposure of screen film very little activation of the emulsion occurs from the action of X rays; nearly all of it is effected by light. Significant protection of the film can be obtained simply by masking it from the fluorescence of both intensifying screens, usually by means of opaque plastic tape. This undoubtedly simplifies preparation of the cassettes but is bound to diminish the contrast and thus the legibility of the printed legend ultimately obtained. However, it may not be unacceptable. At present some manufacturers of intensifying screens will supply their products with a lead mask already in place on each of the paired screens. The position of the masks is specified by the customer at the time of ordering and their dimensions are appropriate for use with the majority of commercially available actinic markers.

Non-screen film must be effectively masked against X radiation. In this case a lead strip is placed directly on the appropriate edge of the film by the radiographer before making the exposure. Some exposure holders have a lead blocker already in position.

ANTERIOR PROJECTIONS

Reference was made in an earlier section to the mirror-imaging of printed information which occurs when an observer views anterior projections from their correct anatomical aspect. This is true of actinic markers as of others.

The effect can be avoided in printing equipment if the titling paper or plate is reversed right to left in the window of the unit before marking posteroanterior or anterior oblique projections. This manoeuvre of course is not applicable to a photographic marker since—if the card were merely reversed—the lens would 'see' only its blank aspect. Many photographic markers overcome the difficulty by means of a flip switch which places a mirror so that the lens 'reads' a reflection of the data on the card.

Actinic markers were discussed in Chapter 11, with reference to daylight film-handling systems.

IDENTIFICATION OF DENTAL FILMS

The presentation of dental films requires special notice since these should not be marked directly with pencil or by any other means. For convenience of handling they are usually prepared for diagnosis by mounting the series relevant to the examination of a particular patient on a cut-out card or a translucent plastic sheet. The films should be arranged anatomically in accordance with the dental formula given below, with which no doubt the student is already familiar.

$$
\begin{array}{c|c}
& \text{Upper} & \\
8-1 & 1-8 \\
\hline
8-1 & 1-8 \\
& \text{Lower} &
\end{array}
$$

R   L

When the radiographs are placed in this way the observer is looking at the dental images as he would look at the teeth themselves, that is from their outer or buccal aspect. This aspect is also the tube aspect of each film.

Dental films are stamped with a circular embossment in one corner. This is convex on the surface which faces the X-ray tube during the exposure and consequently these radiographs should be fixed in their mount so that the 'pip' is towards the operator. It is usual when making dental X-ray examinations to insert film in the mouth so that the embossed corner is coronal in direction rather than apical; and as each is taken to place it on the appropriate clip of the developing hanger in the correct anatomical position with the embossed projection facing the radiographer. This order should be maintained in the darkroom during processing.

If this technique is observed subsequent preparation of the films is a simple process of transferring each to a similar situation on the mount. However, if they should have become disordered it is not difficult to identify the upper and lower jaws if it is remembered that in respect of the lower jaw:

1   the bone trabeculae make a horizontal pattern;
2   usually the shadow of the mandibular canal can be seen;
3   the molars have two roots.

In radiographs of the upper jaw the following evidence may be sought:

1   air-filled cavities, due to the nasal translucency in the central incisor region and the maxillary antrum in relation to the distal teeth;
2   triple roots to the molars.

DENTAL MOUNTS

Mounts are frequently of the slide-in type similar in principle to some photographic mounts. Films can be slipped into position behind apertures of an appropriate size in a rigid card. These cards are available in a number of formats which hold from 1 to 14 dental films arranged in the main horizontally; some of the apertures may have the long axis vertical to conform with common radiographic practice in examining upper incisor and canine teeth with films so placed. Space is available on the mount for completion with the patient's name, the date and perhaps other details such as his hospital number and the name of the referring consultant.

Another type of mount is a plain, thin sheet of cellulose acetate, one surface being matt and the reverse aspect glossy. Held up to any source of light, for example even the window of a dental surgery, it transmits a diffuse regular illumination such as would a piece of ground glass. These sheets are available in sizes suitable for containing either one or two dental films or a number sufficient for examination of the whole mouth. Alternatively the material can be purchased in greater area—approximately 600 mm × 700 mm—and cut as the user requires.

Radiographs can be fixed in position on this mount by means of an ordinary manuscript stapler. However, this method is not ideal since it may be difficult to put the staples where none will obscure radiographic detail. A better device is a special dental mount cutter.

This little machine has a cutting head under which the cellulose acetate sheet is placed. On depression of an operating lever, four semicircular incisions are made. These are appropriately spaced so that the corners of a standard sized dental film can be inserted through them and the film thus maintained in any desired position on the front of the mount; the pages of a photographic album are often similarly ordered to accept a standard size of print. The cutting head can be rotated to allow the format of the radiograph to be either vertical or horizontal. The patient's name and other details can be written easily with a lead or 'Stabilo' pencil or a ball-point pen on the matt surface of the mount.

PREPARATION OF STEREORADIOGRAPHS

Radiographs which are taken as a stereoscopic pair present special problems of identification, mounting and viewing, particularly as there is no standard practice in regard to their marking and there are currently several methods of viewing these films.

The theory and technique of stereoradiography are not properly within the scope of this book but a simple re-statement of principle may be useful to the student at this point. Our normal, three-dimensional vision depends on the fact that the retina of each eye has a slightly different viewpoint of any object at which we look. In stereoradiography a pair of radiographs is taken. These are identical to each other in all features—and this must include factors of speed and processing—except that between the two exposures the X-ray tube is moved under conditions which make its focal spot correspond in turn to each eye of an observer looking directly at the patient. These films are then viewed simultaneously in the following way.

(a) The right eye looks only at the radiograph taken when the tube was shifted in a direction which is defined as the right.

(b) The left eye looks only at the radiograph taken when the tube was shifted in a direction which is defined as the left.

The two images become fused in a single impression which appears to the observer to be three-dimensional. He has an awareness of depth and 'reality' in the appearances recorded, which enables him to differentiate the levels of structures otherwise superimposed on a plain radiograph. Stereoradiographs are necessarily viewed under particular conditions, often by means of special equipment. In their correct presentation for radiological report we must consider first how properly each of the pair of films is to be identified, and secondly how they should be mounted and viewed together.

MARKING STEREORADIOGRAPHS

In addition to the customary identification of the patient, a stereoradiograph preferably should carry two markers. One of these must indicate the anatomical right and left while the other refers to the right or left shift of the X-ray tube: this specifies equally the eye with which the film is meant to be viewed; it is erroneous to believe that the designation is equated with the patient's right and left. All confusion will be avoided if the second of these markers in fact is a complete legend and states 'R stereo' or 'L stereo'.

Where such legends are not available, the radiographer may adhere to the convention that the first letter on the radiograph is anatomical in reference and the second visual. Thus, a left shoulder taken with a right shift of the tube should carry the letters LR in the upper right corner; the film which resulted from the left shift would be marked LL in the same place.

If only one marker is available it can be used to perform both functions. That is to say, the letter R is used for the right tube shift and placed on the right of the patient; it is then changed for the letter L which is put on the patient's left during the exposure from the left shift of the tube. This is satisfactory when the examination relates to the trunk and head, but should it be of a limb the system must result in one of the pair of films being unmarked. The left tube shift cannot be indicated when a right limb is examined nor can the image be anatomically signed; and vice versa for the other side.

However, it may be felt that the absence of a marker is less confusing than the appearance on some of these films of both L and R, particularly to an observer who is not trained in radiology and perhaps is unaware that a stereoradiographic study has been made. A preference for either of these practices can be well justified and students meet different methods current in individual departments.

IDENTIFICATION WITHOUT MARKERS

While we may properly require stereoradiographs to be marked by the radiographer at the time of exposure, the circumstance is neither impossible nor altogether unknown that such a pair of films may require identification at a later stage, because markers have been omitted, or are not visible, or appear to have been incorrectly used.

To make such identification the only essential is to have firm evidence of the tube aspect of the films concerned. When this is obtainable, the processed dry radiographs should be held to some light source with their tube aspect facing away from the examiner; they are placed one in front of the other so that their edges register. It will be seen that the images are not coincident but are laterally out of alignment. The film on which the image is further to the left is that taken with a left shift of the tube and intended for viewing by the left eye. Conversely the image which has moved to the right indicates the right stereoshift and should be viewed by the right eye. It is to be emphasized that for this determination to be correct the tube aspect of each radiograph should be turned away from the investigator.

VIEWING STEREORADIOGRAPHS

In order to have perception of depth, various methods are available for viewing stereographs. However, before considering these, some attention should be given to the direction from which the films are viewed and the significance of this on the impression received.

In the process of ordinary photography the details which appear in an image can only be those that are on the same side of the subject as the camera. From a stereoscopic pair of photographs we can obtain one view only: that is, a front view if the camera was in front of the subject.

However, this is not true of radiography. The ability of an X-ray beam to penetrate matter results, as we know, in recording on the film all layers of the subject. Detail in a radiographic image is composed of structures both near to and further away from the X-ray tube. Thus, in an anteroposterior projection taken stereographically we have the choice of ultimately viewing the subject either from the front or from the back.

If we look at the anteroposterior projection from the front, that is from the same point of view as the X-ray tube, we describe the effect as *orthoscopic*. If we look at such a radiograph from the back, that is in a direction counter to that of the X-ray beam, we call the image *pseudoscopic*. There is nothing complicated about this procedure. The reversal of direction is obtained, as would be expected, simply by turning over each of the films and looking at them from the other side.

We may take, for example, the anteroposterior projection of the sacro-iliac joints made stereoradiographically. If we look at this pair of films as though we were occupying the position of the X-ray tube the pubic symphysis will appear nearer to us than the sacrum. If we reverse the aspect of the radiographs which faces us, so that we are now examining them from somewhere underneath the X-ray table, the patient's sacrum seems closer than the region of the symphysis.

In summary we can say that an orthoscopic image is obtained from the same direction as the exposure was made; while a pseudoscopic image represents a viewpoint counter to the direction of exposure.

Similarly to other radiographs, it is usual to view stereoradiographic films from the anatomical aspect. This means that anteroposterior projections will be examined orthoscopically and posteroanterior projections as a rule pseudoscopically. However, the ability to obtain both viewpoints from a single projection can be useful. Confirmation of the depth of a lesion which continues to be a little doubtful may sometimes be obtained if further observation is made from the aspect not employed before.

In stereoradiography, transposition of the subject, as in a mirror image, will occur if the film intended for viewing by the right eye in fact is seen by the left eye, and vice versa. This will make an orthoscopic image of the right limb appear as a pseudoscopic image of the left limb and is clearly rather a dangerous occurrence, particularly in relation to the head and trunk. It is caused either initially by incorrect marking of the stereoradiographic pair or later by mounting them on the wrong sides of the viewing apparatus.

Films which become reversed in aspect as well as being interchanged in position as regards right and left are probably more dangerous still. They remain in their proper presentation—orthoscopic or pseudoscopic as the case may be—but are again a mirror image in appearance, the right side of the patient seeming to be his left.

Stereoradiographs may be viewed with either a binocular stereoscope or direct vision.

THE BINOCULAR STEREOSCOPE

Stereobinoculars are similar in appearance to opera glasses. The films to be viewed are placed side by side on conventional illuminators, the right stereoradiograph being on the observer's right and the left one on his left. Prisms in the binoculars reflect and also refract the light, the latter phenomenon assisting in the convergence of the images. However, it must be remembered that it is a reflection of the radiographs which is seen and if anatomical transposition is to be avoided their normal viewing aspect must face away from the observer.

DIRECT VISION

With guidance and practice many people can 'see' stereoradiographs in three dimensions without the aid of special viewing equipment and without incurring any sensations of strain. For those who can master it this is a quick and economical method and further has the advantage that the films can be read in any place where no more than conventional X-ray illuminators are available.

The radiographs to be examined should be placed side by side on the viewing area, their edges touching. The right stereoradiograph is put on the observer's left: he will look at it with his right eye. The left stereoradiograph is put on the observer's right: he will look at it with his left eye. Since no optical instruments are involved, other than the eyes, the normal viewing aspect of the radiographs should be presented to the observer.

He will begin the manoeuvre by standing at some convenient distance away from the illuminator and looking first at his own forefinger which is extended in front of him at arm's length and in the midline between the radiographs. He should not at this stage focus his eyes on his finger but should stare into the distance. A dual image will be apparent, and after a little time a third image which is smaller than the others and at a nearer distance.

When this is seen the observer should attempt to superimpose the images by converging his lines of sight; patients in the orthoptic department are familiar with this type of exercise, and in those who have had to practise it the ability seems to remain within easy recall. When he is successful in perceiving only the one, slightly reduced image the observer should remove his finger and keep his gaze on the radiographs, on which he should now focus. There should be no difficulty in seeing a single image of these and in obtaining the impression of depth.

Fig. 14.6 illustrates the positioning of the radiographs, the convergence of the observer's lines of sight and the production of the stereoscopic image in a plane within the shaded parallelogram.

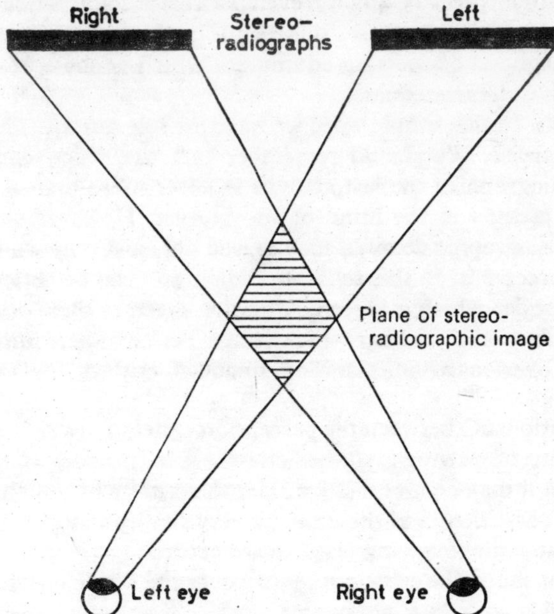

Fig. 14.6. Method of viewing stereoradiographs with unaided sight.

DOCUMENTARY PREPARATION

In preparing radiographs for diagnosis, if the first necessity is correct identification the second is that the films should be properly documented: that is, they should be accompanied by their envelope, the patient's request form, radiological history and any previous radiographs. Record-keeping systems vary to some extent between departments and it is not within the scope of this book to describe them fully nor attempt their evaluation. Students in the course of training no doubt have the opportunity of becoming thoroughly familiar with the practice in their own hospitals and of appreciating how valuable a really efficient system is. Frequently adhesive coloured labels or printed numbers may be put on radiographs and their envelopes so that in the reporting room those of a particular examination can readily be related to others of a specific date. Colour coding of this kind can be adapted to the indexing of pathology or to the indication of other information which any centre may find desirable.

VIEWING CONDITIONS

It has been said, perhaps with some truth, that while thousands of pounds are often spent on highly refined apparatus in order to produce radiographs of impeccable quality, even perhaps at some paticular instant in a rapid physiological phase, these same radiographs may ultimately come for diagnosis on viewing equipment which is not up-to-date and sometimes is quite inadequate.

Diagnosis. In this simple word we have the sole purpose of the whole complex exercise. We should remember that the effectiveness of any medical radiograph in the last analysis is never more than a subjective impression created in the mind of an observer. However delicate and precise is radiographic detail, it may as well not exist if he who is to read it cannot perceive it. In this sense no radiograph can be better than the conditions under which it is seen. Attention given to these conditions is a real contribution to radiographic quality. Perhaps their importance is sometimes overlooked in planning financial outlays for radiological departments.

The relationship between the perception of detail in a radiograph and the conditions of viewing is studied elsewhere in this book (Chapter 12). At this point it may be useful to consider the criteria by which we would judge these conditions and these can be very simply stated. In a good X-ray illuminator the following features are needed.

1   The light should be even in intensity over the whole viewing surface.
2   It should be as 'white' as possible.

3   The source of light should not heat the radiograph even if this remains over it for a considerable period of time.

4   The facility of varying the brightness of the illumination should be available.

Most reputable illuminators at the present time provide a diffuse regular lighting of a suitable standard. For radiographs of medical subjects the light source is most likely to be two 15 watt fluorescent tubes. A reflecting surface, for instance white enamel, is placed behind the light source.

Some types of illuminator may be powered by a group of four or six standard pearl lamps of 40 to 60 watts. These do not show the tendency to flicker which may sometimes be associated with lighting from a fluorescent tube, nor is there any delay in the appearance of the illumination when the unit is first switched on. However, they are probably less satisfactory than fluorescent tubes. Lamp bulbs inevitably become hot in use and the viewing box requires adequate ventilation and perhaps has to be larger if it is to remain cool. Further, the tone of the light tends to be warmer; it has not the blue-white 'daylight' quality provided by some fluorescent tubes which is especially suitable for viewing the radiographic image.

Fluorescent tubes of course can vary in the 'colour' of white light produced. This point should be borne in mind when replacing them, particularly if they are not obtained from the original suppliers of the illuminator but are requisitioned from the electrician's stores in the hospital. In a single illuminator one tube should be the twin of the other, and, where a number of illuminators are banked together on a wall or desk to make a large viewing area, all must match. A disconcerting difference of appearance results when two radiographs of a series are mounted adjacently in lighting of dissimilar quality. This is particularly prone to mislead should a strict comparison have to be made, for example to assess the progress of a lesion in the chest or between a pair taken of the mastoid regions. Ideally, all the illuminators in a hospital should be alike, but these optimum conditions are rarely achieved and maintained.

To compensate for inequalities which may be due to ageing of the tubes, incorrect replacement or even to the presence of strong cross lighting, a 'light trimmer' device is available on certain viewing units which are composed from 2, 3 or 4 individual panels. This gadget provides for matching both intensity of light and its colour value.

In the appreciation of detail in underexposed or overexposed areas of a radiograph the usefulness of varying the brightness of illumination has been described in Chapter 12. This may be done in three ways.

1   A variable switch on the illuminator may alter the intensity of light

over the whole viewing area. This has the advantage that some positions generally are arranged to give lower than 'normal' brightness. These assist visualization of a radiograph which may suffer from some degree of underexposure, for example a study of the chest made on the ward with a portable unit.

2   A spot-light operated by a hold-on switch may be mounted in the viewer and provide a localized illumination of high intensity. In certain viewers which are intended mainly for industry and are otherwise powered by two parallel rows of conventional hot filament bulbs, this may take the form of a Photoflood lamp situated in the centre of the field. Adjustable masks can be closed down to the area of extreme brightness in order to avoid dazzle. Sometimes the film may be moved about on a counterbalanced carriage in order to bring any area of the radiograph over the central lamp. Alternatively the spot-light may be outside the main field of illumination; it is sometimes found for example on the right hand side of the front frame of the viewer.

3   An entirely separate source of high intensity illumination may be used in conjunction with illuminators which do not themselves provide for any variation. This may be a thoroughly organized piece of apparatus with a built-in variable iris diaphragm to alter the diameter of the field from about 10 cm down to less than half a millimetre or nil. On the other hand a much simpler arrangement often gives adequate service, for example an Anglepoise lamp or even a plain unshaded pearl bulb.

In a radiological reporting room a number of illuminators are often grouped together on a wall to form an area where a series of radiographs may be examined and more easily compared without the recurrent need to change their position which a single illuminator entails. In operating theatres a smaller row is quite often used in a similar way and in this case the illuminators are usually mounted so that the front panel is flush with the wall surface. The seal may be water-tight to facilitate hosing of the wall, and even gas-tight and the switches spark-proof as a precaution against risks of explosion from inflammable anaesthetic vapours.

It is important when a number of illuminated panels are arranged like this that independent switching for each of them should be provided; otherwise if only one or two films are being examined there will be considerable dazzle from the unused areas. This is likely to impoverish radiographic quality.

The fronts of X-ray illuminators are necessarily of a ground glass or 'pearl' character. They may be either glass itself or Perspex. Because of the ease with which it acquires a static electric charge Perspex is not suitable for illuminators used in the operating theatre. In the X-ray department it is of course hardier than some glass but more difficult to keep free of dust. A fluid designed to prevent the formation of static electricity is available for cleaning this type of panel. All illuminators should be regularly cleaned if they are not to lose efficiency.

VIEWING FLUOROGRAMS

Many 100 mm fluorograms are viewed without magnification. In this case, if a standard X-ray illuminator is used it is better if a mask can be provided in order to prevent dazzle from the large brightly lit area behind the film. This mask can be a very simple device; perhaps a 35 cm × 43 cm sheet of opaque card or thin plywood in which an aperture 100 mm × 10 mm has been cut. Built-in masking devices no longer appear to be a feature of illuminators designed for medical radiography, although they are usual in industrial models which must provide a high intensity light source for viewing much greater densities.

Equipment for enlarging 100 mm cut film is available and its use may be desirable in some cases, particularly when the observer is long sighted. Two types of enlarger are shown in Figs. 14.7 and 14.8.

In Fig. 14.7, the 100 mm image is projected onto the back of a fine grain opal glass screen to the dimensions of a full sized radiograph. It can easily be viewed by several people simultaneously. In a double model of this kind two 100 mm fluorograms can be analysed side by side, or one miniature can be compared with a direct radiograph placed on the companion screen. This facility if obviously helpful when progress of a case must be assessed.

Smaller models give magnification of the order of 1·5 to 1·9. Fig. 14.8 shows a typical example in which three 100 mm films can be examined together; alternatively the slide at each side can be used to cover one or two thirds of the illuminated area if these are not required. The magnifying glass can be moved into position over any one of the films or moved away from the field altogether if the operator has no need of it. This device includes an 'In' and an 'Out' tray for films that are waiting to be read and those on which the report has been completed.

Other small viewers may accept either a single 100 mm radiograph or a roll of 70 mm film.

Projectors are available for 70 mm film which can satisfactorily enlarge the image either up to about 150 mm square or, if preferred, up to full size. When the intention is to read miniature radiographs by projection rather then directly from a viewer, it is necessary to provide a suitable screen in the reporting room. This need not be elaborate or expensive. For example a sheet of white card of an appropriate size could be fixed to an empty area of the wall and the reader seated at a table some convenient

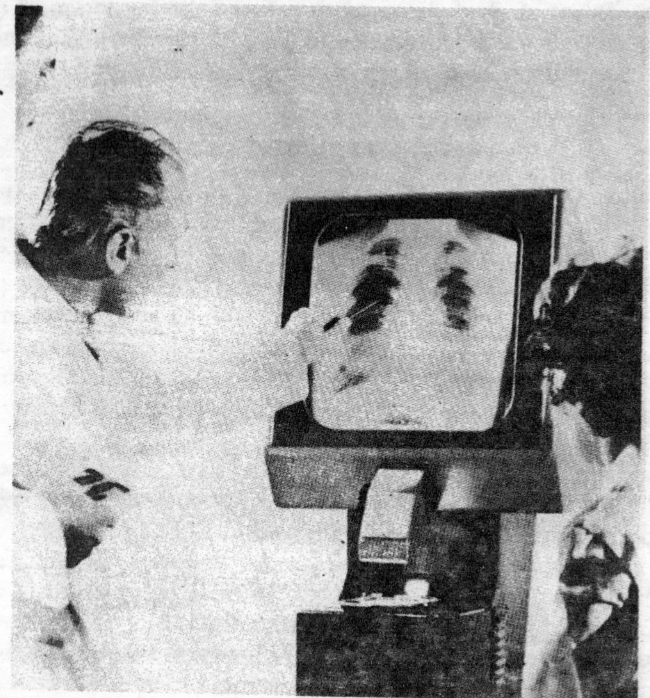

Fig. 14.7. A projector giving full-size enlargement of a 100 mm fluorogram. *By courtesy of N.V. Optische Industrie, de Oude Delft.*

distance away, with the projector beside him. However, viewing screens apart from this do-it-yourself variety are of course available and in some cases may be supplied with the projector.

CINEFLUOROGRAMS

The equipment necessary for viewing cinefluorograms is not essentially different from that used for other forms of cinematography.

A useful addition is the facility to project a loop of film. This means that a length of film which shows a self-contained sequence of events— for example the cardiac cycle as it is demonstrated in angiography—is joined end to end and may be continuously projected, the finish of each cycle being immediately followed by its beginning through as many repetitions as the observer wishes. This type of study is an obvious aid when interpretation is difficult and in all teaching.

The projection of 35 mm cine film presents some problems. Properly

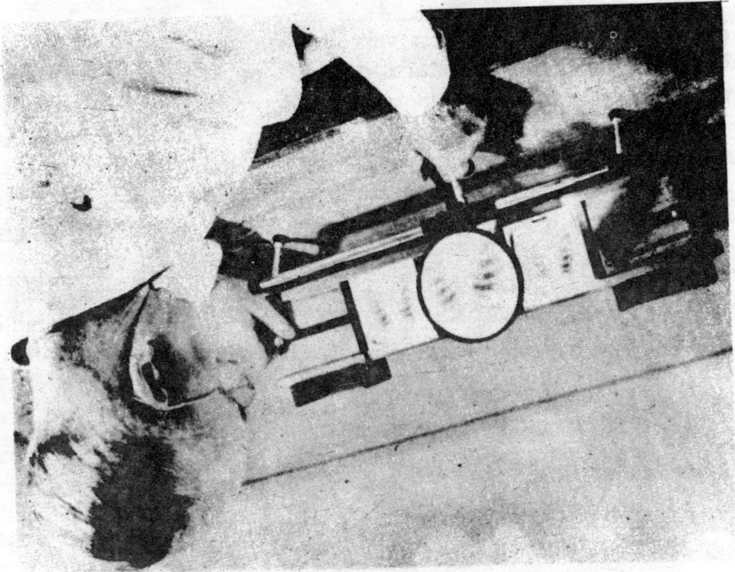

Fig. 14.8. A viewer for examination of up to 3 × 100 mm fluorograms simultaneously. *By courtesy of Picker International Ltd.*

it requires bulky equipment of the kind suitable for cinemas. Apart from the difficulty of handling this in the X-ray department, the use of such projectors is controlled in some countries by legislation. Because of these features the viewing of 35 mm cinefluorograms is usually by means of an apparatus intended for editing such film.

Unlike the upright arrangement of the conventional projector, in this machine the film travels *horizontally* between two spools. As normally the vertical axis of each frame runs lengthwise on cine film, the optical system of the editor turns the image through 90 deg. It thus appears in correct aspect to an observer seated in front of it; he is spared the necessity of himself adopting a horizontal position.

Films can be run in either direction through the editor at any speed from zero to 24 f.p.s. The motion can be halted or reversed as the observer wishes. A counting device makes it possible to give to any interesting frame or sequence a numerical index, by means of which, once noticed, its position on the reel can readily be found again.

In some 16 mm projectors the minimum rate of projection is 16 f.p.s. This means that the camera's speed of taking must be at least this, and if a slow-motion analysis is to be made it will in fact have to be higher, with concomitant problems of radiation dose and electrical load. The possibility of operating the film editor at very low running speeds offers some advantage in making the production of slow motion studies technically easier. For example, a film exposed at no more than 16 f.p.s. might be shown at 5 f.p.s. with the effect of slowing down the motion by 70 per cent. This machine undoubtedly possesses increased tendency to flicker compared with conventional types of projector, although perhaps it is not unduly obtrusive in radiographic subjects and consequently of little importance.

The image is projected by the editor on to a metal screen, painted white, which is about 200 mm × 250 mm in size and is a self-contained part of the unit. It is not easy for more than one or at most two persons to look at this screen together, since the best position for viewing is to be seated directly behind the editor at 90 deg. to the projection area. However, this screen can be removed and thus a longer throw and a bigger image obtained if examination by a larger group or more prominent demonstration of detail becomes necessary. In this event a conventional cine screen at some appropriate distance would be used; the screen might be, for example, about 100 cm × 100 cm.

The editor is normally powered by a 12 volt, 100 watt lamp and in a darkened room this gives adequate illumination of the small screen. However, when the intention is to enlarge the image to some further extent the strength of the lighting is insufficient: 250–300 watts at least would be required. The lamp housing is cooled by a small fan beneath the unit: cooling is likely to become a problem if a much higher power of lighting is sought.

Paramount in maintaining their efficiency is regular cleaning of all viewing instruments, whether projectors and illuminators or screens. Perhaps particular emphasis of this is required for the X-ray department where only occasional use may be made of such equipment. Once apparatus has become very dusty its restoration to freshness is much more difficult. For glass, other than front-surfaced mirrors, a lint-free cloth and methylated spirit are effective. A soft-haired brush is also useful for this work.

SPECIALIZED ILLUMINATORS

In the course of various types of specialized radiographic experience the student is likely to encounter X-ray illuminators which have certain different features to make them suitable for particular work. There are small ones, for example, which are intended for the examination of a dental series; or we may contrast the needs of 35 cm roll film used in certain serial changers for angiography.

Again, a demonstration or conference room may require a viewing unit working on the paternoster system, and perhaps motor driven, on which a very large number of radiographs can be mounted prior to their use in illustrating a lecture.

In sorting rooms, or whenever measurements must be made or lines drawn on a radiograph, for example in procedures designed to localize a foreign body, it is of some advantage to have an illuminated panel horizontally placed and flush with a working surface.

It will be appreciated by the student that the specially adapted features of any of these are quite apart from the fundamental design of all good viewing equipment. In this chapter our discussion has been mainly directed towards an understanding of these essential principles.

Chapter 15
Light Images and Their Recording

This book began with a reference to the production of an optical image, by means of visible light and a lens. It is necessary now to consider optical images a little further, so that we may understand the processes of recording the visible light images which are produced from a phosphor when an X-ray beam irradiates it, in the effect known generally as fluorescence (see Chapter 5, p. 90). The terms *fluorography* and *photofluorography* are descriptive of the procedure of using a camera—of which there are several suitable varieties—to record a fluorescent image.

All cameras require a lens, or optical system of similar effect which will form an image—in this case, of the appearances on a fluorescent screen—in accordance with certain principles of optics. It is these principles with which we are now concerned. Fluorography will be further considered in the next chapter.

THE FORMATION OF LIGHT IMAGES

When light falls on an object three main effects may occur, to a greater or lesser degree.

1   It may be absorbed.

2   It may be reflected; that is, it will reappear on the same side of the object as it originated.

3   It may be transmitted; that is, it will pass through the object or material in question. In the context of photographic optics the last two are of immediate significance; particularly of course the transmission of light through glass since it is upon the characteristics of this that the ability of a lens to form images depends.

REFRACTION

When a ray of light is transmitted through one medium into another of different density—for example from air into water or glass—its direction is generally altered. This is not true of the *normal* ray, that is for a beam at right angles to the receiving surface. In all other cases the beam appears to bend as it passes from one medium into the other. The phenomenon should be known from many practical instances occurring in everyday life, for example the apparent distortion of a stick thrust at an angle into clear water. The effect is illustrated diagramatically in Fig. 15.1. In a general statement we may say that light passing obliquely from a rare into

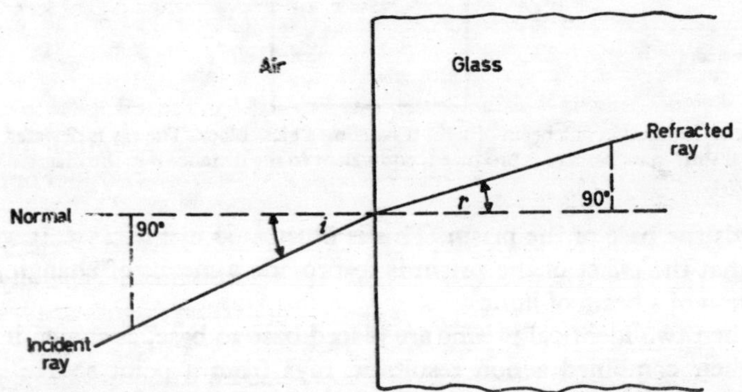

Fig. 15.1. Refraction of a ray of light passing from a rare medium (usually air) into a denser one such as glass. The ray of light is bent nearer to the normal (a line at right-angles to the surface on which it is incident); the angle *r* is smaller than the angle *i*. *By courtesy of Ilford Ltd.*

a denser medium is bent *towards* the normal: rays are reflected *away* from the normal when their passage is from a dense into a rarer medium. These effects are known as *refraction.*

When refraction is studied in more detail by means of light passing through a glass block which has parallel sides it is found that the oblique beam is refracted twice. As we would expect, on entering the glass it is bent towards the normal at the point of incidence: on leaving, the deviation of the ray is away from the normal. This state of affairs is depicted in Fig. 15.2.

It will be noticed that the effect of the second part of the process is to balance the first. This means that though it has been shifted laterally by its passage through the glass, the light leaves the block in the same direction as it entered.

A somewhat different result is obtained when the experiment is applied not to a rectangular block of glass but to a triangular prism. Here the refracting surfaces of the glass are not parallel but at an angle to each other. In these circumstances the light is bent as before on entering the glass and bent again on leaving it but in the same direction, that is

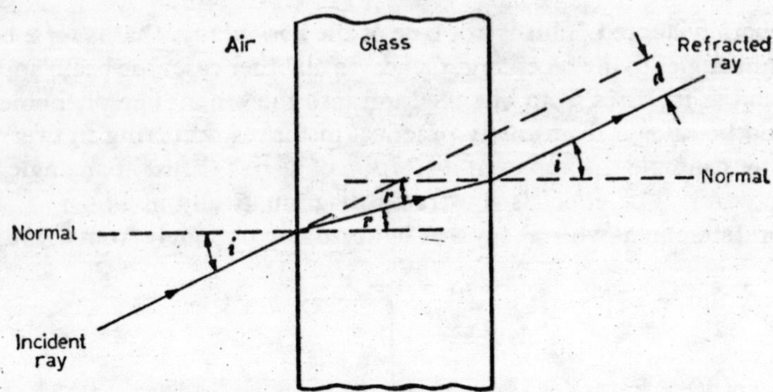

Fig. 15.2. Refraction of a beam of light traversing a glass block. The ray is deviated twice. A lateral shift in its passage is produced, equivalent to the distance *d* in the diagram. *By courtesy of Ilford Ltd.*

towards the base of the prism. This is illustrated in Fig. 15.3 It will be seen that the effect of the prism is to provide a means of changing the direction of a beam of light.

When two identical prisms are placed base to base, as shown in Fig. 15.4 their combined action results in rays from a point source being brought together again at another point some distance from the prism.

This is the way in which a simple converging lens operates. It can be considered as a series of prisms. (Fig. 15.5). Any light reaching such a system may conveniently be considered as having emanated from a large number of point sources covering the surface of the object, each such point being similarly imaged. It can be depicted here only two dimensionally.

REFLECTION

When a surface reflects light it may do so in a diffuse way or directly. To our present study of optics only the latter is important.

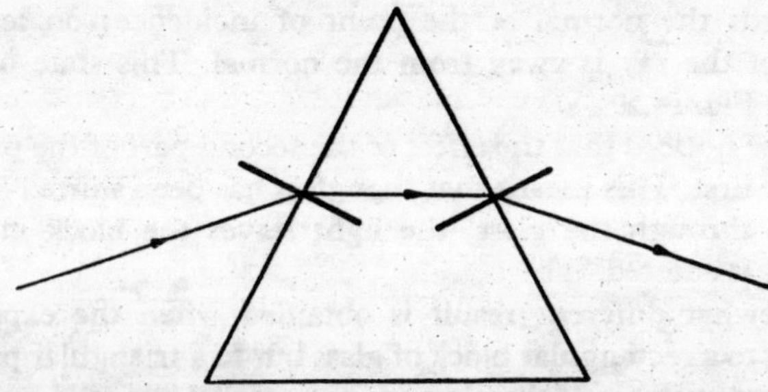

Fig. 15.3. Refraction of a beam of light traversing a triangular prism. In this case the direction of the beam is changed. *From The Science of Photography (H. Baines) by courtesy of The Fountain Press.*

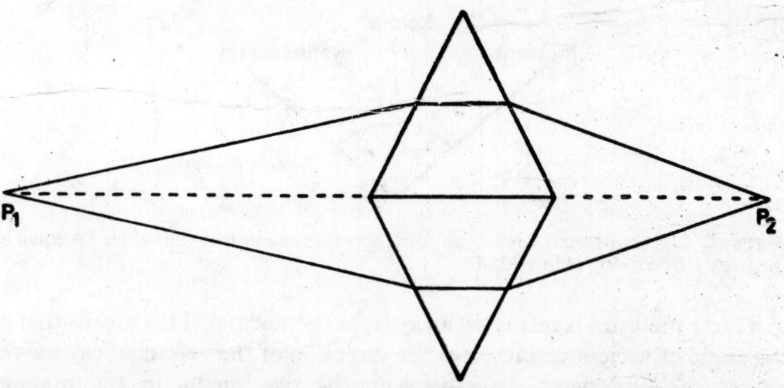

Fig. 15.4. Two identical triangular prisms placed base to base will bring light rays from a point source (P$_1$) together again at another point (P$_2$) some distance beyond the prisms.

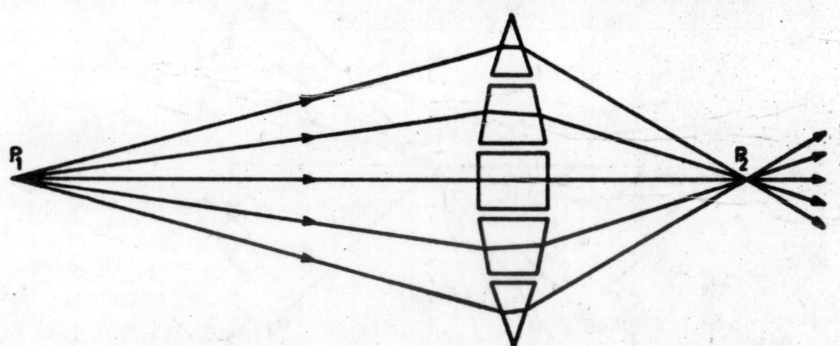

Fig. 15.5. A simple converging lens shown as a number of prisms. From a source P$_1$ light rays are refracted by the lens, resulting in their focus at a point P$_2$.
By courtesy of Ilford Ltd.

DIRECT REFLECTION

Direct reflection is the type of reflection which occurs in a mirror. The light is not scattered but redirected along a definite line on the same side of the reflecting surface as its origin. The effect is illustrated in Fig. 15.6 which shows that the angle of the incident ray with the normal is equal to the angle of the reflected ray.

This kind of reflection is sometimes termed *specular reflection*.

TOTAL INTERNAL REFLECTION

Total internal reflection is a type of reflection which occurs in certain specialized circumstances. It has been said that light passing from a dense

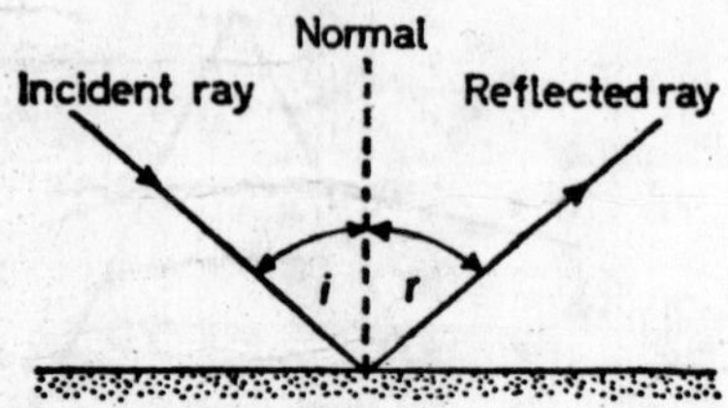

Fig. 15.6. Direct or specular reflection, such as occurs in a mirror. The angle *r* is equal to the angle *i*. *By courtesy of Ilford Ltd.*

to a rarer medium is refracted away from the normal. This means that as the angle of incidence increases the direction of the refracted ray moves nearer the boundary plane between the two media in the manner illustrated in Fig. 15.7. Ultimately, for a certain angle of incident ray, the

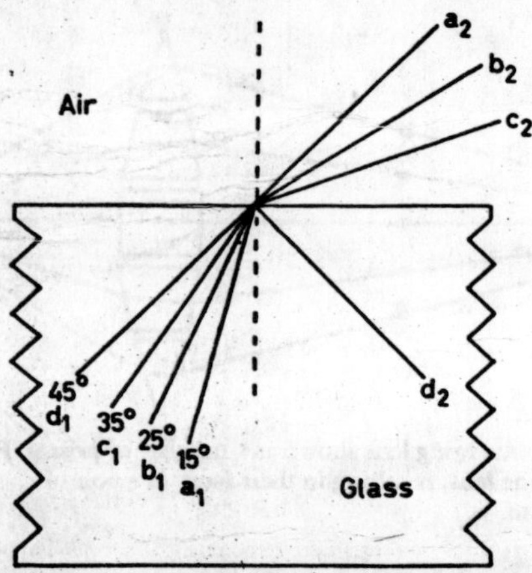

Fig. 15.7. Total internal reflection. In the figure, a number of rays of light a_1, b_1, c_1, d_1, are passing from a block of glass into air. They are at different angles of incidence. As this angle increases, the direction of the refracted rays a_2, b_2, c_2, becomes nearer to the boundary between glass and air and eventually passes it. This has happened in the case of the ray d_1, which is internally reflected along the line d_2.

line of the refracted ray will be the boundary line between the media. When this is so the angle of incidence is termed the *critical angle*. When the angle of the incident ray is greater than the critical value then total internal reflection occurs.

For glass the critical angle is of the order of 40 to 42°; it depends on the refractive index of the glass concerned. The significant point at present is that light striking the boundary at 45° will be totally reflected in the manner shown in Fig. 15.7. Figure 15.8 illustrates the employment

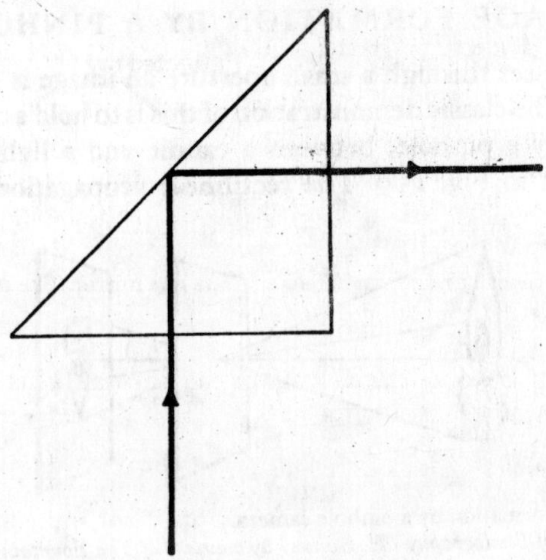

Fig. 15.8. Total internal reflection by a right-angled prism.

of this property of glass in a right-angled prism such as is used in some document copying cameras; the reflection rectifies a lateral inversion caused by the lens and thus gives right-way-round copies.

IMAGE FORMATION BY A MIRROR

The image of an object which is obtained in looking at a plane mirror is a *virtual image*. No light from the object actually passes through the mirror: the image gives the impression that it is beyond the glass but it can be observed only from the same side as the object originating it. Virtual images are produced by divergent beams and cannot be projected on to a screen.

However, not all mirrors reflect a virtual image. In contra-distinction to this term, the image formed by a *concave* mirror is called *real*. Real images are produced by convergent beams of light and they can be projected on to a screen: their formation is an important aspect of mirror optics, since a suitable mirror system may replace a conventional lens in some circumstances. A relevant example of this is found in the Odelca mirror camera used for fluorography.

The experiences of everyday life make us all familiar with the fact that a mirror image, whether virtual or real, is laterally reversed, right appearing as left.

IMAGE FORMATION BY A PINHOLE

When light passes through a small aperture an image is formed beyond the aperture. The classic demonstration of this is to hold a card, perforated at its centre by a pinhole, between a candle and a light screen in the manner shown in Fig. 15.9. The rectilinear propagation of light in all

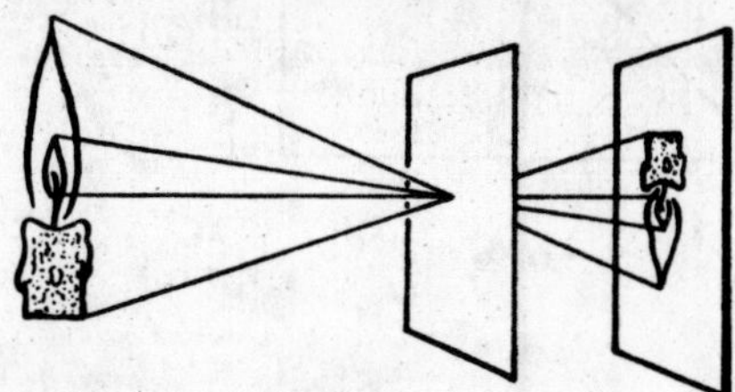

Fig. 15.9. Image formation by a pinhole camera.
From The Science of Photography (H. Baines) by courtesy of The Fountain Press.

directions results in the inversion of the image; the lines in the diagram represent some of the image-forming rays.

A pinhole is a simple way of forming an image. However, it has practical limitations which prevent it from being a very serviceable device. The sharpness of the image produced is related to the size of the pinhole, assuming a given distance between the pinhole and the screen. A relatively large hole admits more light and results in a brighter image but it becomes ever more poorly defined. If the size of the aperture is reduced, initially a sharper image results but eventually diffraction from the edges of the pinhole begins to impair definition. There is an optimum size of pinhole which gives an image of maximum sharpness. Even assuming a hole of this ideal size, the definition obtained with a pinhole device is never really good, nor are short exposures possible owing to the very limited brightness of the image.

IMAGE FORMATION BY A LENS

A lens is a system of one or more pieces of glass which causes regular convergence or divergence of light rays passing through it. A lens which consists of only one piece of glass is described as *simple*. Except for those found in the most elementary cameras, photographic lenses are of the *compound* (or *complex*) type: they consist of several components, each of which may consist of a number of pieces of glass cemented together.

Fig. 15.5 shows a simple converging lens as a number of prisms. Light rays radiating from a point source P_1 are refracted and—providing that the angles of the prisms are appropriate—are brought together again at a point P_2 to form a sharp, bright image: they are described as coming to a *focus*.

Simple lenses may be either *positive* or *negative*. Positive lenses converge light to a point on the side of the lens remote from the source. Negative lenses diverge light but we need not consider them here.

Simple lenses are not necessarily all the same shape. A number of them are listed below and Fig. 15.10 illustrates their cross-sectional appearances.

DOUBLE-CONVEX. This is perhaps the 'typical' lens. It has two convex surfaces.

PLANO-CONVEX. One surface is plane and the other convex.

DOUBLE-CONCAVE. Two surfaces are concave.

PLANO-CONCAVE. Comparable with the plano-convex, this lens has one plane and one concave surface.

MENISCUS. This lens has two curved surfaces, the centres of both curves being on the same side of the lens: more simply, we can say that it is crescent-shaped. Meniscus lenses are often used in inexpensive 'snapshot' cameras.

LENS AXIS

The term *lens axis* refers to the line which contains the centres of the curved surfaces of a lens. In Fig. 15.10 it is represented in each case by the dotted line.

Camera lenses, although they are often complex and may contain both negative and positive components, must in their overall effect be positive. For this reason we may now concentrate our attention on the behaviour of a thin, simple, positive lens.

FOCAL LENGTH

When light from a point on a very distant object, such as the sun, reaches a lens the rays may be regarded as being parallel; the object is said to be at *infinity* in respect of the lens. The plane on which the image of a distant object is formed is termed the *focal plane* and its intersection with the axis of the lens determines the *principal focal point*. More simply we can say that the principal focal point is the focus for parallel light. The distance again from the principal focus to the lens is the *focal length* of the lens. Fig. 15.11 illustrates these features.

Rays which emanate from points on the object above the lens axis come to a focus in the focal plane *below* the lens axis; that is, the image is inverted by the lens just as was the image formed by a pinhole.

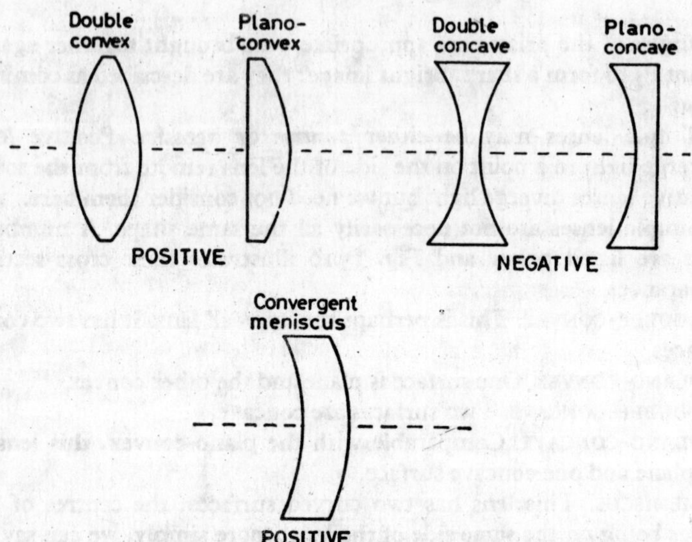

Fig. 15.10. Types of simple lenses.

The focal length of a lens is extremely significant in determining its suitability for any particular purpose, since it has a marked influence on the scale of reproduction of the image, and the angle of view (that is, the amount of the subject included on the film); it is also an important factor in the relative brightness of the image.

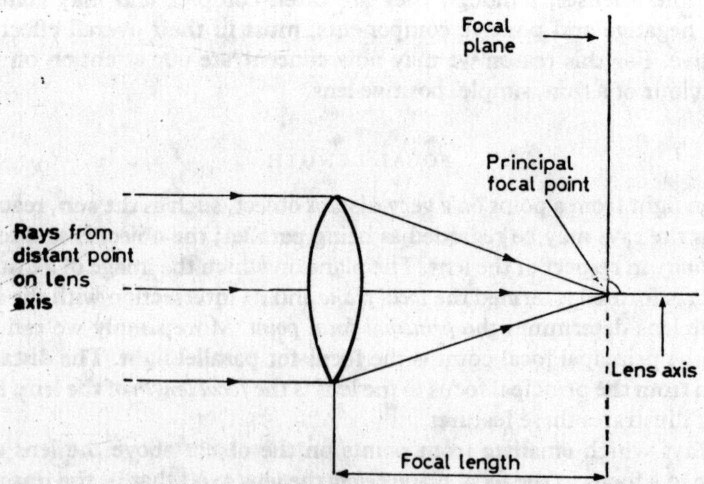

Fig. 15.11. Image formation by a simple positive lens.

RELATIVE APERTURE (F-NUMBERS)

The brightness of an image formed by a lens must depend upon two factors:

(a) the amount of light transmitted by the lens;

(b) the area over which the light has to extend.

Assuming the lens has perfect transparency, (a) is proportional to its size, or more accurately to its area: this is proportional to the square of the lens diameter. (b) is the area of the image and this becomes greater as focal length is greater, increasing with the square of focal length.

It will be seen that these two factors work in opposite ways to each other: a lens having a large diameter produces a bright image; a lens of long focal length implies an image of diminished brilliance. From this we can say that image brightness is proportional to:

$$\left(\frac{\text{lens diameter}}{\text{focal length}}\right)^2$$

However in this particular form the expression would be awkward to handle. Almost always the diameter of a lens is smaller than its focal length and consequently the function becomes a fraction. To avoid such an arithmetical inconvenience we invert the formula and consider the ratio of focal length to lens diameter. This function $\frac{\text{focal length}}{\text{lens diameter}}$ is called the *relative aperture* or f-number of the lens. It is written usually as a small f followed by an oblique stroke and a numerical value: thus f/8. In Europe the relative aperture of a lens often is expressed simply as a ratio: thus 1:8. Both forms of statement mean the same thing.

We need to remember that as we have inverted our original expression f-numbers increase as image brightness becomes less. A lens of f/8 is one which has a diameter one-eighth of its focal length. The student should have little difficulty in remembering this if it is observed that the oblique stroke indicates 'divided by': for example, we may write one quarter with equal intelligibility as 1/4. The f/8 lens might have a diameter of 5 mm and a focal length of 40 mm; or it might have a diameter of 1 inch and a focal length of 8 inches. In either case an image of similar brightness results—theoretically we can say that these lenses have comparable speed. However, the image produced by the second is much larger than the first.

The f-number is a generally accepted and useful statement of the speed of a lens. One having a relative aperture of f/2·8 is 'faster' than another of f/5·6 because it admits more light. However other factors can be significant, since it is the amount of light *transmitted* by the lens which really is the relevant quantity. Our original statement assumed a lens of perfect transparency, capable of transmitting 100 per cent of the light received. In practice there are likely always to be some losses due to absorption and reflection, especially if the lens is compound in type and has several components. A complex lens may in fact lose up to 50 per cent of incident light.

DEPTH OF FOCUS

It is convenient to consider image formation in terms of light rays emanating from a point or a number of points on the object studied. It is assumed that the lens is capable of rendering such a point as a point on the image. In practice however perfect resolution is unattainable. Even with sharpest focusing a point on the object appears in the focal plane as a small circle of light to which is given the name—perhaps inappropriately—of the *circle of least confusion.*

It might appear from this that it is impossible in any circumstances to obtain an image which looks completely sharp. This would be so were it not for the fact that the human eye is satisfied with something less than pinpoint definition. There is a limit to the smallness of detail which the eye can perceive: when this limit is reached the image appears sharp because the eye cannot appreciate any further increase in sharpness. We can say that it will accept as a true point a circle of confusion of which the diameter is no greater than a thousandth part of its distance from the eye.

At a distance of not less than ten inches—this being considered the minimum normal viewing distance—the average correctly functioning human eye will accept as perfectly sharp a circle 1/100 inch in diameter. The circles of confusion may be less than or equal to this maximum without affecting the appearance of the image to an observer under general conditions. Obviously this implies some latitude of focus. Fig. 15.12 illustrates how points immediately in front of and immediately behind the plane of sharpest focus appear sharp because the circle of confusion is within the limits above defined. The distance between these front and rear boundaries constitutes *depth of focus.*

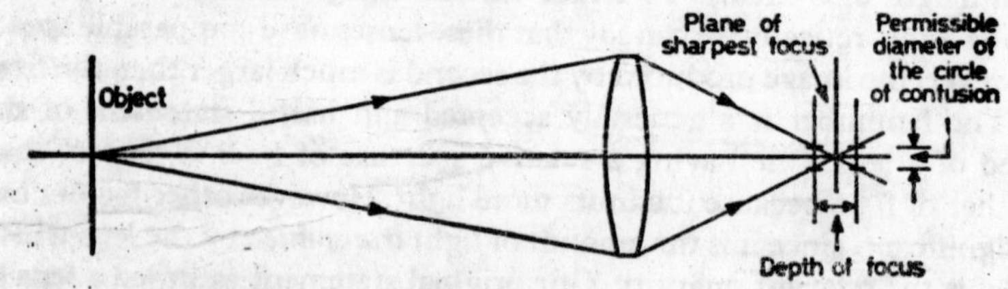

Fig. 15.12. Depth of focus. *By courtesy of Ilford Ltd.*

From a practical point of view depth of focus means the distance through which the recording film may be moved without the image of a flat object becoming appreciably unsharp. It is related to the f-number and the focal length of the lens. Depth of focus increases with larger f-numbers (i.e. smaller relative aperture) and in normal circumstances with greater focal length. This characteristic of the lens is not of any direct practical significance to the average photographer but it is of course important to the manufacturer since it indicates tolerance levels for the positioning of the sensitive material in the camera in relation to the lens. In most miniature cameras depth of focus may be very restricted because they commonly possess lenses of wide relative aperture and short focal length: this is one of the features which require such cameras to be precision built.

ABERRATIONS OF LENSES

Lenses are not perfect instruments. They do not in all circumstances form a completely faithful image of the physical aspects of an object. The defects which they may display are termed *lens aberrations*. A simple lens will exhibit a number of aberrations but photographs can be successfully taken with it in an inexpensive camera because its relative aperture is kept small. Aberrations as a rule become more intrusive in their effect as aperture increases and that is why the 'fast' lenses of sophisticated cameras must be highly complex structures. Different kinds of glass are combined and radii of curvature accurately computed in order to correct errors of reproduction inherent in a simple lens.

Lens aberrations fall into certain defined categories of which two important groups are:

1　chromatic errors;
2　spherical errors.

CHROMATIC ABERRATIONS

The way in which glass may refract light varies with the wavelength (colour) of the light concerned: not all wavelengths are brought to a focus at the same point. Shorter wavelengths are refracted by a simple lens more sharply than long and consequently the focus for blue light is nearer to the lens than the focus for red light. White light, as we know, contains both these—as well as other—colours. The effect is that the image will appear to lack definition in all parts of the lens field. This is chromatic aberration.

Chromatic aberration can be reduced if the lens is constructed of two types of glass in a special way. A lens so constructed is called an achromatic lens, or more briefly an *achromat*.

SPHERICAL ABERRATION

Spherical aberration again results in unsharpness of the image and is due to peripheral rays coming to a focus nearer the lens than do those passing centrally. It can be reduced to a minimum by a special construction of the lens.

Coma is a special type of spherical aberration affecting rays which strike the lens obliquely.

CURVILINEAR DISTORTION

Unlike other aberrations, the presence of curvilinear distortion affects the shape of the image but not its sharpness. Furthermore, curvilinear distortion is not diminished by reduction in aperture. It causes the image of a square object to appear with its sides bowed either outwards (*barrel distortion*) or inwards (*pin-cushion distortion*). The effects are illustrated in Fig. 15.13.

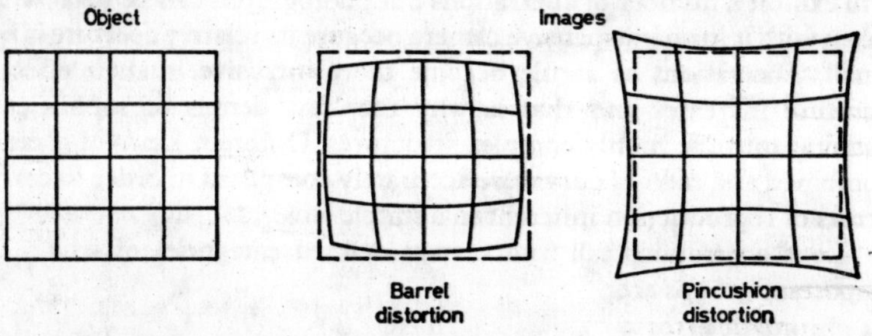

Fig. 15.13. Curvilinear distortion. *By courtesy of Ilford Ltd.*

Curvilinear distortion is due essentially to an alteration in scale of the edges of an image. If the scale is too small at the edges we see barrel distortion; if it is too large, pin-cushion distortion results. The error can be corrected by constructing the lens of two separated elements and placing a limiting diaphragm between them.

CURVATURE OF FIELD

Curvature of the field is a defect which causes the plane of sharpest focus to be not flat but saucer shaped. The effect is illustrated in Fig. 15.14.

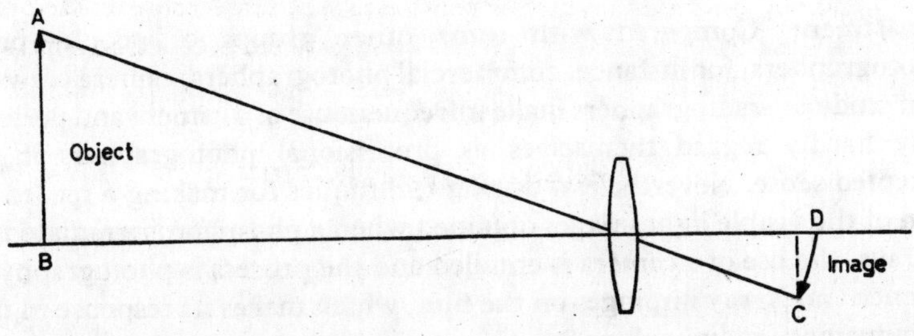

Fig. 15.14. Curvature of field. *By courtesy of Ilford Ltd.*

In practice this means that an image sharp at the centre is unsharp at the edges and vice-versa. In the case of a simple positive lens a suitable meniscus shape will flatten the field to some extent.

In some instruments a curved focal plane cannot be avoided and arrangements may be made to bend the film slightly to follow the field. This is true of the mirror focusing system employed in the 'Odelca' 70 or 100 mm cameras for photofluorography. Students who have seen this apparatus operated or are in practice familiar with its use will perhaps have noted the convex platten which holds the film in place.

ASTIGMATISM

Broadly speaking we can say that a lens which exhibits astigmatism fails to render horizontal and vertical lines sharp at one time. This is not a fully accurate statement, since it is strictly applicable only to lines which respectively are radial and tangential to the lens axis: however, it certainly expresses the effect on the observer's eye and is an acceptable conclusion for general purposes.

Astigmatism is an important defect and is associated with curvature of the field. Early attempts to correct astigmatism in a lens tended to increase the curvature of the focal plane: a flat field was obtained only with the introduction of astigmatism. However, progress in the manufacture of optical glasses has made this no longer true; lenses can be constructed which do not exhibit astigmatism. Such a lens is described as an *anastigmat* or an anastigmatic lens.

CAMERAS

Many people have cameras who never need to use one professionally and many varieties of camera exist, of which only a few are likely to be found operating in association with an X-ray tube in a radiodiagnostic department. Compared with some other groups of people—press photographers, for instance, commercial photographers, camera crews in film studios—radiographers make infrequent use of a camera and perhaps may hardly regard themselves as professional photographers in an accepted sense. Nevertheless, during techniques for making a record on film of the visible light images obtained when a phosphor is irradiated by X-rays, the use of a camera is entailed and the process is photography in essence: no X-ray impinges on the film, which makes its response in this circumstance to light alone.

Professional operators of any equipment naturally are expected to have at least an adequate working knowledge of what they employ. In the next few pages we shall consider certain important basic features of a camera, which should include the five characteristics stated below.

1 A camera must not admit any extraneous light.

2 It must have a lens at one end and at the other a means of supporting a light-sensitive material in some suitable frame at right angles to the lens.

3 The lens must be focused or capable of being focused in the image plane occupied by the film.

4 It must generally be possible to 'aim' the camera by the use of a viewfinder. In radiographic practice the 'viewfinder' may be quite different from the devices usually signified by the term: for example during modern cinematography of the fluorescent X-ray image the 'view' taken is seen and selected through observation of the image intensifier or the television monitor screen.

5 There must be a means of controlling both the amount of light admitted by the lens and the duration of its passage.

It is convenient to consider (5) first. Two features of the camera take part in this: they are the *diaphragm* and the *shutter*.

THE DIAPHRAGM

The diaphragm of a camera is a device which alters the aperture of the lens, thus also altering the amount of light which it admits (see p. 441). All professional photographers—and many amateurs—need to alter lens aperture, for reasons associated with the provision of flexibility of focusing, the control of exposure and the reduction of lens errors (some aberrations are more significant when the lens is at full aperture than when the aperture is reduced).

Although more than one variety of diaphragm exists, many cameras have the type known as an iris diaphragm. This, as its name must suggest, is analogous in operation to the way in which the human eye adapts itself to light. It consists of a number of light metal blades or leaves which are equally spaced round the lens in a circle and can overlap: this construction is shown in Fig. 15.15. Open, they form a virtually circular aperture centred on the axis of the lens.

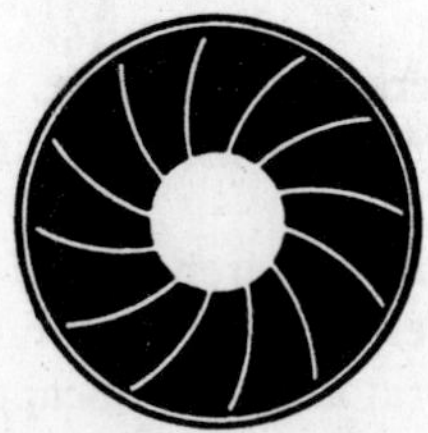 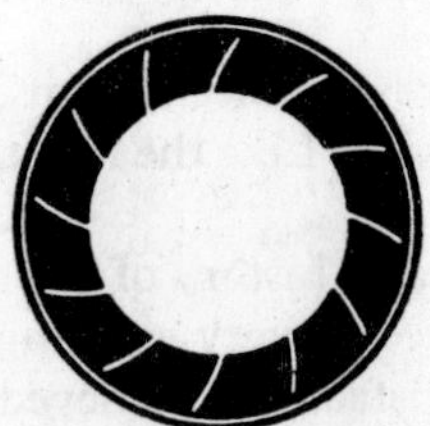

Fig. 15.15. An iris diaphragm.

The components are closed by rotation of a ring in the lens mount, the circle which they form becoming then decreased in diameter in a continuously variable fashion; the actual extent of the aperture is dependent on the degree of rotation of the ring. When the aperture of a lens is reduced by operation of the diaphragm the lens is said to be stopped down.

Alteration of the diaphragm aperture in order to reduce the effective diameter of the lens necessarily affects exposure time, because less light can enter the lens during any given period of exposure. For the film to reach the same density, a longer interval is required when the lens is stopped down that when it is used at full aperture. It is consequently important to provide the operator with some means of knowing what the aperture is, or rather of attaching to it some specific and reproducible value.

This can be done by means of the f-number (see page 441), which is a statement of the relative aperture of a lens: an f-number which is numerically low indicates a wide lens aperture and conversely a high f-number tells us that the lens aperture is small.

It is usual to calibrate the diaphragm of a camera by a series of f-numbers, such that each requires twice the exposure time of its immediate forerunner. A series in use in the United Kingdom is typified by the following run: f2.8; f4; f5.6; f8. In any particular camera, the maximum aperture of the lens is usually to be seen engraved on the lens mount.

Cameras in use in radiodiagnostic departments do not usually offer the facility of stopping down the lens by adjustment of a diaphragm. Radiographers have no need of variable focusing effects. A camera recording from an image intensifier, for example, has a predetermined relationship to the intensifier tube and is focused accordingly, at installation. Furthermore, the camera is imaging a two-dimensional subject—another image—and a fixed focus is all that is necessary.

THE SHUTTER

The shutter is the mechanism in the camera which controls the duration of the exposure. Like the lens the function of the shutter is intricate and sensitive.

In the early history of photography the requirements of the camera shutter were not very exacting. Exposures of several seconds' duration could be satisfactorily achieved if the operator simply uncapped the lens by hand and then replaced the cover when he deemed the film to have received an adequate amount of exposure to the available light.

In more recent times the use of much faster sensitive materials and lenses of increased relative apertures has made it necessary to obtain exposure intervals of merely fractions of a second and of course these intervals must be accurately timed, in some cases down to one thousandth of a second (not cameras used during fluorography). Efficiency of this order can be achieved only by a specifically designed, well functioning mechanism.

However, student radiographers need hardly become connoisseurs of camera shutters, of which several types are in existence and use. Some cameras applied to fluorography do not have a shutter: exposure of the film is dependent upon the duration of the X-ray exposure and this is controlled elsewhere in the system than at the camera. For the present purpose, a brief description of two shutters should suffice, one being appropriate to a still camera and the other to a cine camera.

LENS SHUTTER

A lens shutter is one which is situated close to the lens. Most are of the iris diaphragm type: three or four interleaved blades uncover the lens by a rotary action, the moving force being provided by a spring. In some self-setting shutters this spring is compressed and released through a single movement of the exposure button. In others, which must be pre-set, a preliminary 'cocking' action of the exposure mechanism is required. In many modern cameras this is done when the film is wound on and this interlocking device prevents dual exposure of the film. The arrangement has advantages of considerable increase in speed and a finger-touch lightness of release. Consequently there is less likelihood of movement of the camera when the exposure is initiated.

Such shutters may provide for exposure intervals varying in duration from 1 second to 1/500 second. Very often their actual progression is arranged in a manner similar to the standard series of f-numbers, the value of each setting being halved and doubled by its immediate neighbours: thus, 1, 1/2, 1/4, 1/8, 1/15, 1/30, 1/60, 1/125, 1/250, 1/500.

A CINE CAMERA'S SHUTTER

The shutter mechanism of cine cameras operates on a different principle from those employed for still photography. It takes the form of a disc which continuously rotates when the camera is in action. The disc has a cut out or open sector which will allow light to reach the film and a solid or closed sector which will cover the film during that interval of time when the latter is being moved forward, ready for exposure of the next 'frame'. The rotation of the disc is synchronized with the film movement. Camera speed can be controlled to suit different subjects and effects. For example motion can appear to be accelerated if the film is exposed at a slower speed (small number of frames per second) than that at which it is subsequently projected. Conversely, rapid movement can be slowed and in consequence more readily analysed if it is filmed at a high number of frames per second and projected at the conventional rate of 24 f.p.s.

The matter of filming speeds may appear a little confusing to the student. Sixteen frames per second was used originally for silent cinematography because it is the minimum speed which will give a smooth appearance of movement. Later when sound was introduced, a rate of 24 f.p.s. was adopted because this allowed more space for better sound quality. Television uses a framing speed of 25 f.p.s.

In many commercially available cine cameras the shutter-open time is 180°: this means that the pull-down of the film occurs during half a revolution of the rotating disc and exposure occurs during the next half turn. Thus, if the camera is driven at 25 f.p.s. the film is exposed for half of 1/25th (i.e. 1/50th) of a second. Increasing the number of frames per second, as might be required for a rapidly moving subject, necessarily decreases the actual interval of exposure. In terms of cinefluorography this would mean the use of higher milliamperages to obtain adequate density of the film and associated with it would be implications of heavier tube loading and increased patient dosage.

Because of these factors some cameras have been designed specifically for cinefluorography, with improvement of the ratio between the shutter-open period and the film pull-down. The latter is accelerated and the shutter has a 270° clear sector: that is, it is closed for only a quarter and open for three quarters of the period of one revolution. At 25 f.p.s. this would result in an exposure interval of approximately 1/30 second, with consequent lightening of the tube load and perhaps patient dosage. A typical 35 mm camera planned for cinefluorography has a lens aperture of f/0·75, a 270° shutter and a speed variable from 0 to 50 frames per second. This is an instrument capable of a very satisfactory performance.

The use of the phrase 'slow' or 'fast' shutter should be noted. A 90° shutter is faster than one of 270° because it is bound to give a shorter interval of exposure.

FOCUSING

Certain very simple cameras are of the type known as *fixed focus* and no focusing adjustment by the operator is needed. However, such cameras cannot be used closer to a subject than about 3 metres. In a more sophisticated camera which has a faster lens (larger relative aperture), the position of the focus—and consequently the focal plane where the image is sharp—depends upon the distance of the subject from the camera. If such a camera is to be properly useful, it must make provision for altering the distance between the lens and the film in order to maintain the latter in the plane of sharpest focus, or else a means of altering the focal length of the lens to achieve the same effect.

Focusing is performed in a number of ways depending on the type of camera concerned. Commonly, the lens is mounted on a rotating ring which gives it an axial forward or backward movement. The ring is calibrated with distances and this type of focusing mechanism no doubt is familiar to most people from personal experience. It is found on any miniature camera and others in general use.

THE LENS

The lens no doubt is the most important feature of any camera and to a large extent determines its suitability for a particular type of work. The optics of image formation by a lens and some aspects of lens performance have been considered. It is unnecessary to discuss these facts further, nor is detailed knowledge of the construction and use of different lenses required by the student radiographer. However, in this section are listed some varieties of lens, together with a little comment on their characteristics. It may be noted as an attractive feature of high quality miniature cameras that a ready interchange of lenses is possible. Thus the one instrument may be made suitable for a wide variety of work by the selection of the appropriate lens.

'Normal Focus' Lens

The term *normal focus* is applied to a lens of which the focal length is equal to the diagonal of the film it is intended to cover. It gives an angle of view about equal to that of the human eye when it is wandering inattentively without movement of the head. Such a lens is likely to be used at a reasonable distance from the subject, neither very close to it nor remote from it, and thus gives the appearance of a normal perspective. The angle of view provided by a lens is determined by the focal length and itself determines the amount of the subject which will be included in the film.

Wide Angle Lens

A wide angle lens is capable of covering a film which has a diagonal longer than the focal length of the lens. Such lenses usually embrace a field of about 75°, though some have been successfully constructed to include angles of as much as 180°. Because they are often used in confined spaces and close to important objects, they tend to give a steep, exaggerated perspective and are sometimes employed to make deliberate, though possibly false emphasis of some feature of a subject: for example, a small room can appear majestic and spacious by the use of such a lens.

Wide angle lenses are valuable for work in confined conditions where the camera-subject distance is limited, though they must be used with care if the unpleasant effects of distortion at the edges of the field are to be avoided. Their relative aperture is generally small, for example f/16.

Long Focus Lens

A long focus lens is designed to cover a film having a diagonal markedly shorter than the focal length of the lens. It gives a concentrated narrow angle of view and is useful when a large image must be obtained of a subject which the photographer is unable to approach closely; for example it could be of value for photography in the operating theatre. A *telephoto* lens is a long focus lens of special construction which enables the camera body, i.e. the distance from the lens to the film, to be much shorter than the focal length of the lens would normally necessitate.

Varifocal Lens

A varifocal lens is probably better known as a *zoom* lens. It is often used to direct attention in cinematography or television since the camera appears to move in close to the subject. The principle of its operation is that the focal length of the lens is altered by varying the separation between its components.

Chapter 16
Fluorography

Elsewhere in this book fluorography has been described as a process of applied photography. The radiant energy which initiates the process unquestionably is an X-ray beam. Its role—once it has passed through the body of a patient—is to stimulate a phosphor, upon the surface of which a fluorescent image will result. This image may be photographed by a suitably situated camera, from the lens of which all other light than that from the fluorescent screen has been excluded. We are about to consider now some cameras which may be applied in this way and the circumstances of the employment of each.

The term *fluorography* means simply the process of photographing the image which appears on a fluorescent screen. Students may perhaps encounter another word in the same context: *photofluorography*. This expression, which appears both tautological and superfluous, is employed by some writers and speakers to make a needless distinction: they use *fluorography* for the techniques involved in recording the appearances which originate from an image intensifier tube; and *photofluography* when the camera operates through a special, mirror optical system in place of a refractive lens and produces a miniature radiograph. The most familiar—although not the only—application of miniature radiography is to examinations of the lung fields of relatively large groups of people, in the procedure known as mass miniature radiography (MMR).

AN OPTICAL SYSTEM FOR IMAGE INTENSIFIER FLUOROGRAPHY

An optical system is normally necessary to view the image on an X-ray intensifier tube and this requires particular arrangements if the image is to be observed and recorded simultaneously. Typically, the system includes a gadget called a light distributor, which is fitted to the output phosphor of the intensifier tube.

The operation of the light distributor depends upon a mirror of a

452

light-splitting type: this is a partially silvered mirror which reflects some portion of a beam of light and allows another portion to pass through it. The distributor consequently gives two outputs of light—a reflected beam and a transmitted beam—for a single input.

In the equipment, the light from the image intensifer tube passes through an optical system which includes a light distributor; the image intensifier is thus providing the input. The customary closed-circuit television camera-tube is permanently linked with one of the output channels of the distributor, for fluoroscopic viewing; the other output channel permits a suitable fluorographic camera to be attached for recording purposes. The arrangements allows the fluoroscopist to record what he is seeing at any stage of an examination and at the same time to continue to observe what is being filmed.

A more complex light or image distributor makes available not two but three channels of light. This would permit television viewing together with fluorography by means of one or other of two cameras, fitted respectively to each of the spare output channels: for example, a cine camera and a single-shot camera might be regarded as an appropriate fluorographic armament.

CAMERAS FOR FLUOROGRAPHY

CINE CAMERAS

When a cine camera is used to record images from an image intensifier tube the process is *cinefluorography*. It implies recording on a continuous roll of film, moving at a minimum speed of 16 frames or pictures per second.

Sometimes, radiographic records made at speeds slower than 16 frames/second are called cine films, but this is an inaccurate terminology: properly, they are rapid serial radiographs. The eye's persistency of vision is such that it will accept as continuous a succession of images which replace each other at a rate of 16 or more per second. Below this figure, the lag is too great for the eye successfully to merge each image into the next. Serial radiographs projected at a rate faster than that at which they were exposed result in an acceleration of the movement and—if the motion was rapid—in an appearance of jerkiness.

Radiographic examinations calling for cinefluorography are those which investigate rapidly dynamic physiological actions and effects, particularly the flow of blood through the chambers of the heart. During angiocardiography, exposure rates much greater than 16 frames/second are employed: typical instances are 48 frames/second and 100 frames/second, but speeds as high as 200 frames/second have been used.

Rapid cinefluorography is a highly demanding procedure for an X-ray generator and tube, as the greater is the camera's framing speed the shorter must become the interval of the X-ray exposure. A reader, who pauses to consider the minimum exposure rate of 16 frames/second for cinefluorography and performs the little arithmetical exercise of dividing 1 second by 16, will face the inescapable fact that an exposure time greater than 0·06 seconds 'won't go into' the period available. In fact, an exposure time appreciably shorter than this would be necessary because the action of the camera's mechanical parts, together with other factors, such as the phasing of the generator and the operation of interlocks and relays in the X-ray generating circuit, give rise to a very brief interval of 'dead time' in the total film-cycle. This 'delay' prohibits the interval of exposure of the film from being greater than about 30–40 per cent of the framing interval. Typically, an exposure time of 5–6 milliseconds (0·005–0·006 sec.) has been associated with an exposure rate of 48 frames/second. Consequently, X-ray generators suitable for cinefluorography must offer high output (130–200 kW), short minimum exposure times and high exposure-repetition rates.

Cinefluorography may be successfully performed using either a 16 mm camera or a 35 mm camera. In some instances the smaller lens may be faster and the reduction in radiation dosage which this implies may be an argument for the camera's use. However, the main—and perhaps the only significant—advantage of the 16 mm camera is that it permits the use of high framing speeds, such as 200 frames/second. So rapid a sequence, whilst appropriate to examinations of the cardiac cycle, necessitates extremely short exposure intervals; if the patient is an adult, it becomes questionable whether adequate radiographic densities can be obtained without a generator of exceptionally high output. Generally speaking, such high framing speeds are not widely used.

Thirty-five millimetre film offers approximately 4 times the recording area, relative to a 16 mm film. A fine grain emulsion combined with a slow fine grain developer should result in good detail.

Some features of a camera suitable for cinefluorography were described on p. 449 in connection with the design of the shutter. If the camera is photographing the image presented on a televison monitor—as distinct from the presentation on the output phosphor of an image intensifier tube—it is essential that the camera be driven at a speed which is a multiple of the frequency with which the picture appears on the monitor and is correctly phased with it. If the phasing is wrong, an unexposed bar will appear on each frame of the film, due to the fact that the shutter was open during a blank interval on the television screen. Synchronisation and phasing of the camera can be achieved if it is driven by a phased synchronous motor operating from the same mains supply as the television system, but the limitations imposed by the phasing may preclude cinematography at high speeds. This is one of the reasons why a cine camera is better placed at the end of the intensifier tube than incorporated in the television link.

Cine fluorographic equipment is often pulsed in operation. This means that the X-ray tube is not continuously energised during filming but passes current only during those intervals when the camera shutter is open. In the alternating periods, during which the film is wound past the lens to obtain the next picture area or frame, the shutter necessarily is closed. Energising the X-ray tube at these times cannot affect the emulsion, because of the closed shutter, and consequently results in unnecessary irradiation of a patient.

Pulsing of an X-ray beam, to synchronise its production with the open phases of a camera shutter, implies the use of a grid-controlled X-ray tube. A special pulsing unit associates a blocking voltage on the grid with the operation of the shutter, to ensure that the X-ray tube passes no current except during those intervals when the camera shutter is open.

SINGLE SHOT AND SERIAL CAMERAS

Several types of camera are available for single shot photography of the appearances seen on an image intensifer tube. They are commonly employed equipments for record purposes during image intensifier fluoroscopy, of the gastrointestinal tract for instance. The use of a camera in this circumstance has several important advantages, relative to exposing full-sized radiographs by means of the serial changer on the fluoroscopic table. These advantages include·

1   lower radiation dose;
2   lower film costs;
3   simpler, and therefore faster procedure, with reduced demand on personnel.

Some of these fluorographic cameras are capable of providing a framing frequency of 1–6 (or even as many as 12) frames per second and thus may be as applicable to the dynamic actions of blood vessels as to those of the oesophagus. The term 'single shot' by itself as a description of such cameras is possibly misleading, but it is used as a rule to distinguish them from cine cameras: more properly, these are serial cameras with both a single and sequential operation.

Systems for image intensifier fluoroscopy permit the introduction of a camera for recording purposes by one or other of two methods. They are:

1   the camera may record the image directly from the output phosphor of an image intensifier tube;

2   the camera may receive the image from a special television monitor, offering high resolution.

The first of these approaches is the more generally employed, as radiographic quality should be better: the image on the anode phosphor is at its sharpest and brightest and it is free from the scanning lines and 'noise' inherent in television systems. (*Noise* is the term used in electronics for the intrusion on a television signal produced by extraneous variations in current through any of a number of components; it is inevitably present in some degree, although in good equipment it is minimal.)

The cameras about to be described are associated with fluorography from the output phosphor of an image intensifer tube and are best classified according to the format of the film which is appropriate to each. Whilst quite a variety of models is available, certain features apparent in most categories of camera should be noticed. These features include:

1   separate supply and take-up magazines or cassettes;

2   automatic identification of the patient (for example by the use of an IBM or similar card);

3   automatic recording of other data, such as the serial number of each shot in a sequence of exposures;

4   incorporation of various safety mechanisms, to indicate and prevent operation of the camera under incorrect conditions, such as absence of—or very little—film in the supply magazine, or a failure to attach either magazine. These safety mechanisms incorporate monitoring devices (usually presented as coloured lamps which become illuminated) as well as interlocking circuitry which prohibits a camera from being used unless it is functionally ready. The monitor lamps may be mounted either on the body of a camera or on a separate control/programming console.

We may notice also that these cameras require no shutter. Exposure times are controlled through the operation of the X-ray generator, of which the exposure-switching characteristics and abilities must significantly influence the performance required of the associated camera. Here let us assume that switching is ideally rapid and efficacious. The maximum duration of any interval of exposure is necessarily limited by the exposure rate. (Compare the similar situation during cinefluorography, which is described on p. 449). A typical progression of maximum available exposure times is seen in the table below.

440 milliseconds at 1 frame/second

210 milliseconds at 2 frames/second

138 milliseconds at 3 frames/second
105 milliseconds at 4 frames/second
70 milliseconds at 6 frames/second.

Preferably, the operation of these cameras should be associated with a system for automatic control of radiographic density. When exposures are to follow each other quickly in a series, there cannot be any smooth procedure of the examination if the operator must adjust exposure conditions before each shot.

105 MM CAMERA

The 105 mm camera uses a perforated roll film, 150 mm in width. On a 45 metre roll of film, the supply cassette of the camera offers the capacity for some 430 exposures. The capacity of the take-up magazine varies in different models: in one of two cameras currently on the market this capacity is 60 frames of film (or exposures) and in another it is 150.

The body of the camera will have an in-built film cutter. This enables the film to be divided and the magazine withdrawn as a daylight operation, so that any particular length of film may be processed and examined at any time. The control module often provides indications of the amount of film in both the supply and take-up magazines. When planning a particular filming sequence, the operator should make certain that:

(a) there is sufficient film in the camera for the projected number of exposures;

(b) the sequence will not result in a length of film too great for the capacity of the take-up cassette.

The lens characteristics of the available 105 mm cameras vary a little between different models. Typically, the focal length is of the order of 320 mm–480 mm, whilst the maximum relative aperture (f-number) might be f/5, f/6·3 or f/7·2. It may be useful here to remind the reader of the significance of these quantities and ratios.

In essence, focal length influences the dimensions of the image and the amount of the subject included in the view. Generally speaking, images from a lens of longer focal length, relative to another of shorter focal length, (1) are larger and (2) include less of the subject. The f-number, which is the ratio between the diameter of a lens and its focal length, makes a statement regarding the amount of light admitted by a lens: the lower the f-number the greater is the amount of light admitted and the lens is commonly described as being 'faster'.

These fluorographic cameras are usually associated with a programme selector which permits the following determinations.

1　Change of mode between a single exposure and a run of exposures in sequence.

2　In the sequential mode, a choice of rates for the advance of the film through the camera.

Typically in (2), one might select any of the following: 1 frame (exposure) in two seconds; 1, 2, 3, 4 or 6 frames per second.

3　Selection of the photographing period in seconds. This might be a relatively sophisticated system, like that associated with a rapid large-film changer (such as the AOT or Puck), which would allow the sequence of exposures to occur in three stages, with a variable pause between the second and third stage.

100 MM CAMERA

The 100 mm camera exposes separate sheets of film, each 100 mm × 100 mm. In some respects, cut film is a more convenient material than roll films, since it may be handled, processed, read and filed in much the same way as are large-sized radiographs. Furthermore, this particular format is compatible with copying systems which miniaturize radiographs for filing purposes (see p. 85).

A manufacturer or supplier of 100 mm cameras may offer two versions:

1　a model which makes either a single exposure or a sequence not faster than 2 frames/second;

2　a high speed model of extended scope, offering maximum framing speeds as high as 6–12 frames/second.

The capacities of the film magazines for these cameras are various, being lower in the simpler instruments: typical of these are a supply cassette capable of holding 70 films and a take-up cassette which can receive 20 sheets of film. The more complex cameras necessarily require higher film-capacities: these are found in a supply reservoir of 150 films and a collection magazine for 100 films.

As with the others, lens characteristics of the 100 mm cameras are not all the same and may depend in particular on the type of image intensifier with which the camera is linked: 322 mm and 400 mm are typical examples of the focal length of these lenses, which respectively have maximum relative apertures of f/5·2 and f/6·3.

High speed 100 mm cameras (those with maximum exposure rates of 6 frames/second or more) are usually associated with a remote programme selector or operating module fitted to the generator's own control desk. If so, this—as usual—will carry indicators of the camera's functioning readiness (pilot lamps, film counters for each magazine, etc.), which otherwise are placed on the body of the camera.

70 MM CAMERA

The 70 mm camera is another which uses roll film, in this case unperforated and 70 mm in width. Each reel of film contains about 600 exposures (45 metres of film). Like the others, these cameras have detachable supply and take-up cassettes, to enable the camera to be loaded easily and a run of film to be removed at any time for processing and reading. Typically, the capacity of the take-up cassette is some 4 to 5 metres (around 60 exposures).

In typical examples, we find relative apertures of $f/5 \cdot 1$ and $f/4 \cdot 5$, together with focal lengths of 300 mm and 210 mm.

Exposures may be made singly and—in many instances—serially at a frequency of up to 6 frames/second. Again we may expect to find a separate unit for programming of the camera: this unit will include a selector of the exposure rate and the usual monitor lamps to indicate various stages of readiness (or unreadiness) in the camera's operating condition.

THE ODELCA MIRROR CAMERA

The Odelca mirror camera is a specialised unit which photographs a full-sized fluorescent screen on a small film (100 mm or 70 mm), thus producing a miniature radiograph of the subject X-rayed. The camera has been applied particularly to mass miniature radiography of the chest.

In some parts of Europe, notably in the Netherlands and Germany, attention has been given to the use of the 100 mm camera for examinations of the gastrointestinal tract and the skeletal system; even for angiography and intravenous urography, when the camera is associated with a programme selector of a kind similar to those of other film changers.

The use of a small film greatly reduces the cost of a radiodiagnostic examination, whilst the thin, single-sided emulsion husbands the world's silver resources; but even so, the Odelca mirror camera is not employed widely in the United Kingdom at the present time.

THE CAMERA UNIT

Figure 16.1 illustrates the essential arrangement for obtaining a miniature fluorogram of the chest. A patient is positioned in the customary way in relation to a fluorescent screen in front of which there is a secondary radiation grid, although this is not shown in the diagram. The fluorescent screen is at one end of a light-tight tunnel, at the other end of which is a camera. A sheet of clear lead glass, on the surface of the screen distal to

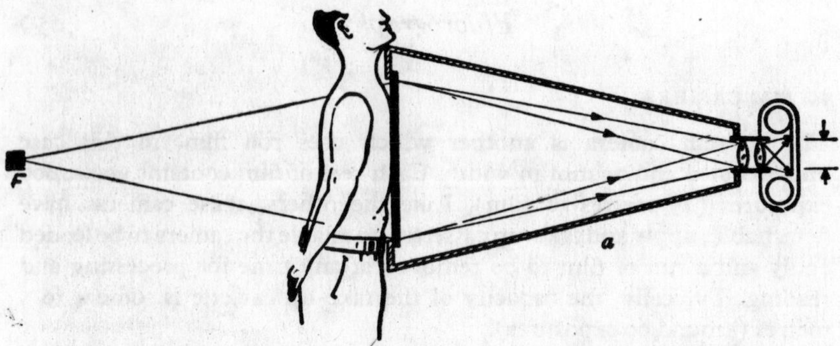

Fig. 16.1. *By courtesy of The Centrex Publishing Company (Philips Technical Library)*

the patient, means that no X-rays affect the film. A side-arm, or some equivalent arrangement, links the X-ray tube to the screen and necessarily also to the camera, through the agency of the enclosing tunnel. All three components move together, as one unit, vertically upwards and downwards on a pair of supporting columns, the operation being controlled by a single release lever; this capability of movement is to provide for patients of differing heights and facilitate radiographic centering.

A general view of a fluorographic unit in use for mass radiography of the chest is shown in figure 16.2.

THE CONCENTRIC MIRROR LENS

For the sake of simplicity in illustrating a principle, the camera depicted in Figure 16.1 is of a conventional type for 35 mm film and has a refractive lens. In practice, such a camera is not used. The image on the fluorescent screen is photographed by means of a special optical system which employs a concave focusing mirror: it is simpler in construction and much faster—about four times faster—than the lens of the miniature camera in use in Figure 16.1.

The mirror system effectively has a greater focal length than a lens of similar application and this means that larger film formats may be used (100 mm and 70 mm in place of 35 mm). Both these facts—higher speed and greater image-size—are advantageous for radiography, the first because of reduced radiation dose to a subject and the second because subsequent radiological interpretation is more easily made.

Mirror optical systems used in fluorography depend on a spherical mirror; this is a curved mirror of which the reflecting surface is defined as part of the surface of a sphere. This is shown in fig. 16.3. As might be

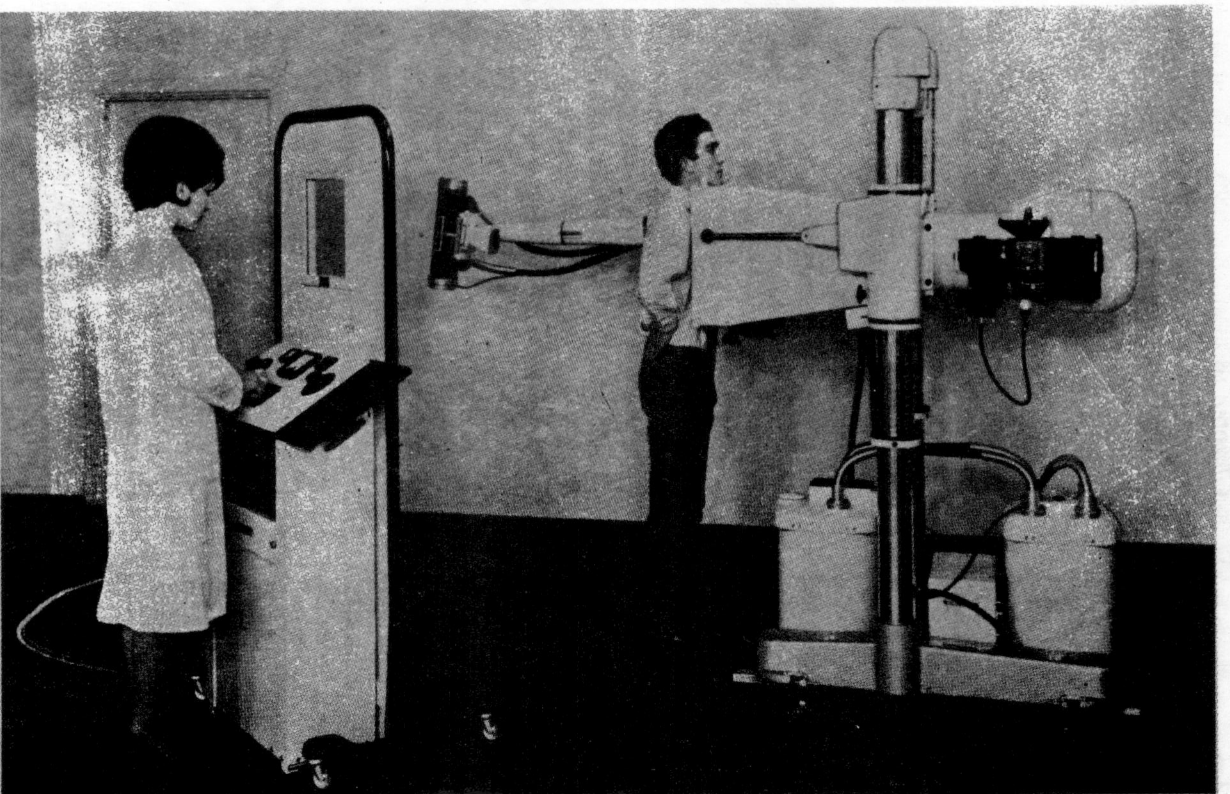

Fig. 16.2. A camera unit for fluorography of the chest, using roll film. *By courtesy of Picker International Ltd.*

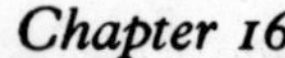

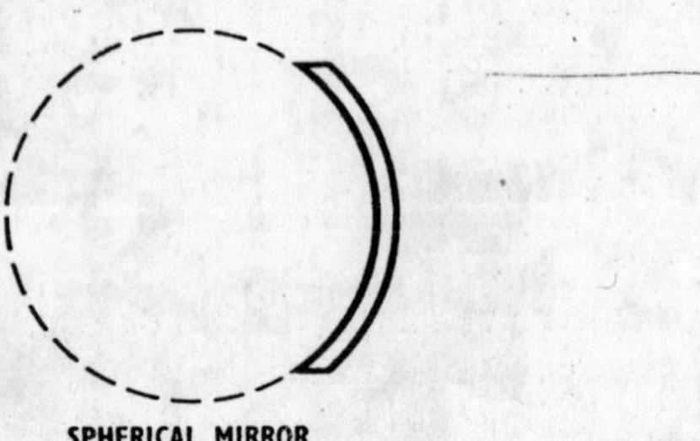

Fig. 16.3. Diagram of a spherical mirror. The reflecting surface is part of the surface of a sphere. *By courtesy of Kodak Ltd.*

anticipated the image formed by such a mirror is subject to spherical aberration (Chapter 15). In the Bouwers concentric mirror system, now widely employed, this is corrected by means of a low power lens which has a spherical error opposite to that of the mirror; the two elements possess a common centre of curvature and the general scheme is depicted diagrammatically in Fig. 16.4a. In Fig. 16.4b a cone lens has been added

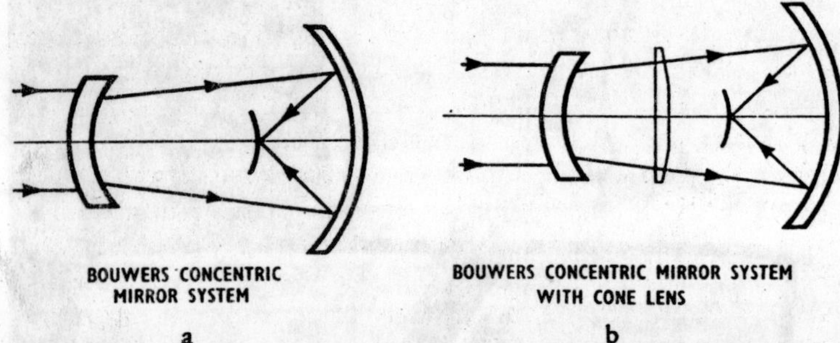

Fig. 16.4. (a) The Bouwers concentric mirror system used for fluorography in place of a refractive lens. Light from the fluorescent screen (depicted as parallel arrowed lines) passes through a correcting lens; this lens eliminates spherical distortion produced by the mirror. The mirror reflects and converges the light on a convex focal plane.

(b) The Bouwers concentric mirror system with the addition of a cone lens to improve resolution. *By courtesy of Kodak Ltd.*

for improvement of the system's resolving power. It should be noted that the focal plane is curved (Chapter 15; curvature of field.)

With this arrangement definition over the whole area of the field and the resolution obtained are so good that on high powered magnification the fine structure of the secondary radiation grid can be seen to be recorded on the film. The thickness of the lead elements is 0·07 mm.

It will be appreciated from Fig. 16·2 that the spherical mirror is of a size comparable with the fluorescent screen. A large mirror increases the speed of the optical system.

EXPOSURE CONTROL

The Odelca mirror camera used for fluorography does not require a shutter. Exposure is effected in the X-ray generating system and its duration controlled usually by a photo-electric timer.

The full operation of this type of radiographic timer is not within the intended scope of this book and no doubt the student will study its detail in another connection. In resumé we may say that the essential difference between this timer and others used in radiographic practice is that the photo-timer does not mark a specific physical period but terminates exposure when the film has received a pre-determined energy which will give it on development a certain density. If the subject is thin and a high tube tension is selected, then the actual time of exposure will be short. If converse conditions obtain, then the interval is bound to be longer—how much longer can only be appreciated by observation of a milliampere-seconds meter and some requisite mental arithmetic, since the radiographer receives no direct indication of the *time* of exposure. With this type of apparatus the exposure interval cannot be pre-set but can be only recorded.

The photo-electric cell on which the fluorographic photo-timer depends receives part of the light from each apical area of the lungs. It is this quantity which determines the duration of the exposure. Within certain obvious limits of over- and under-exposure, there is a considerable range of individual opinion on the densities which constitute a well exposed radiograph of the chest. To allow for variations in the criteria of the examining radiologist or chest physician, or for a change in film speed, a density control is incorporated in the photo-timer. An adjustable knob can be set to any chosen position in a scale numbered perhaps from 0 to 10: these figures are arbitrary, unrelated to any form of densitometric calibration, and there only for convenience.

This selector knob is easily accessible but once its position has been decided it should not be subjected to frequent alteration by the operator. To use the density control to increase the exposure obtained for an obese patient is to make nonsense of the photo-timer's principle and purpose. Equally incorrect is the assumption that the presence of photo-electric timing will produce a satisfactory radiograph in any circumstance. The operator has still to make a proper selection of tube kilovoltage: in doing this the presence of the grid, the relatively slower response of the fine grain emulsion and the limitations of the optical system should be remembered. Tube tensions appropriate to fluorography usually are above those in general employment for direct radiography of the chest. A well established practice, though one perhaps not very commonly employed, is to relate their determination to the anteroposterior diameter of the thorax and a known satisfactory exposure for a 'normal' or average subject.

A timer called the Iontomat also is in use for the automatic control of fluorographic and indeed other radiographic exposures. The principle is the same as that just described but a distinguishing feature of its operation is that the radio-sensitive element is not a photo-electric cell but an ionization chamber. It should be noted that this is passing current in proportion to the quantity of X-rays incident upon it, whereas the photoelectric cell responds to light. However, the foregoing discussion on exposure control is equally applicable to either device.

FILM IDENTIFICATION

Proper film identification is an important part of all radiographic procedures. It has been said that an undated radiograph is without value; even more obvious is the necessity to attach to each film the correct patient's name or record number. In the case of a miniature radiograph the latter may be more practicable. The length and nature of a name cannot be foreseen and the legend preferably should appear large enough for reading without the aid of a magnifier; figures also have the advantage in mass surveys that they can be serially printed in advance on an appropriate number of cards. However, from the operative aspect of providing fluorographic units with an automatic means of film identification it is immaterial whether a name or a number is recorded.

The method adopted is photographic; that is selected details from a record card are photographed by the camera at the same time as the fluorescent image—in fact under automatic control it occurs immediately on completion of the X-ray exposure. For this purpose the patient's card must be placed in front of the camera in a suitable relationship to the fluorescent screen and illuminated for an appropriate interval. A card tray is provided below the fluorescent screen and can be pulled forwards by means of a handle to permit the card's insertion.

The card is a standard size, in Europe and in the United Kingdom, but only a limited area, 90 mm × 20 mm, is actually recorded on the film. This rectangle, known as the *identity frame*, may occupy the top left or right hand corner or the top middle portion of the card, as shown in Fig. 16.5. Its position is indicated on the card by a heavy black line. Though different sizes of cards may be employed through the provision of an

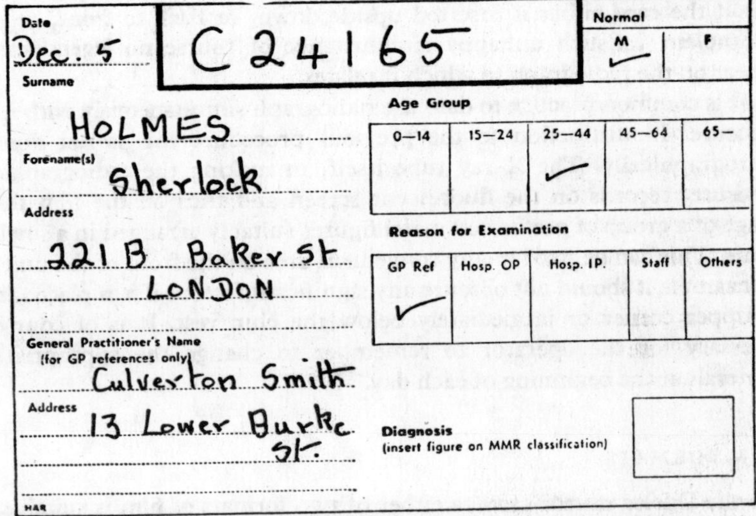

Fig. 16.5. Identification card for use with a fluorographic unit. Only details printed in the upper central frame are recorded on the fluorogram.

appropriate card holder, the dimensions of the identity frame are fixed: within it should be written or printed prominently the patient's number or name.

In use, as each patient presents with his card it is placed in the tray and the latter pushed into the closed positon for exposure. Illumination of the card is provided by a small fluorescent tube within the holder and in order to obtain a constant density from the card's exposure, irrespective of film speed, the operation of this light is usually through the discharge of a suitable capacitor in the feed unit.

The legend, whether number or name, appears on the radiograph in a central position along its lower border, that is in the subphrenic area of the chest where it is easy to read and unlikely to obscure any feature of diagnostic significance.

The camera unit incorporates a number of important electrical interlocks to ensure that it is impossible to take a radiograph which is not positively related to the person examined. The function of these means that:

1   no film is transported from the magazine to its correct position in the focal plane unless there is a card ready for exposure in the holder;
2   no subsequent exposure can be made until the card is changed.

It is evident that in this equipment considerable thought in design and executant skill have been devoted to the end that film identification shall be a fool-proof procedure. However, sad experience must add the observation that it is possible to obtain a radiographic exposure from the unit if the card either is inserted upside down, or back to front, or is incomplete. In such unhappy circumstance of course no legend can appear on the radiograph to which it relates.

It is common practice to date the radiograph simultaneously with its exposure. In distinction to the previous procedure this is not done photographically. The X-ray tube itself, in making the radiographic exposure, records on the fluorescent screen and thus on the film the image of a group of perforated metal figures suitably arranged in a small frame. This can be fixed in any convenient area on the front of the unit; for example it should not obscure any significant feature if it is placed in an upper corner or immediately below the chin rest. It is of course necessary for the operator to remember to change the appropriate numerals at the beginning of each day.

FILM FORMATS

For the Odelca mirror camera either of two formats of film is suitable, provided that the camera is equipped with an appropriate cassette and magazines. The formats in question are a roll film, 70 mm in width, and a cut sheet film, 100 mm × 100 mm in area.

The roll film is obtainable in a spool containing 30 metres and sufficient for 450 exposures; this is appropriate for the examination of very large numbers of people at one time. In radiodiagnostic departments, if it is encountered at all, the Odelca camera almost certainly is associated with the 100 mm cut film, which is supplied in packets of 50 sheets; that is, 50 exposures may be made before the cassette is reloaded. This is an appropriate capacity for handling such groups of patients as those referred by their general practitioners, those attending some outpatient clinics, or members of a hospital's staff needing a 'routine' chest survey.

Because of the higher radiation input which fluorography requires and to avoid the possibility of incurring further dosage from a subsequent 'recall' examination on a large film, it is not usual to survey on these camera units either pregnant women or anyone occupationally exposed to ionizing radiation. Both the dose factor and the usually longer intervals of exposure make children also—up to the age of about 14 years—unfavourable subjects for examination by this method.

Compared with the 70 mm format, the larger 100 mm film is advantageous for radiological interpretation, since these radiographs may be read directly quite easily by most observers, without recourse to magnification. No doubt not only radiologists but medical records officers may have some preference for the 100 mm sheet film, which is much simpler to handle and to file—perhaps within a patient's case notes, for example—than are rolls of miniature film containing the radiographs of many patients at once.

THE ROLLER SEPARATOR CASSETTE

The type of cassette which the camera unit incorporates is dependent on the size of film to be employed. As the 100 mm cut film is the one most likely to be found in a radiodiagnostic department we shall refer only to the roller separator cassette, which is appropriate to it. A separator cassette includes:

1 a supply magazine into which sheets of unexposed film are loaded in a darkroom and from which they are automatically fed to the focal plane in the camera;

2 a take-up magazine into which each film automatically passes upon completion of the exposure.

A system of dark-slides, which are usually self-operated, makes it possible to withdraw either magazine as a daylight operation, without risk of fogging films whether these are within the withdrawn magazine or the other.

The supply magazine of the separator cassette is mounted above the camera unit and the take-up magazine is situated below. Figure 16.6 shows the supply magazine being withdrawn from the separator cassette. Figure 16.7 shows the take-up magazine beneath the camera unit and the action of its removal.

In the present context we need not be closely concerned with the operation of a roller separator cassette but may content ourselves with a reference to figure 16.8. This is a schematic diagram of a fluorographic mirror camera, with a roller separator cassette and magazines in position. The diagram includes the following salient features.

1 The relative positions of:
(a) the secondary radiation grid;
(b) the fluorescent screen;
(c) the patient-identification device;
(d) the optical system;
(e) the concave focusing mirror which replaces a lens.

2 Films in the supply magazine are pushed forward successively by a spring-loaded plate.

3 A system of rollers drives each sheet of film in turn downwards to the focal plane of the camera, where it is held stationary and is curved slightly by a convex platten or pressure plate.

Chapter 16

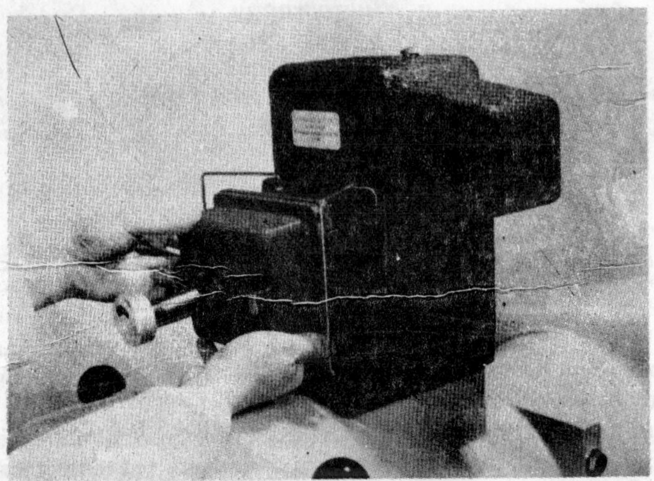

Fig. 16.6. The supply magazine being withdrawn from the cassette for 100 mm film, in use on an Odelca fluorographic camera. *By courtesy of Picker International Ltd.*

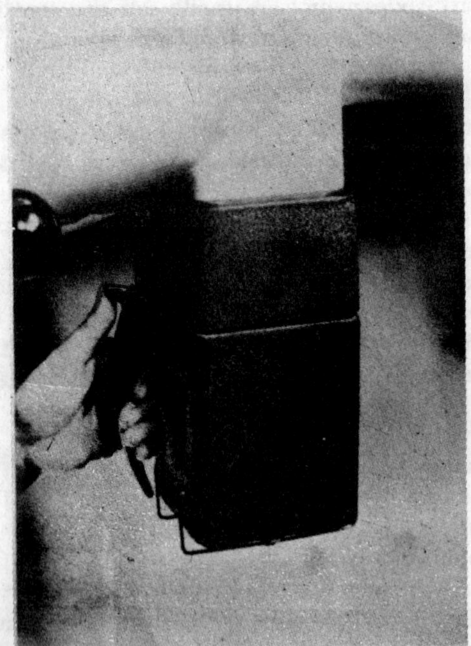

Fig. 16.7. Withdrawing the take-up magazine (100 mm film) from an Odelca fluorographic camera. *By courtesy of Picker International Ltd.*

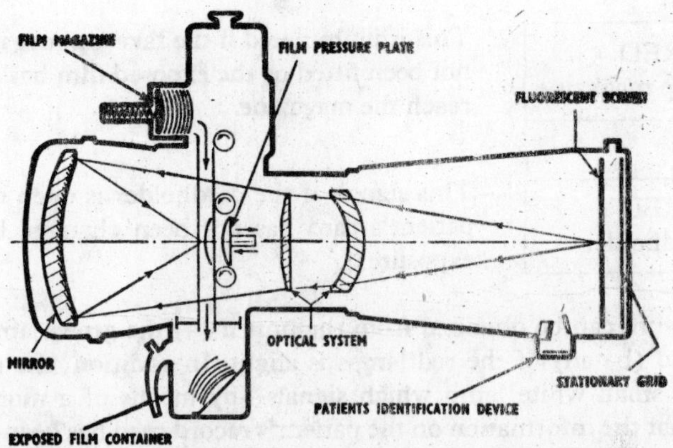

Fig. 16.8. Diagram of a fluorographic camera using 100 mm cut film.
By courtesy of Picker International Ltd.

4   After exposure of the film, the platten withdraws and allows other rollers to drive the film downwards again, to an orderly arrival in the take-up magazine. At any convenient time the take-up magazine may be removed and its contents processed, with no interference to unexposed film in the other magazine.

THE MONITOR UNIT

A self-contained monitor unit (not shown in Fig. 16.2) is a standard accessory to the 100 mm camera unit employing the roller separator cassette above described. This monitor is wall mounted near the camera, in a positon where the operator may easily see it. It is associated with certain interlocks in the camera unit and its function is to warn the operator of omissions or errors creating conditions unsuitable to the use of the camera.

The monitor has a vertical row of four pilot lamps, the uppermost one being green and the others red. They operate in the following way.

GREEN	This lights up when the film is in the pressure frame and the camera is ready for exposure.
RED **Supply magazine**	This becomes illumined when the supply magazine is empty or not in place.

<table>
<tr><td>RED
Take-up magazine</td><td>This is illuminated if the take-up magazine has not been fitted or the exposed film has failed to reach the magazine.</td></tr>
<tr><td>RED
Cardholder</td><td>This signals if the cardholder is open or if the patient's card has not been changed between exposures.</td></tr>
</table>

No exposure can be obtained from the unit if (a) the green lamp is *not* alight and (b) any of the red lamps is alight. In addition, the monitor carries a small white lamp which signals—by means of a momentary flash—that the information on the patient's record card has been printed on the film; usually this occurs immediately after the X-ray exposure.

An important purpose of such monitoring systems—both here and elsewhere in X-ray and other advanced equipment—is to eliminate as far as possible the occurrence of an operational error because of some human oversight. It is equally significant that these devices offer warning of an operational defect, such as—in this case—exhaustion of film in the supply magazine, or failure of a film to transport, or an 'open circuit' condition in the identifier.

SENSITOMETRIC RESPONSE OF FLUOROGRAPHIC FILM

COLOUR SENSITIVITY

Elsewhere in this book (see p. 96) reference has been made to an important link between the colour of light emitted by an activated phosphor and the spectral response of the film, on which the fluorescent image therefrom is to be recorded. This is no less significant during fluorography than during radiography with an intensifying screen.

In the case of fluorography, the emission which we must consider is predominantly green light and consequently the emulsions employed for fluorography are either orthochromatic or panchromatic; the wider spectral sensitivity of the latter implies a more rapid response and thus affords a reduction in both exposure times and radiation dosage.

However, it must be remembered that neither of these types of film may be handled safely in the lighting often found in radiographic darkrooms. Orthochromatic emulsions require a dark red light. If they are fast they should not be exposed even to this for more than a few seconds. Panchromatic material should be manipulated in total darkness, though it may withstand *indirect* illumination from a dark green lamp for a similarly limited period of time.

This means that in a general radiodiagnostic department such materials probably have some nuisance value. They are troublesome to manipulate because of reduced visibility and they impose lighting requirements which may be inconvenient to meet, since special installations may be entailed. Furthermore, these materials may require particular processing.

CONTRAST AND SPEED

In distinction to normal radiographic film which is directly influenced by radiation contrasts in the subject, fluorographic film can be affected only by the contrasts available in the screen image: these inevitably have a shorter range. Consequently, fluorographic materials should have high contrast if changes in the luminosity of the screen are to be made readily apparent.

At the same time, emulsion speed is of some importance, in view of both the limited brightness of the fluorescent image and the desirability of using short exposure intervals when examining dynamic structures, such as those within the thorax and abdomen. Up to a point, the resolving power of these materials is of slighter significance than their speed and contrast; the limits of resolution are unlikely to be with the grain size of the emulsion but rather will be found elsewhere, in the optical system or in the structure of the fluorescent screen.

STRUCTURAL CHARACTERISTICS

Since these emulsions are exposed, not to penetrating radiation, but to light which is meeting the sensitive surface from one aspect only, they are single sided. In the case of roll film, the base is 0·13 mm in thickness and permanently grey dyed as an anti-halation measure. The 100 mm cut film has a somewhat thicker base (0·2 mm) which is blue tinted and has an anti-halation backing, which clears during development.

PROCESSING EQUIPMENT AND PROCEDURE

The processing of fluorographic film needs particular attention and exactitude of method. This is because the negative is a miniature and may require enlargement if its appearances are to be interpreted satisfactorily; the smaller the format, of course, the stronger is the reason to employ some optical enlargement and the greater will be the degree of enlargement necessary. In these circumstances, any processing imperfection (such as surface scratches and splashes or a 'dirty' appearance of the emulsion) is enlarged equally with the detail of the image, tends to be distractive and—at its worst—may intrude on the reading of radiographic information.

The extent to which such defects are unacceptable depends necessarily on the degree of their occurrence and on their perceptibility, which increases very rapidly with magnification. The common sense conclusion, at which no doubt the reader has already arrived unaided, is that any processing artifact appears worse on a 35 mm cine film than on a 100 mm single shot fluorograph.

It is not particularly easy to put lengths of roll film through a standard, manually operated, X-ray film processor. It has had to be done on occasions and undoubtedly is feasible, but in the interests of efficiency and success a department which intends to process fluorographic film should have an automatic processor capable of accepting such film. We shall consider now the equipment and methods available.

CUT FILM

MANUAL PROCESSING

If it is to be manually processed in a standard X-ray film processor, fluorographic cut film in a format of 100 mm × 100 mm is relatively easy to manipulate, provided that suitable processing hangers are available. A typical hanger for the purpose is seen in Fig. 16.9. A stainless steel frame, similar in its general style and overall dimensions to a hanger used for full-sized radiographs, is sectioned to provide a separate slot for each of nine miniatures.

Such hangers are suitable for use in a conventional X-ray film processor, having 2-, 3-, 5- or 10-gallon (9, 13, 22, 45 litres) tanks and are really the only specialised equipment required for an an efficient manually operated procedure.

However, so prevalent in hospitals at present are rapid automatic systems for processing radiographs, that perhaps the very application of a manual processor requires from us some remark. Users should note that only some varieties of cut fluorographic film are suitable for processing manually: operators should make certain that the emulsion used and the developer's formulation are compatible with the procedure and with each other. The manufacturer's instructions on the subject should be strictly followed, from the mixing and the use of the developer, to the temperature of the working solution and the period of the films' immersion.

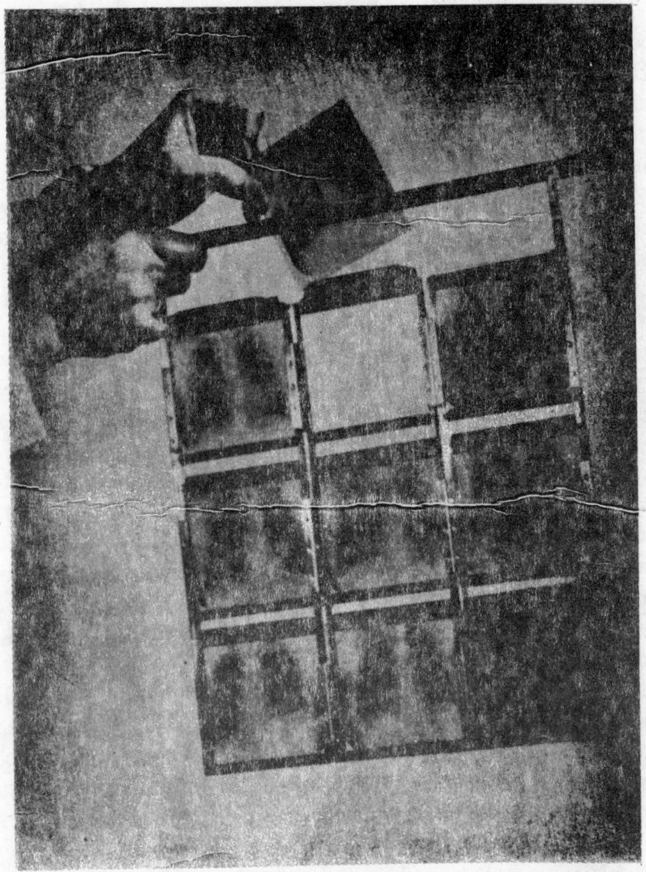

Fig. 16.9. A processing hanger for 100 mm fluorograms.
By courtesy of Picker International Ltd.

The recommended duration of the development time usually allows the user a considerable latitude: for example, it might be stated as 4–5 minutes. This is to permit some manipulation of density and contrast to meet a selected norm; it should not be employed as a sanction to develop films by sight, the operator determining visually when the films 'look as though they were dark enough'. The procedure should be standard, once it has been agreed. For the purposes of this book the proper norms are difficult to define: in most radiodiagnostic departments the criteria applied are wholly subjective and results are judged in terms of acceptability to the radiological eye.

AUTOMATIC PROCESSING

In radiodiagnostic departments within the United Kingdom the use of automatic equipment for radiographic processing is widespread. Many practitioners of fluorography probably expect—and are likely to prefer—to use their customary processing method, for fluorograms as well as for other radiographs, if reliably good image quality can be assured. In a general diagnostic X-ray department, where 100 mm fluorograms may form only a small part of the total processing load, it is understandable that a requirement to install special equipment either might be regarded as uneconomic or even might be impossible, because of lack of adequate space for an extra processor.

However, not all conventional X-ray film processors (particularly the bigger processors) are successful handlers of 100 mm cut film. The small sheets of film may fail, at some point in their travel, to negotiate any of several large racks of rollers and 'disappear' in the processor. It is necessary then to mount a search for them, which will entail switching off and opening the processor; and afterwards the careful examination of every rack of rollers in turn, until all the casualties are found. In a busy darkroom, this is an exercise which nothing recommends; nor are complaints of the occurrence confined to the darkroom, since not only the fluorograms, but other radiographs simultaneously involved, may have to be repeated.

Attaching a leader to a small film (see p. 482) reduces the likelihood of its 'loss' in the processor, but this is not a practical procedure when many such films have to be processed, as is usually the case for 100 mm fluorograms. Anyone purchasing a processor which will have to take both full-sized radiographs and 100 mm fluorograms should make a careful choice.

If difficulties are encountered with a department's existing equipment, or when the fluorographic load is a significant part of the work of a processing area, a special processor should be acquired. Typically, such a processor is suitable for any film of small width and can accept a maximum length of perhaps 180 metres. Thus, it is designed to receive both 100 mm cut film and cine or other roll film of various formats.

Like its larger brethren, a processor of this type transports the film by means of rollers in a number of racks. In a typical instance the processor operates from a cold water supply. It uses its own hot air—from the drier—to heat the wash water, a feature which might simplify a small darkroom's ventilation problem.

The processor described in the paragraph above may be highly automated. Whenever such a processor is switched to accept a new width of film, it makes an automatic adjustment of the processing conditions. It is programmed to prevent its starting unless all processing data are correct; for example, solution levels and temperatures. In addition to displaying a read-out of any such mishap, the processor is able to indicate to a probing service engineer the locations of faults in its systems. This sophisticated characteristic (not unusual in electronic equipment) is designed to reduce expenditure in various categories: this includes the engineer's time and consequently maintenance costs to the hospital, as well as delay and inconvenience to patients and others concerned in the service.

A choice of four transport speeds in this processor is available. They are adjustable by means of a switch and are of the following order: 1 metre/minute; 1·5 m/minute; 2 m/minute and 3 m/minute. In the case of 100 mm cut film for fluorography, the suggested transport speed is 1·5 to 2 metres/minute. For cine fluorography, a higher speed (3m/minute) is suitable for obtaining satisfactory density and contrast. Choices of transport speed depend upon the type of film to be processed, as well as on features of the equipment itself; 5 and 6 m/minute are typical values which may be encountered in the case of other processors. A manufacturer's recommendations always should be followed in relation to the use of an equipment and its chemistry and the type of film involved.

A typical processor has integral replenisher tanks for developer and fixer, each of 30 litres capacity. An automatic feeder for 100 mm fluorograms is available, which presents films one at a time to the processor in their order in the cassette. This is a daylight operation, although a darkroom is necessary to load the feeder.

Whatever, the method of processing, darkroom facilities are required for reloading the roller separator cassette. In carrying out this procedure, the sheets of cut film should be placed in the magazine so that the emulsion's surface will face away from the X-ray tube. It is good practice, upon removing the films from their wrapping, either to drop them as far as possible singly into the magazine, or—more quickly—to separate them by running the ball of the thumb over the edge of the pack (practised card players have the right knack). This is to assist the introduction of a thin layer of air between the films. Particularly in a damp atmosphere, individual members of a box may tend to adhere to each other and if more than one is taken up by the camera mechanism normal operation of the unit is prevented.

ROLL FILM

Darkroom manipulation of roll film is often more difficult, for two reasons.

1 The material may be panchromatic and thus impose total darkness on the operation.

2 Those who are more practised in handling conventional radiographs may be mildly disconcerted by long lengths of roll film. A reel of film can become unwound easily enough, sometimes with a freedom which escapes control; festoons of film on the darkroom floor are not readily rescued without damage, in the absence of any light by which to see what you are doing, and the result is a scratched emulsion or even a torn base.

Short lengths of roll film (not more than 3 metres) can be processed in a typical, manually operated X-ray processor. The film is wound—emulsion side outwards—on a processing frame which in effect is a conventional processing hanger. The hanger then is put through the different sections of the processor, in the usual way but for the absence of any safelight.

However, all this may be more easily said than done and the method has significant disadvantages, which include the following.

1 It is inappropriate for long runs of film.

2 Identification of the emulsion surface can be confusing, especially in total darkness. (An old trick is to touch a licked finger to an unimportant part of the film, such as the first inch or two of the roll: the emulsion aspect should feel a little tacky, compared with the reverse side.)

3 If the operator incorrectly identifies the emulsion surface and winds the film so that this aspect is innermost, the junctions at which the film and processing frame come in contact will fail to develop: the finished film will appear striated.

The simplest form of equipment particularly designed for processing lengths of roll film, and offering manual control of the cycle, is described as a spiral processor.

SPIRAL PROCESSING OUTFITS

A number of spiral processors are available. These vary in elaboration, details of design and the size of film for which they are appropriate. However, in general they consist of similar components.

1 A spirally grooved spool which is large enough in circumference to accept a suitable run of film, for example lengths of 7–30 m.

2 A loading device to facilitate winding the film on to this reel and rewinding it on to its original spool when necessary.

3 A set of circular processing dishes or tanks, usually four, of a size to accommodate the reel.

4 A lid to fit these dishes.

5 A spin drier.

Figs. 16.10 and 16.11 illustrate the Hansen unit which probably exemplifies the most refined of these systems.

The spool and loading unit. In this equipment the core of the spool is made up of three loose rings. The upper flange of the spool can be placed on the core so that all of these rings are between it and the opposite flange; or alternatively so that only one or two of the rings separate the two halves of the spool. This is illustrated in Fig. 16.12 and it can be seen that the device makes the reel adaptable to four different widths of film. Each of the flanges of the spool consists of a large number of toothed radii, the serrations of which are aligned with each other. The diameter of the reel is 292 mm.

The spooling unit is motor controlled and on completion of processing can further be used for winding the film back on the small spool which it will hereafter occupy for projection in the case of a cinefluorogram. This facility is helpful in keeping considerable lengths of film under control, in performing the operation quickly and in ensuring that the film is wound at an even and acceptable tension.

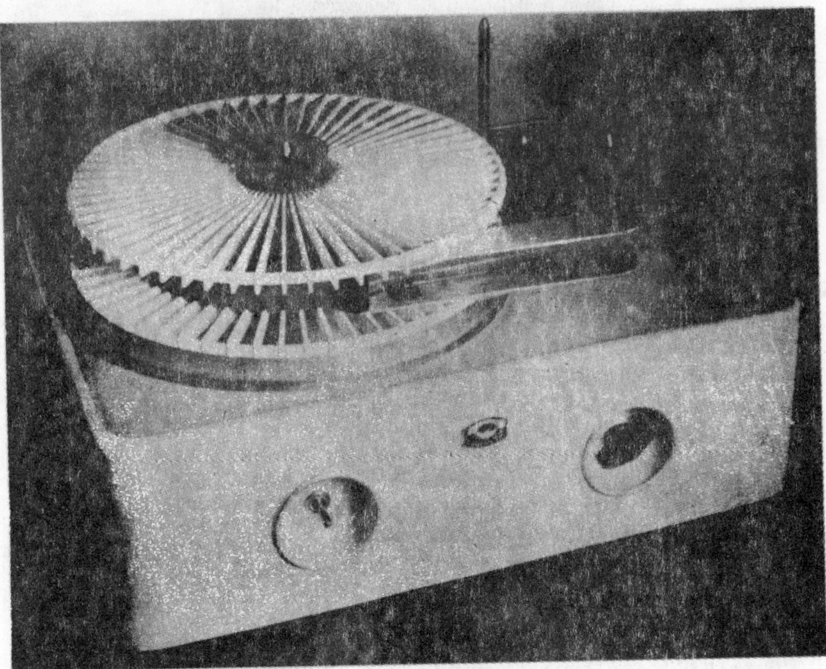

Fig. 16.10. The Hansen spiral processing reel and loader.
By courtesy of NV Optische Industrie de Oude Delft.

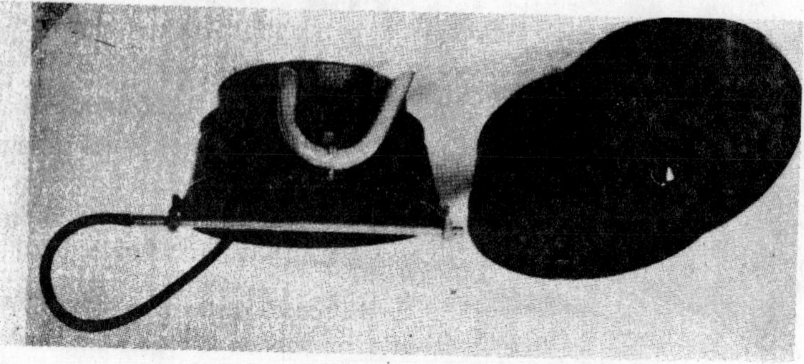

(a)

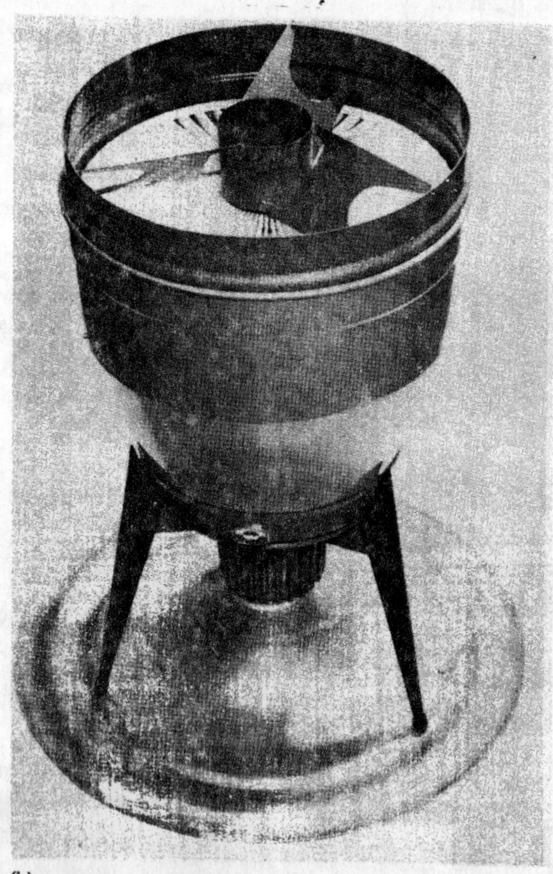

(b)

Fig. 16.11. Processing tanks and spin drier for the processing reel shown in position on the loader in fig. 16.10. *By courtesy of NV Optische Industrie de Oude Delft.*

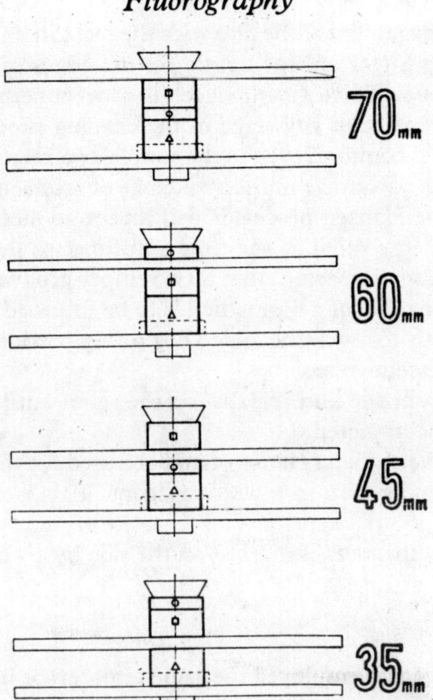

Fig. 16.12. Elevation diagram of the Hansen processing reel showing how the separate components of the centre section can be varied in position to alter the width available between the flanges of the reel. *By courtesy of NV Optische Industrie de Oude Delft.*

In operation the processing spool is first adjusted for the size of the film concerned and is then placed on a turn-table, with which it engages and will synchronously rotate. The film guide is a metal channel, the sides of which are adjustable in separation to accommodate the different widths of film. A needle at the free end of the guide engages a spiral groove on the rotating turn-table and causes the guide to move outwards in an ever widening orbit.

In its starting position the guide is swung inwards as far as possible towards the core of the spool. The roll of film is placed on an adjacent spindle. A small right-angled fold is made at the free end of the film and it is then fed down the guide until it passes beyond the extremity of the latter. By means of a variable control the motor is then started at a gentle speed. The synchronous rotation of the spool and movement of the guide will engage the film in the teeth of the former and feed it continuously on to the reel.

Successful engagement of the film with the reel can be detected aurally and by touch if a finger is kept lightly on the edges of the film at the entrance to the guide. Once the film is felt to move it need not be handled further by the operator at any stage in the ensuing procedure. The 'no touch' technique is common even to the simplest spiral processing outfits and offers obvious advantage in the avoidance of artefacts.

The reel of the Hansen processor will accept 30 metres of film. It is possible to put on the spool at one time a number of shorter lengths of film provided adequate spacing, that is two empty grooves, is maintained between them. The end of a film which is to be followed on the spool by another is less likely to touch the folded beginning portion of its successor if it is cut in a crescent shape.

Once in position, the film remains on the spool until processing and drying have been completed.

The processing tanks. The Hansen tanks are used for the following.

1 Preliminary immersion in a wetting agent. This is not an essential procedure.

2 Development; this tank is marked on the side by a white disc.

3 Rinsing.

4 Fixing.

5 Washing.

If a wetting agent is employed the same tank can be used for this and for rinsing.

The quantity of solution required in each tank during the first four stages will depend on the width but not the length of the film being processed. It is obviously important to respect the manufacturer's instructions in this and to be sure before processing is begun that the quantity of solution which has been prepared is correct for the film concerned. Apart from the waste of materials it is not serious if too large a quantity is made up: but if too little is prepared only part of the spool may be covered by the solutions and thus along one or other edge of the film an unprocessed band will result.

The spiral drier. The drier has a fan and in most cases a heater as well so that the air which is blown through the film spiral is warm. The reel is placed on a central spindle, upon which the current of air causes it to rotate. Water is flung off the surface of the film by centrifugal force as well as being evaporated by the passage of the warmed air.

Drying time averages about 1 hour. Its actual duration will depend on a number of factors which are significant whether fluorograms, radiographs, or indeed other photographic films are considered. These have been discussed in Chapter 8 and are restated briefly at this point.

1 The water-absorbing properties of the particular emulsion.

2   The degree to which the film was hardened in the fixer.

3   The length of time it was washed.

4   The ambient temperature and humidity of the atmosphere.

The interval required for complete drying will be minimized if the following points are observed.

1   The fixing solution is fresh, so as to ensure optimum hardening.

2   Washing is not unnecessarily prolonged nor the temperature of the water too high. Both these conditions result in increased swelling of the gelatin and consequently prolong the period of drying.

3   Efficient removal of excess water from the film surface before drying is begun. This means the use of a wetting agent as a final rinse. Immersion for about 1 minute in such a solution not only shortens drying time but prevents the formation of drops and consequently drying marks on the films.

4   The film is dried in a well ventilated room.

5   The drying apparatus both circulates and warms the air in the vicinity of the film. Most modern driers do this but some models may have a fan only.

AUTOMATIC PROCESSORS

Roll films applicable to fluorography—especially certain panchromatic emulsions in 16 mm and 35 mm formats for cinefluorography—may not be suitable for the automatic processors (and their chemistries) which inhabit X-ray departments. Such emulsions require either professional laboratory processing or manual processing by means of one of the systems which we have just described.

On the other hand, there are plenty of fluorographic materials available which are compatible with the chemistry, processing cycles and machinery of several standard X-ray processors, of the roller transport type. For a busy, general radiodiagnostic department, its appropriateness to a processor which is already functioning in the department might easily be a decisive factor in the choice of a particular fluorographic material. Images of high diagnostic quality can be obtained from these emulsions, even when they are processed through the rapid cycles and in the fast developers which many X-ray departments employ for virtually all radiography.

When roll film—particularly a narrow film—is put through an automatic processor not specifically designed for it, a leader is usually necessary. This may be a conventional sheet of X-ray film (in a small size, for reasons of economy) which is attached to the end of the roll film. The two films should be spliced edge to edge with a piece of chrome tape on either side, in the manner shown in Fig. 16.13. A 16 mm film will be narrower than the splicing tape and the latter's projecting portion should be cut away; the unwanted section is marked with a dotted line in the diagram.

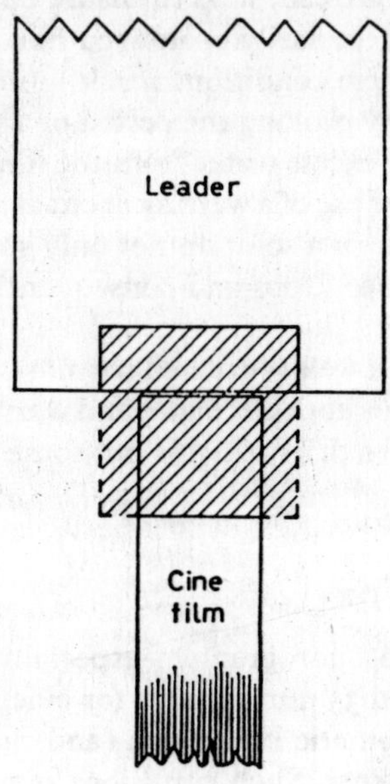

Fig. 16.13. Method of splicing a leader before processing a cine film. If the splicing tape (chrome) is wider than the cine film, remove—before processing—the sections marked by the dotted line.

If the roll film is kept over to one side of the automatic unit, other radiographs may be processed simultaneously provided that they are not so large as to overlap the smaller width of film. Safelights of course must be appropriate to the more sensitive film: the roll film is likely to be orthochromatic and the safelighting then should be dark red.

In a general radiodiagnostic department, when the through-put of film is assessed for replenishment purposes, the occasional cine film may be ignored, owing to both its narrowness and the thickness of the emulsion layer.

When a long length of narrow roll film is fed centrally through an automatic processor, a build-up of solution on the rollers may occur at the edges of the roll. Radiographs of conventional width, which follow the narrow film through the processor, may carry typical artifacts as a result of this. Several 'cleaner' sheets of film should be fed to the equipment before it is put to further use for wide films.

The automatic processor which has been described earlier in this chapter (p. 474), in connection with 100 mm film, is designed for all films of small width; this includes, of course, all roll film as well as cut sheets.

GRAININESS IN FLUOROGRAMS

As we have seen, at a much earlier stage of this book (p. 5), photographic and radiographic emulsions have a crystalline, granular structure. The images which are formed upon them—by light or X rays or both—similarly consist of a large number of small grains (grains of silver), which—in some circumstances—may produce an appearance of graininess when the image is viewed. This point was discussed in an earlier chapter, where it was said that graininess is unlikely to become significant for an observer, unless he is studying an enlargement. Consequently, in relation to medical radiography, the possibility of graininess in an image can be discounted to a large extent.

However, in fluorograms we have a category of radiograph which commonly may require optical enlargement, if an observer is to appreciate detail satisfactorily.

Image sizes obtained from the various fluorographic formats are of the following order:

Format	Image size
105 mm roll film	effective 100 mm diameter
	(90 mm across width of film)
100 mm cut film	95 mm diameter
70 mm roll film	65 mm × 65 mm
35 mm roll film	18 mm × 24 mm.

It is apparent that the smallest format is certain to require an enlarged display, whilst the larger formats are less likely to do so. Observers may satisfactorily interpret images on even 70 mm film without recourse to a magnifying glass, if the circumstances are such that one reader is viewing these films. Where it is necessary to make a display to a group of people simultaneously, magnification of the fluorographic image becomes essential. It is obvious that the larger the group and the smaller the format (for example, a 16 mm film projected in a lecture hall), the greater will be the degree of magnification required. Equally, certain short sighted observers may need to use magnification for any of the formats mentioned, and in almost any viewing circumstance.

Equipments for viewing fluorograms are described elsewhere in this book (Chapter 14). Our concern now is to establish that fluorographic images frequently are viewed under optical enlargement. If the degree of enlargement is sufficiently great, an image will lose coherence. In the extreme, it becomes no more than a meaningless distribution of 'dots' or grains on the surface of the emulsion; but much lesser occurrences of the effect may spoil recognition of image detail and thus constitute a significant hindrance to radiological interpretation.

A number of factors, as was stated in Chapter 2, affect graininess. One of these is the grain size of the emulsion and it is easy to appreciate that when the average grain size is large then the particulate structure of the emulsion will become apparent more readily than when the grains are small.

However, this is not the only significant factor. Other important influences are found in the developing solution and the degree of development. It is easier to understand the effect of these if we keep in mind that when we complain of a certain film that it is grainy it is not the individual particles of emulsion which are troubling the eye. These in fact are much too small and even at magnifications of 100 diameters would not become intrusive or perhaps even visible.

Graininess is due to the tendency of silver particles during development to cluster. These aggregates, since they are bigger than the individuals which compose them, can often be detected at quite low levels of magnification. They become perceptible because light percolates unequally through the groups and creates on the film areas of uneven density which are interpreted by the eye as a granular appearance. The student should understand that *grain* and *graininess* are not synonymous terms. Grain size is an important factor in the production of graininess, since materials which have a large average grain size generally show greater graininess.

In processing these fast, coarse-grained films, attention may be given to reducing as far as possible the tendency of silver particles to form these aggregates. For this purpose certain developers known as *fine grain* are available.

FINE GRAIN DEVELOPERS

The reasons why variations in graininess are obtained in different developing environments are perhaps not fully understood, nor need they concern us closely in the present context. We can accept as a practical fact that aggregation of the silver particles occurs more easily when the process of development is rapid; this implies an active, highly alkaline developer. It follows that fine grain developers are solutions of low energy. There are a number of types of such developer but those in most general photographic use are normal Metol-hydroquinone or Phenidone-hydroquinone developers in which the sodium carbonate has been replaced by an alkali of lower activity, for example borax. They have a pH value between 8 and 9. Usually their content of sodium sulphite (the preservative) is much increased.

One of the characteristics of sodium sulphite is that it is a weak solvent of silver bromide and during the relatively long period of development, which the lowered activity of the solution requires, this substance may dissolve a proportion of small, less sensitive halide grains. It has been thought that the solvent action of sodium sulphite on silver bromide may take part in inhibiting the production of graininess, perhaps by preventing the intermingling of developing centres in different crystals of the emulsion. However, the mechanism and facts of this are not known with certainty.

While it may seem desirable in principle to process fluorograms, particularly cinefluorograms, in fine grain developers, the following aspects of their use must be remembered.

1 They are generally, although not invariably associated with some loss of emulsion speed.

2 They produce images of comparatively low contrast. This is to the advantage of decreased graininess as the latter is more apparent when contrast is high, but it is to the disadvantage of detail perception in the fluorogram and of its suitability for projection.

3 The development time required to produce a given contrast may be impossibly long in an X-ray department, unless the film is given special processing (either manually controlled or automated).

4 The preparation and maintenance of separate tanks of developer in a general radiographic processing room inevitably complicate the work and they are to be avoided for practical reasons, unless there are strong arguments of another kind in their favour.

The determination of an appropriate film/developer combination for fluorography is seldom simple, though it is easy enough to state what may be needed to obtain images of optimum quality. Together, the materials should offer:

1 high resolution;

2 good contrast;

3 adequate density, for acceptable levels of radiation input;

4 freedom from grain.

Having set down these criteria, we find ourselves at once at the edge of a quicksand of decisions. Germane to these decisions is a question which we might ask: what quantity is implicit in any of the four requirements just stated? If we could quantify these characteristics in medical radiographs, attach to each a numerical label, we would have taken a firm step towards accurate evaluations of different materials.

Unfortunately, the appearances present in medical radiographs cannot readily or usefully be quantified, because their analysis finally is made subjectively by the human eye. When we see degraded images, we recognise that resolution may be too low, or contrast too poor, or density insufficient, or grain obtrusive; conversely, when all these qualities are moved to the other limits, everyone would agree that the images are 'good'. However, we cannot realistically determine a single level or quantity for any of these criteria, when for all viewers in all viewing conditions an image would pass the line between acceptibility and unacceptability. Our assessments are mainly opinioniative.

When it is necessary to select a film/developer combination for fluorography, first thoughts on the subject will be governed by the type of fluorography to be undertaken and the film format to be used. After that, individual elements of experiment and experience are likely to shape a practitioner's arguments and determine a choice. The following considerations are relevant.

The graininess inherent in a faster emulsion might be combated successfully if the material were processed in a fine grain developer. However, this could entail a loss of emulsion speed sufficient to cancel the original advantage for which the emulsion was chosen. In these circumstances the combination would offer no improvement in effective speed over a slower film of finer grain in association with a standard X-ray developer; indeed the latter might be the preferable partnership since the resolution obtained with the finer grained material would be superior, contrast would be higher and processing easier.

Differences in contrast increase the difficulty of comparing such film/developer combinations. Processing to a high degree of contrast in an X-ray developer may permit visualization of details which are not apparent when a fine grain, low contrast developer is used; but there is equal likelihood of this treatment's producing a grainy pattern in the image, particularly in the case of a narrow film of which magnification must necessarily be higher for comparable viewing.

It is very clear that there is not an ideal 'right' answer to the problem created by these opposing forces. In order to summarize the matter we can high-light the pinnacles of the argument as follows.

A fast film processed in high contrast, X-ray developer results in:

1 maximum speed, therefore diminished dose to the patient and least electrical load on the X-ray tube;

2 maximum image contrast;

3 maximum graininess.

A slow film processed in a fine grain developer results in:

1 maximum detail but high radiation dosage and severe electrical load;
2 lower contrast in the image;
3 minimum graininess.

Depending upon the camera available, the characteristics of its lens and shutter speeds and the type of work which it is intended to undertake, practical cinefluorographic techniques are likely to be found with some intermediate combination of these materials. It must be recognized that the ultimate choice can hardly be made theoretically but only from experiment and experience in the conditions obtaining and with the equipment at hand.

IMAGING WITH VIDEO TAPE AND VIDEO DISC RECORDING

Earlier sections of this chapter have been concerned with cameras and films which may be used for record purposes during fluoroscopy with an image intensifier. Such cameras, with their associated films, are not the only instruments which may be so employed. Recording and storage systems are available which depend on television applications. These do not use film and are neither photographic nor fluorographic, as we have defined the word. However, it may be argued that video images—since they are radiodiagnostic images—cannot be kept apart from the readers of this book; and even that video recordings of fluoroscopy are within the scope of a chapter on fluorography (especially if we follow Humpty Dumpty's policy of making words mean what he chose them to mean, neither more nor less!).

MAGNETIC TAPE RECORDING

Video tape recording of the fluoroscopic image is a process which is similar to the magnetic recording of sounds, familiar to us in its application to dictation machines and cassette players. In this case, two large video heads (the reel diameter is 26·7 cm) carry a chromium dioxide tape, 2·5 cm in width; the tape width affects resolution, narrow tapes being worse resolvers of a video signal than are wide ones. The video tape includes two audio channels for the synchronous recording of—say— reporting notes and the patient's heart sounds or speech; or a spoken commentary may be added later, if so wished. Any of these tracks may be erased independently, or all may be erased simultaneously, as required. After erasure a video tape of course can be used again, although—like other magnetic tapes—its life is not indefinite; in time its recording quality must deteriorate and a new tape is needed.

Many control aspects of video recorders hardly differ from those of their commoner audio brethren; these include facilities to record, stand-by, playback and rewind. Typically, playing time might be 110 minutes, with a tape speed of 21 cm/second and a high re-wind speed of 1·5 minutes for 1 hour of playing time. Additional features incorporate slow-motion replay, either forwards or backwards, and also single frame advance and reverse. There is a photoelectric end-of-tape cutoff, to prevent tape being pulled from either reel.

A video recorder can be attached to any installation for an X-ray image intensifier with closed circuit television. As the television signal is fed to the recorder through cables, it is not essential for the fluoroscopic table/image intensifier and the recorder to be immediate neighbours; this has an advantage in adding no extra weight to the fluoroscopic equipment.

The main advantage of a video tape recorder is not to formulate permanent records but in its ability to provide an instant replay of an examination or of any phase of an examination. A fluoroscopic sequence can be studied at once and as often as may be required, without the occurrence of either the delay entailed in radiographic processing or any added inconvenience and radiation risk to a patient; the next stage of a procedure may be planned quickly from information contained in a 'scout' survey made on video tape.

In some equipment, a video recorder is used to check immediately the content of fluorographs or radiographs exposed directly by means of a table's serial changer. An arrangement of this kind is sketched diagramatically in Fig. 16.14.

In giving the examining radiologist instant reassurance that he has obtained the exposures required for diagnosis and record, such equipment potentially accelerates a procedure and may allow patients to leave an X-ray department more quickly after examination. From everyone's viewpoint, this might be a saving grace in a department topographically cramped.

VIDEO DISC STORAGE

Image storage by means of video discs offers several possibilities during television fluoroscopy. The storage medium is a magnetic disc, 10–15 cm in diameter. It is made from high density nickel cobalt, applied to a substratum of aluminium, and carries a variable number of tracks, from 1 to 4. During use, the disc is driven by a motor and rotates synchronously with the mains supply (3000 rev./min. at 50 Hz). If the disc recorder is to

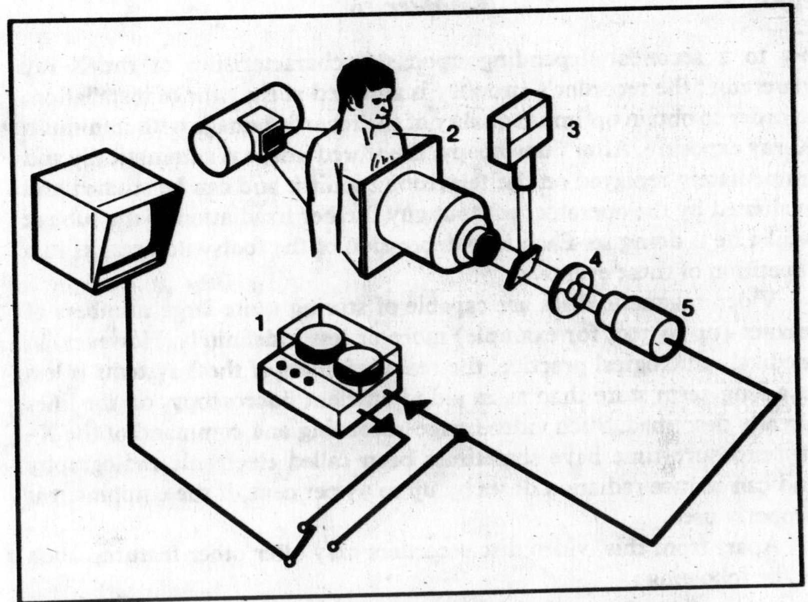

Fig. 16.14. A sketch to depict the use of a video tape recorder for the purpose of immediately checking fluorographs/radiographs exposed during image intensifier fluoroscopy.

1   Video tape recorder
2   Spot film device (serial changer)
3   Fluorographic camera —
4   Iris diaphragm to reduce the light for the TV camera tube and avoid over-exposure
5   Television camera tube.
By courtesy of Siemens Ltd.

be manually operated, this is done through a remote control box; but sometimes an automatic mode is adopted which gives automatic storage of the last television picture of a fluoroscopic examination (last image hold).

An arrangement of an automated kind is often used as a safeguard in preventing over-irradiation of a patient during television fluoroscopy by an inexperienced operator; C-arm mobile units are especially risky, as the fluoroscopist may not be radiologically educated (for instance, ortho-paedic surgeons and endoscopists often use these equipments, although a radiographer should be present whilst they do so).

Examination during very short periods of X-ray exposure is achieved through simultaneous video recording of a single 'picture'. Interfacing logical circuitry permits continuation of the fluoroscopic exposure only for as long as is required to record the video image. This period may be o·3 to 2 seconds, depending upon the characteristics of the X-ray generator; the recorder's circuitry is adjusted at the time of installation, in order to obtain optimum quality of the recorded image with minimum X-ray exposure. After fluoroscopy, the stored image is automatically and immediately replayed on the television monitor and can be studied and evaluated by the operator, without any further irradiation of the subject whilst he is doing so. Each new depression of the footswitch results in a repetition of these events.

Video magnetic discs are capable of storing quite large numbers of images (up to 300, for example) more or less indefinitely. However, in medical radiological practice, the real usefulness of these systems is less as a long-term store than as an aid to efficient fluoroscopy, on the lines already described. Such video image-recording and command of the X-ray exposure-time have sometimes been called electronic radiography and can reduce radiation doses by up to 95 per cent, if the equipment is properly used.

Apart from this, video disc recorders may offer other features, such as the following:
— automatic storage of the last television image of the fluoroscopic examination (last image hold);
— storage of any television fluoroscopic 'picture' (by means of manual, push-button control);
— by the inclusion of a second television monitor, simultaneous display of any stored image with the 'live' fluoroscopic image (for instance, during orthopaedic surgery, viewing of lateral and anteroposterior projections together would be possible);
— again with the use of a second television monitor, simultaneous playback of any two stored images;
— storage and immediate replay of several hundred dynamic images at variable rates (this almost cinematic facility includes the ability to stop the 'action' images at any time and view them singly or alternatively to display them in slow motion).

Chapter 17
Some Special Imaging Processes

XERORADIOGRAPHY

Like many another radiographic procedure, xeroradiography was first attempted within a few years of the discovery of X-rays, passed into disrepute for lack of adequate technology and was revived decades later as a realistic idea. Xeroradiography is not a process requiring any specialized X-ray equipment: it is merely a different method of recording an X-ray image. It depends upon the photoconductive behaviour of a selenium plate and substitutes a photoelectric process for the photochemical one associated with the use of a film.

THE XEROGRAPHIC PROCESS

THE LATENT IMAGE

The xerographic process depends on certain characteristics of an aluminium plate coated with a thin layer of vitreous selenium. These characteristics are:

1 the plate is an insulator in the dark but may become conductive when exposed to light or X rays;

2 if the plate is given a superficial electric charge, it is capable of retaining this charge for a period of hours;

3 in the charged condition, exposure of the plate to light or X rays effects conduction in the exposed areas.

Subsequent to any exposure of a charged plate to an X-ray beam, areas of the plate which have not been irradiated remain charged; areas which have been irradiated present diminished charges, correspondent with the pattern of incident radiation. As a result, losses of charge are found across the surface of the plate which are proportional to the radiation doses received at the points of interest and are in a distribution which duplicates the various blackenings which might be obtained on a radiographic

491

emulsion. The responses of the two image-recording media are depicted diagrammatically in Fig. 17.1.

It is seen that the exposed selenium plate contains a latent image, constituted from electric charges; this is comparable with the latent image formed in a photographic emulsion by undetectable chemical changes.

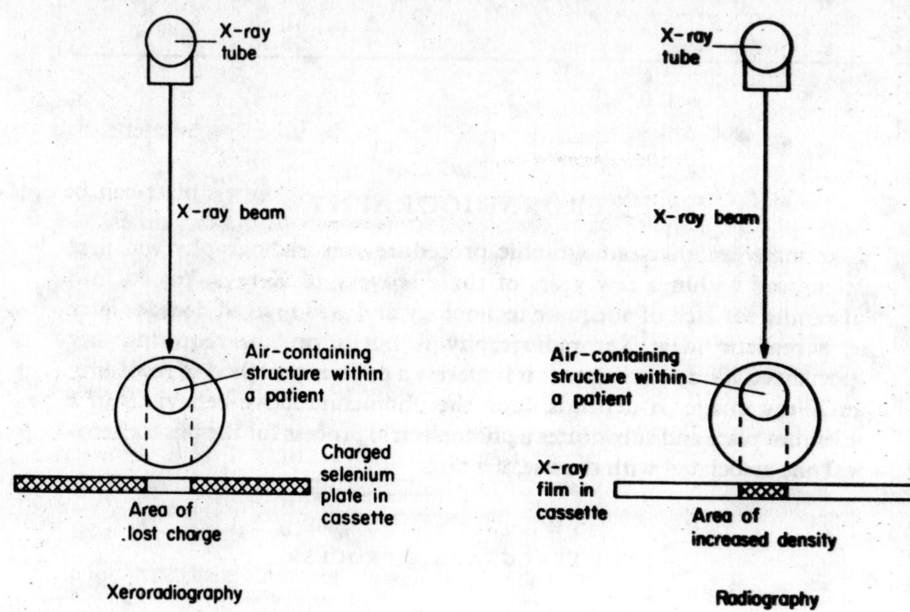

Fig. 17.1. Photoelectric and photochemical responses.

DEVELOPMENT OF THE IMAGE

Development of the latent image is a process which makes it visible. The most usual—although not the only—method of making the xerographic image visible is to spray the plate with an aerosol of powder; during this time the plate must continue to be protected from light in a dark box. The powder—which essentially is a cloud of charged particles—is attracted and adheres to the plate in a manner dictated by electromagnetic lines of force created near the surface. These occur because of:

1 the charge differences on the surface which we have already considered;

2 a voltage which is applied to the back of the plate during development. In this way the latent charge-image becomes a visible powder-image formed by the deposited powder. The distribution patterns of the powder

follow faithfully the electrostatic charge patterns on the plate, as these in precedence followed the radiation patterns of the X-ray exposure.

The production of a powder image on a selenium plate cannot remain as the final stage of xerographic processing. Such images necessarily are unstable: they would be readily marred by handling, by a breath, a sneeze or a breeze. Some more permanent form of record is required and this could be obtained from either of the next following processes:

1   photographing the powder image;
2   transferring the powder image to a plastic-coated paper and heat-sealing it to achieve a permanent fusion.

The second of these methods is the one widely used in commercially available equipment for xeroradiography.

Once a 'fixed' record has been obtained, the selenium plate can be discharged, cleaned and—with proper care—used again many times.

PROCESSING EQUIPMENT

Equipment for processing xeroradiographs needs to provide for the following operations:

1   charging of the selenium-coated plate (sensitization, usually performed immediately before use of the plate for an X-ray examination);
2   protection of the charged plate from light during all stages of its use (cassette-loading);
3   submission of the exposed plate to a powder aerosol (cassette-unloading and development);
4   transfer and sealing of the image to a sheet of suitably prepared paper (fusion);
5   complete discharge of the selenium plate (described as cleaning and relaxation);
6   storage of the cleaned plates ready for re-use (their safekeeping is important, as the vitreous selenium surface is delicate and may easily be damaged by handling).

To fulfil these various functions two machines are necessary, each dependent on the other: they are called respectively the conditioner and the processor. These equipments do not require any special lighting conditions and normally are arranged to stand side by side in almost any convenient working area which possesses a twin-socket 'domestic' power supply and is near to the X-ray room to be used.

THE CONDITIONER

The stages of processing for which the conditioner is responsible are:

1   plate storage;

2   cancellation of any remnant charge on an individual plate, which has been automatically abstracted from the store for next use;

3   sensitization of this single plate;

4   insertion of the sensitized plate in a cassette;

5   automatic release of the loaded cassette to the operator.

During normal use of the equipment, the plate is moved automatically by the conditioner's transport system and the operator should not need to handle it. In fact there is a requirement to avoid touching the plate—unless there are compelling reasons to do so—in order not to mark the sensitive surface layer.

In appearance the conditioner approximates to a large box mounted on a stand to bring it to a convenient working height (in fact, to equal the processor's height). It is almost a metre in length and is about half a metre in width and in depth. Fig. 17.2 indicates the internal arrangements of the

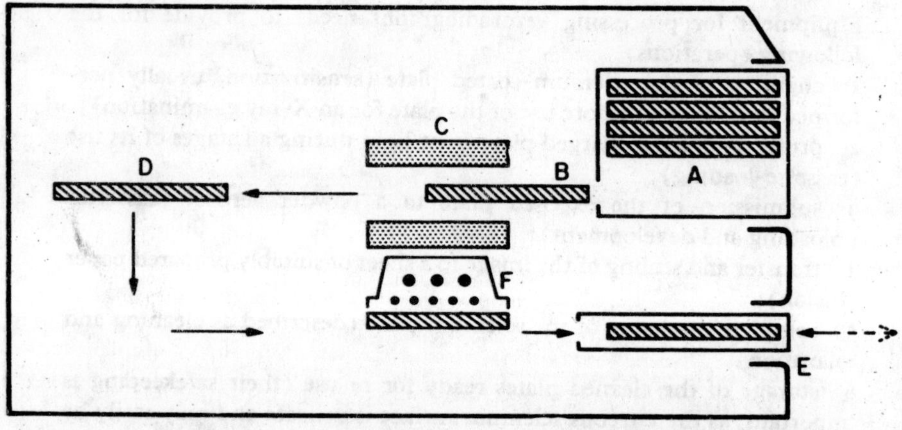

Fig. 17.2. Diagram (not to scale) illustrating the main features of the conditioner for xeroradiography.

A—a storage box inserted in the conditioner and containing 5 xerographic plates.

B, C—a plate (B) passes from the storage box through a small oven (C) which removes any residual charge from it; the plate passes then to a storage elevator (indicated at D).

E—insertion of an empty cassette initiates the charging process.

F—an ionizing device which charges the surface of the plate after it leaves the storage elevator and before it enters the open cassette.

conditioner, including two cavities or slots at the front end: in one of these, the operator loads a storage box containing five xerographic plates; and in the other, an empty cassette is placed to initiate the charging process. The cassette is a slim plastic box, rather less than 2 cm in depth and 40 cm × 26 cm in its other dimensions. At the time of writing, this is the only size of cassette commercially available: it carries a plate which is 34 cm × 23 cm.

The interval of time from the cassette's insertion in the conditioner to its ejection, loaded and ready, is of the order of 15 seconds. Initially, the conditioner requires a warming up period of about 30 minutes, but once this is completed it is maintained with stand-by characteristics and—so long as it remains connected to a live power supply—is immediately available whenever required.

Apart from the usual on/off switches, the equipment has one other external control. This is a thumbwheel switch which permits the operator to influence the contrast of the xeroradiograph by altering the level of the surface charge given to the plate: a high surface charge increases image contrast (and slightly increases density). The qualities of the xero-radiographic image are discussed more fully on p. 496.

THE PROCESSOR

The processor superficially looks much the same as the conditioner but is larger, being 130 cm in length and 64 cm in width; it stands 103 cm high, unaided. Like the conditioner, it includes—must include—a transport system for the plate: in this case it is necessary for the finished print and the xerographic plate eventually to go separate ways, the plate to a storage box and the processed print to a chute for delivery to the operator.

In summary, the duties of the processor are:

1   to unload the exposed selenium plate from a cassette inserted in a slot at one end of the processor;

2   to transport the plate to a development chamber;

3   to impart a bias voltage to the exposed plate, relative to the earthed body of the development chamber (the polarity of this voltage determines whether the image develops as a positive or a negative);

4   to submit the plate in the development chamber to a spray of powder, metered in short bursts and diffused by the introduction of air to the chamber;

5   to lift a sheet of transfer paper from a storage tray and move it to a position for contact with the powdered plate;

6   to bring the plate and the paper to a meeting or registration point, where a charge of opposite polarity, passed over the reverse of the paper, holds paper and plate closely together and attracts the powder layer to the paper;

7   to remove the paper—now carrying most of the powder—and diverge it to a 'fixing' station;

8　to transport the plate on another route, along which, at various stages, a neutralizing charge is applied to it, it is brushed clean of remaining powder and finally it enters a storage box at the front of the processor;

9　to fix the image on the paper by the application of heat to its surface;

10　finally to eject the finished xeroradiograph through a delivery chute at the front of the processor.

The total progression through the processor, from the insertion of an exposed loaded cassette to the emergence of a finished xerographic print, occupies about 90 seconds. The general arrangements within the processor are shown in Fig. 17.3.

Apart from on/off switches, the processor has two other external controls. These—like that on the conditioner—are thumbwheel switches: one of them allows the operator to select whether the final image will be in a positive or a negative mode; the other, which alters the length of the developing cycle, is the equipment's main control of image density during processing. The density and contrast of the xeroradiographic image are further discussed in the next section of this chapter.

THE XERORADIOGRAPHIC IMAGE

The most striking quality of a finished xeroradiograph is its peculiar contrast. In the second place, radiographers—and indeed others—may find it strange that the product is a print on paper, that this print is made in tones of blue and white and that we may study it, as we do a photograph, in any well lit room, without recourse to a special illuminator.

CONTRAST

The peculiar contrast pattern obtained by xeroradiography resides in a certain enhancement of all the 'edges' of an image, giving an impression of *bas relief*, almost a three-dimensional illusion. The effect of this high edge-contrast is to facilitate the recognition of detail by an observer and it is thus a significant aid to radiodiagnosis; indeed it is one of two important reasons why xeroradiography is medically practised.

Edge contrast occurs as a result of particular factors in the distribution of powder over the charged xerographic plate during development. A powder aerosol is not the only known method of developing xerographic images, but it is the one which results in this edge enhancement and thus is the only development process applied to xeroradiographs obtained for medical diagnosis.

During development of the exposed xerographic plate by a powder aerosol, the powder (properly known as the toner) is attracted to the plate

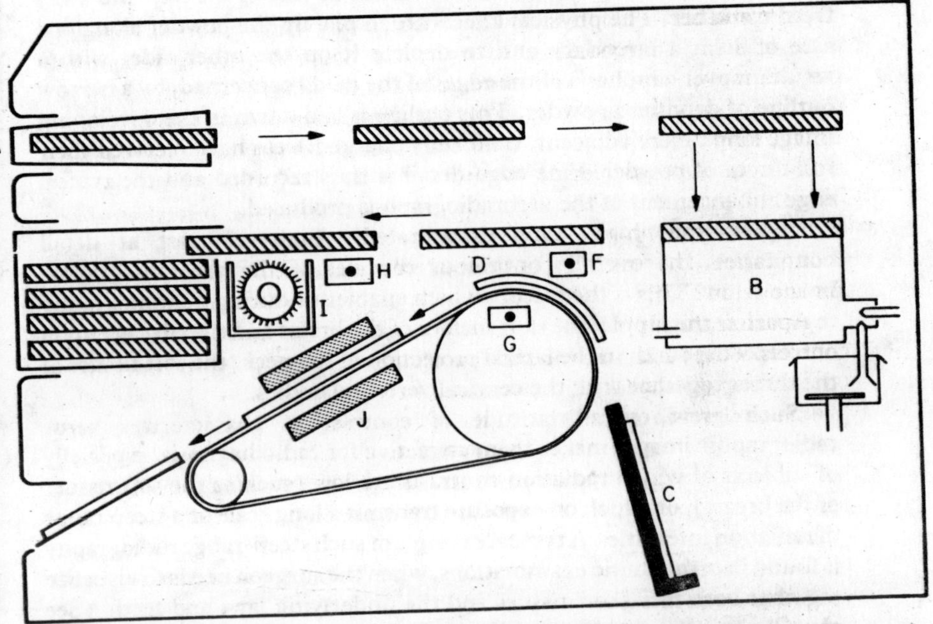

Fig. 17.3. Diagram (not to scale) illustrating the main features of the processor for xeroradiography.

A—the cassette, containing the exposed xerographic plate, is inserted in a slot and automatically unloaded.

B—the plate is transported to a development chamber, where developer powder (toner) is sprayed on its surface.

C, D—paper is removed from the paper tray (C) to a position (D) for contact with the powdered plate.

F—an ion-emitting device, the effect of which is to loosen the powder on the plate, preparatory to its transfer.

G—another ionizing device which gives the reverse side of the paper a charge of opposite polarity.

H—a third ionizing device which loosens any powder remaining on the plate after transfer.

I—a rotating brush which cleans the plate before it enters a storage box.

J—the paper passes through an oven (J) which fuses the powder image to the paper.

under the influence of electromagnetic fields. Of these, the important ones are perpendicular to the plate; they are strongest—and therefore attract the greatest quantity of toner—in areas of discontinuity in the charge pattern; they are weakest in areas of the plate where the charge is uniform. The edges of any well defined structure which is xero-radiographed—for example, a bone trabeculum—create sharp charge-'steps' on the plate's surface. Wherever such a step occurs, there is a small region on either side of it where the magnetic lines of force are closed semicircles and direct the powder towards one side of the step and away from the other. The physical effects are to pile up the powder along one side of such a boundary and to deplete it on the other side, with a resultant over-emphasis of the edges of the detail concerned, by a narrow outline of deposited powder. This outline is laid down in the developing image long before adjacent, uniformly charged areas have received their full quota of powder. Fine edge-detail is thus recorded and the typical edge enhancement of the xeroradiograph is produced.

Apart from high—even exaggeratedly high—contrast at detail boundaries, the overall continuous contrast of the xeroradiographic image is low. This is the feature which enables us during mammography to visualize the nipple, the skin surface of the breast and the rib cage upon one exposure; and, in the lateral projection of the neck, the soft tissues of the throat together with the cervical vertebral bodies.

Such great overall latitude of contrast as characterizes xeroradiographic images makes them attractive for radiodiagnosis, especially of subjects of which radiation contrasts are low (such as the soft tissues of the breast), or which on exposure transmit a long scale or a steep range of radiation intensities. A typical example of such steep-range radiography is found in orthodontic examinations, when the surgeon needs to visualize together both facial soft tissues and the underlying jaws and teeth. (See also Chapter 12 on radiographic contrast.)

The low continuous contrast of powder-developed xeroradiographic images is obtained because—within a few millimetres of the plate and provided that development time is short—the amount of powder which adheres to the plate over large areas is more significantly influenced by the density of the powder cloud, than by the value of the charge in each area. Thus there is a tendency for the distribution of the powder to be uniform; and, although there may be charge differences between areas, the powder makes little distinction of these differences, other than in a narrow region at the boundaries of each area. At such boundaries, as we have already described, strong edge-fields dominate the powder's distribution and lead to emphasized contrast. The matter may be summarized in the statement that the latitude of response given to us by xeroradiography occurs because the process of powder-development is very sensitive to charge differences and relatively less sensitive to absolute values of charge.

DETAIL SHARPNESS

Like other radiographic images, those made xerographically are subject to blur, which is compounded of three constituent unsharpnesses:

1 unsharpness inherent in the geometry of radiographic projection (size of the focal area of the X-ray tube, etc.);

2 unsharpness present because of movement from the subject during the exposure;

3 unsharpness inherent in the recording/processing media applied to the image.

The influences of (1) and (2) are described elsewhere in this book (see Chapter 12): here, we need consider only (3), the unsharpness arising from—and intrinsic to—the xeroradiographic system itself, firstly at the imaging stage and secondly at the processing stage.

If we take first the selenium plate upon which the image is formed by the distribution of electric charges, we find that the resolution of the recorded image is related to the thickness of the selenium layer. A thick coating (possibly—for example—a millimetre or more in depth) is bound to impair resolution, from merely geometric principles. Radiation being propagated in straight lines, as the X-ray beam traverses the active layer, charge patterns on the surface are unable fully to register with the similar patterns arising at a depth and therefore at a distance. This lack of registration between effectively two images is appreciated as blur.

To avoid such a situation, the selenium must be thinly coated. However, the use of a very thin layer may significantly affect the sensitivity of a plate; that is, the plate becomes 'slow' and an unacceptably high level of exposure dose might be required. One xeroradiographic system, which is widely available commercially, employs plates coated with selenium to a thickness of 120–130 microns, which—we may suppose—puts no undue limitation upon either resolution or speed.

The second important factor in the intrinsic unsharpness present in xerographic images exists in the method of development. Powder development of xeroradiographs may limit resolution, depending upon (a) the size of the powder particles and (b) the value of the charge acquired by the particles. It is unnecessary now to consider these aspects in mathematical detail. The situation can be easily summarized if we say of (a) that the production of good detail sharpness depends on the toner having small particles of powder, rather than large ones. In regard to (b), when the particles of powder are diffused in air they become charged by particle-to-particle contact and the processes of friction, negative and positive charges being acquired in about equal numbers. Good resolution is dependent upon each particle carrying a high specific charge and this in turn occurs when the aerosol contains a low concentration of powder.

From what has been said, it must be evident to the reader that those characteristics intrinsic to a xeroradiographic system and affecting image sharpness do not come within the immediate control of the radiographer operating the system. We may expect that the equipment and materials which we use have been carefully planned in awareness of the principles here indicated and that intrinsic unsharpness is not as a rule dominant in our xeroradiographs.

POSITIVE AND NEGATIVE IMAGES

Xeroradiographs may be obtained as either a positive or a negative image, at the choice of the operator. The determination occurs during development of the image and is effected through a control on the processor which alters a bias voltage applied to the selenium plate (see p. 495).

The positive image is the easier to produce. The charge patterns on the plate after exposure are always positive. A positive voltage applied to the plate (relative to the earthed body of the development chamber) enhances the attraction of the charged areas for negative powder particles and results in a deposition of powder which is heavier in areas which have been irradiated less. Consequently, the radiographic appearances are the reverse of those usually seen, skeletal parts being visualized in 'darker' tones than are other tissues. The image is said to be positive and the required development process is described as charged area development.

For a negative xeroradiograph, the circumstances of development must reverse and the highest charged areas of the plate attract the least quantity of powder: this is discharged area development. It is achieved by applying a negative bias to the plate. Positive powder particles, reaching the vicinity of the plate, are repelled from charged areas, especially those highly charged, but are helped by the negative bias voltage to become attracted to areas where the charges are least, that is those areas which have had most X-ray exposure: the familiar, negative radiographic appearances result.

It is generally said that positive xeroradiographs are preferred for soft tissue studies, such as those of the face in the course of orthodontic treatments, and their use for mammography is traditional. On the whole, viewers are able to adapt quite readily to the strangeness of the positive mode.

Harder to recognize is the print's mirror-transposition of the subject. A radiograph avoids this, because it is a transparency and can be viewed from either side, thus correcting such reversal when it occurs. Anatomical marking of all radiographs is important (see Chapter 14) and never more so than in the case of xeroradiographs: the right and left sides of the patient must be clearly and permanently signified.

COPYING RADIOGRAPHS

To copy a radiograph is to produce a second from the first: the second may be smaller in size than the first, it may be the same size or it may be larger than the first. These three descriptions could be classified as follows: (i) miniaturized copies; (ii) facsimiles; (iii) enlargement copies. We have already (in Chapter 4) mentioned the miniaturized copies with reference to the storing of radiographs. A somewhat different need for miniaturized versions is the production of 35 mm copies to be mounted as slides used for projection in lectures, demonstrations and training programmes. In this present chapter we mention later a technique which may be used to obtain such copies by reduction.

We are not here considering techniques for enlargement copies as they do not come within the scope of practice in X-ray departments. Facsimiles, however, are commonly made in diagnostic X-ray departments by means of a relatively simple technique, using materials which are readily available: this matter we propose to describe further.

FACSIMILE RADIOGRAPHS

To be able to provide facsimile radiographs with a minimum of specialized equipment, materials and skills is useful. The additional radiographs may serve in teaching and in disseminating knowledge; may be transferred with a patient to another hospital; may be put in a patient's records; may be used in exhibitions and in film libraries; may eliminate for the patient a repeated examination. So there are good reasons for practising this technique, some of them academic, some of them economic, some of them protective of the interests of the patient, who may be spared wasted time, perhaps extra discomfort and certainly unnecessary radiation dose.

FILM MATERIALS USED FOR FACSIMILES

The method used to make facsimile radiographs in X-ray departments is called copying by contact. The radiograph to be copied is placed in contact with a special film material, the contact being close, even and firmly maintained. These special film materials, called duplicating films, are exposed to light through original radiographs which are to be copied and the results after processing are further radiographs which appear similar to the originals.

The special characteristic of the copying material is that it has been treated to make its reaction to exposure and development opposite to the usual one: instead of being dark with a photographic density where exposure has occurred, this film is dark where exposure has not occurred. When this film is put into perfect contact with a radiograph and is exposed to light through it, the following sequence of events occurs (see Fig. 17.4):

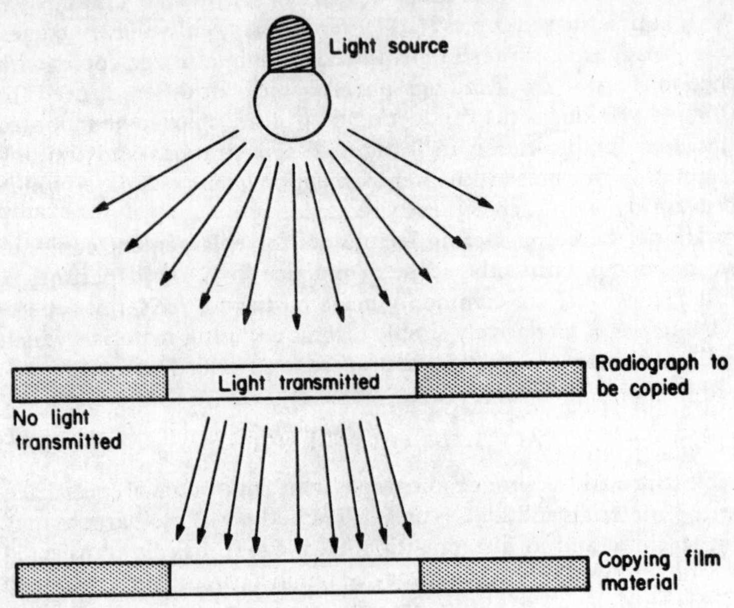

Fig. 17.4. Contact printing on duplicating film.

(i) the dense areas of the original radiograph transmit no light to the new film;

(ii) the new film reacts to this lack of exposure by showing dense areas itself on development;

(iii) the translucent areas of the original radiograph transmit light to the new film;

(iv) the new film reacts to the exposure by itself being translucent and lacking in density after processing.

So the dense and translucent areas of the original radiograph are matched by the densities and translucencies of the copy and the results constitute a facsimile, in tone and in size the same as the first radiograph.

We have already mentioned duplicating film on page 44 in Chapter 2 and have described it as a single-sided material: that is, with emulsion on one side only of the base. The other side of the base has an anti-halation layer to absorb any light which passes at the time of the exposure through the emulsion and the base: this layer is removed during processing. The emulsion side is usually identifiable by a code notch in one corner of the sheet of film, placed there at the time of manufacture in order to aid orientation. For example, Kodak RP/D X-Omat Radiograph Duplicating Film has the notch so placed that when it is in the top right corner of the sheet of film, the emulsion aspect is then facing towards the user: this placing of the notch in the top right corner is commonly encountered.

Duplicating film commercially provided for use in X-ray departments is suitable for processing in the automatic processors and in the conditions of safelighting which are found in their darkrooms. Thus, for example, Kodak state of their duplicating film which is mentioned above that it can be processed automatically in 90-second machines and in those with longer cycles or, if you insist, it can be processed by a manual method. The suggested safelight filter under which to handle the film is Kodak No 6B (which is brown) or Kodak OA (which is greenish yellow). Duplicating film is blue-sensitive as is X-ray film and so the safelighting conditions which are appropriate for radiographic materials are suited also to the handling of duplicating film. Duplicating film must be treated carefully for it is susceptible to damage from strains such as pressure and creasing and to the marks of finger prints: the results of mishandling are artefacts in the image.

THE LIGHT SOURCE AND EXPOSURE TIME

The light source to which the duplicating film is exposed in making a contact copy importantly influences the result obtained: the nature of the light varies the contrast obtainable in the copy. If it is intended that the contrast of the copy should be very similar to or identical with that of the original radiograph, then the light source used to make the contact copy should be an ultra-violet one: Kodak recommend for use with their film a 230–250 volt, 8 watt BLB fluorescent tube. Alternatively it may be wished to use the copying process to obtain a radiograph with contrast which is enhanced beyond that of the original. An increase in contrast up to 30 per cent is said to be obtainable and for this a tungsten light source is used. Kodak suggest for use with their film a 275 watt Photoflood bulb in a suitable holder.

The density of the copy is controlled to match that of the original by varying the exposure time. In considering this matter, it must be remembered that since the response of the duplicating film is the reverse of the usual, *increased density* in the copy is the result of *less exposure* and *decreased density* in the copy is the result of *more exposure*.

The amount of exposure which is required to make a good copy depends upon the following factors:

(i) the mid-range density of the original radiograph;

(ii) the brightness and the nature of the light source used;

(iii) the distance between the light source and the film which is being exposed;

(iv) characteristics of the material being used to make the copy.

DETERMINING THE EXPOSURE TIME

The exposure time required to give a good copy of a particular radiograph can be determined by trial and error but of course this is potentially a wasteful method since you may have to discard a quantity of expensive material. If you do wish to make a test exposure first, the most economical way to do it is to cut a broad strip of the duplicating film and use it placed across the main area of diagnostic interest in the radiograph to be copied.

For their X-Omat Duplicating Film Kodak publish a chart which is shown in Fig. 17.5. To use this chart, the mid-range density of the original radiograph must be assessed and the exposure conditions should

Exposure chart (s.f.d. 1.2m; standard processing) processed either automatically in a Kodak RP 'X-Omat' Processor or manually in Kodak DX-80 Developer, diluted 1 + 4, 4 minutes at 20°C.

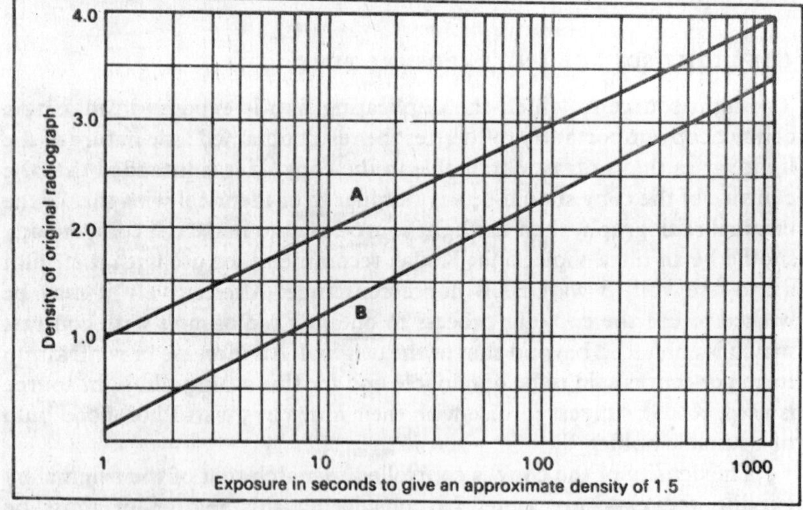

A = 275 watt Photoflood
B = U.V. 8 watt BLB

17.5. Kodak chart for exposure times.

be as indicated in the chart: that is, the light source should be a 275 watt Photoflood bulb or a UV 8 watt BLB fluorescent tube at a distance of 1·2 metres from the film. To take examples from the chart, if the mid-range density of the original radiograph is 1·0 and the UV fluorescent tube is the light source, the suggested exposure is 6 seconds; if the mid-range density is 1·5, the suggested exposure to the same light source is almost 20 seconds.

EQUIPMENT USED

It is essential to use some equipment to hold the duplicating film and the original radiograph in close contact with each other while the exposure is made. The contact needs to be maintained by firm pressure evenly applied over the surfaces of the films: if this condition is not met, the definition in the copy is poor for the image noticeably lacks sharpness of outline. It is also essential for light to reach the duplicating film through the original radiograph while the two are held in contact against a smooth flat surface. There are various possibilities, as follows.

(i) Use a very simple home-made contact printing assembly. It consists of a piece of firm hardboard of size as large as the largest radiograph to be copied, one surface of it being covered with a thin (6·0 mm) layer of polyfoam sheet. A piece of heavy, optically clear glass (6·0 mm plate glass) which is somewhat larger than the hardboard is used as the front for this. The glass should be heavy enough for its weight to keep the two films in contact with each other. For use, the duplicating film is placed on the hardboard, the original radiograph is laid on top of it and the glass is put over both. The light used for the exposure is transmitted through the glass and through the radiograph to reach the duplicating film.

(ii) Somewhat more convenient in use, especially if several copies are to be made, is a photographer's contact printing frame. This is a device specially constructed to hold film materials for contact printing and it is simply a frame with a glass front similar in form to an ordinary picture frame and its glass. The back is hinged and is designed to keep firm even pressure over the whole surface of the glass front. For use, the back is opened and the original radiograph is laid inside on the glass front, the duplicating film is put on top of it and the back is closed. The frame is then turned so that its glass front faces the light source to be used for the exposure.

(iii) A third possibility is to use commercially available printers (or indeed something similar constructed in a hospital workshop). A printer designed specially for radiographic use is basically a box-like structure with light sources inside it. The 'lid' of the box acts effectively as a printing frame and the original radiograph with the duplicating film in contact with it are placed on the glass at the top of the box: Fig. 17.6 shows the arrangements. Within the box there may be up to three light sources available: one white light source for viewing when the radiograph is placed in the printer; one tungsten light of higher wattage for the exposure; one ultra-violet light source for the exposure. Switches allow choice of light source and there is an automatic timer with a range of selections. A press-button switch is operated to start the exposure, which is automatically terminated through the timer at the end of the selected time.

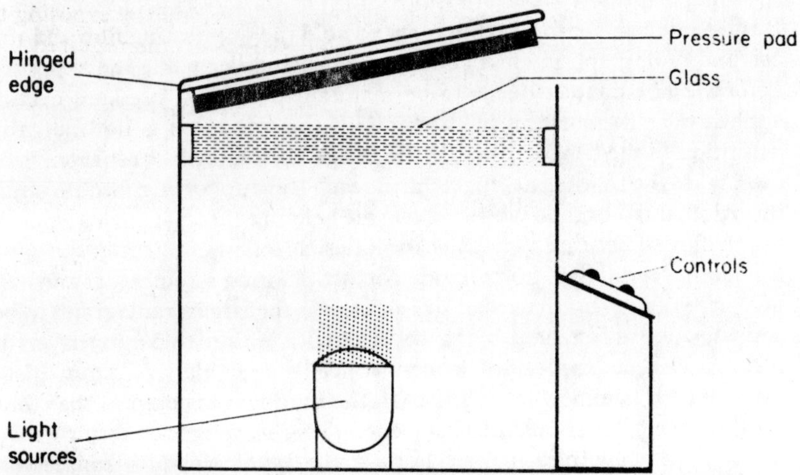

Fig. 17.6. Contact printer.

THE PROCEDURE

The duplicating film, having emulsion on one side only, has one surface which is shiny and reflective (the back) and one surface (the emulsion side) which is matt: the difference between the two surfaces is still apparent after the duplicating film is processed following exposure. A radiologist may be reluctant to view facsimile radiographs which are unexpectedly glossy: the slight shock of this can be evaded if copies are viewed always from the matt side. It is easy to arrange for this as explained below in the steps of the procedure.

(i) The radiograph to be copied is put into the printing frame or printer so that its conventional viewing aspect is against the glass and so towards the light source when the exposure is made. This ensures that the copy, when conventionally viewed, will be seen from its non-glossy aspect.

(ii) Under safelights, a sheet of duplicating film of the same size is placed in contact with the radiograph, emulsion side towards it and in registration with it.

(iii) The printing frame or printer is closed.

(iv) If the hardboard and glass assembly is being used instead of a frame or printer, the hardboard should be placed on the darkroom bench with the polyfoam surface uppermost. The sheet of duplicating film is then put on top of it with its emulsion surface uppermost. The radiograph to be copied is put on top of the duplicating film, the viewing aspect of the radiograph being uppermost: that is, towards the light source and next to the sheet of glass when that is put on top.

(v) Exposure is made either by operating the printer or by exposing the glass surface of the frame or hardboard assembly to the required light source for the required period of time.

(vi) The duplicating film is then removed and is processed. The result is a facsimile radiograph from the original.

COPYING BY REDUCTION

It is not a complicated process to obtain from radiographs reduced versions which will be 35 mm copies mountable as 2 × 2-inch slides. The absence of specialized reduction equipment or of access to a photographic department is not a bar to this procedure since slides can be made using a single lens reflex camera loaded with 35 mm daylight-type reversal colour film: for example, Kodachrome 25 Film (Daylight). Such film is sent for commercial processing and is returned with each frame in a card or plastic mount which is 2 × 2 inches square and is suitable for projection in a standard slide projector. Fig. 17.7 shows arrangements. There are a few practical points to consider, as follows.

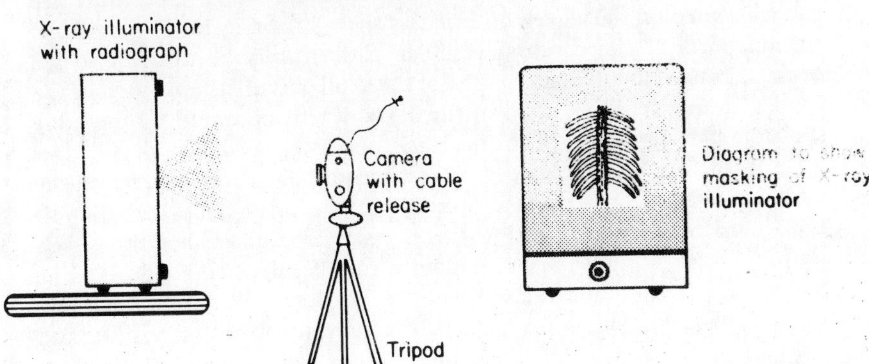

Fig. 17.7. Copying with SLR camera.

(i) The illuminator must be masked as indicated in Fig. 17 7 if the radiograph to be copied is not large enough to cover its whole surface. It is essential that the only light transmitted from the illuminator towards the camera is *through* the radiograph. If the illuminator is not fitted with masks, suitable masking can be arranged with black paper or card.

(ii) If the illuminator is fitted with tubes of colour temperature 6500 K and daylight-type film is used, the resultant slides have a slight blue tint which makes them acceptably resemble original radiographs.

(iii) The camera much be mounted on a firm tripod and the exposure must be made through a cable release so that jarring can be avoided: camera shake is bound to give a blurred image.

(iv) Very little incident light should fall on that aspect of the radiograph which is facing towards the camera and certainly no direct light should reach it. So it is best to undertake the photography in a semi-darkened room.

(v) Exposures should be calculated by means of a suitable exposure meter. The areas of the radiograph to be read with the meter are those of the least density which show perceptible detail.

(vi) Since the film being used is a reversal material, if the resultant reduced copy lacks density in comparison with the original radiograph then the copy has been overexposed. If the reduced copy has density which is too great in comparison with the original radiograph, then the copy has been underexposed.

SUBTRACTION APPLIED TO RADIOGRAPHY

In some angiographic examinations, radiographs taken after the injection of a contrast agent may be unhelpful because other structures are superimposed on the vessels outlined by the contrast agent. For example, certain parts of the cerebral vascular pattern may be difficult to see because bony structures in the base of the skull obscure them: parts of the vessels arising from the arch of the aorta can be obscured by the bony skeleton and soft tissues of the neck and upper thorax.

Subtraction is a technique to remove the obstructive parts of the image and to give a radiographic record in which the bones and the soft tissues are not shown (or are shown only as a faint image) and the vessels outlined with contrast agent remain clear of intrusive shadows. The name subtraction indicates that the process takes away certain radiographic shadows. This removal is achieved by using a positive and a negative image to cancel each other.

We can explain this further in considering Figs. 17.8 to 17.13. Fig. 17.8 can be considered to represent a radiograph of certain metal numerals. As

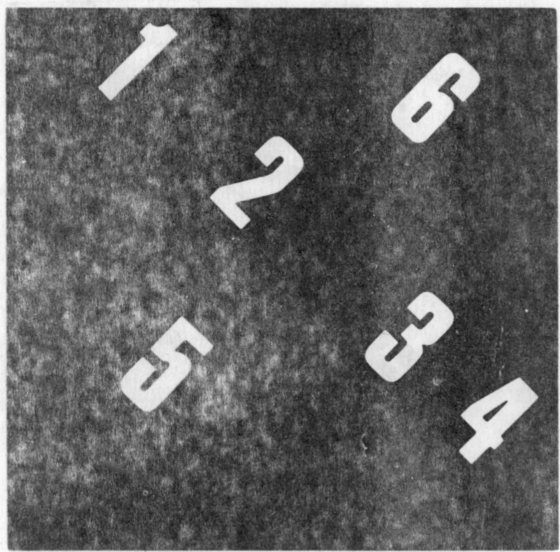

Fig. 17.8. Diagrams to illustrate subtraction.

usual, it is a negative image showing white digits on a dark ground. We call it Film A and describe it as the basic radiograph. Fig. 17.9 can be considered to represent the radiograph that results if Film A is used to make a contact copy on another piece of film which is not a reversal material: as can be seen this second radiograph is a positive image showing black digits on a light ground. We call this Film B and describe it as the radiographic mask.

If Film A (the basic radiograph) and Film B (the radiographic mask) are exactly superimposed, the translucent areas of the one fit over the dense areas of the other and the two images cancel each other. The result is seen in Fig. 17.10 as a radiographic image which is not there! It has been made to disappear by the negative-positive superimposition.

Fig. 17.11 is almost the same as Fig. 17.8. It represents another radiograph which is the same as the basic radiograph with some addition: in our Fig. 17.11 it is an extra numeral and this represents the addition of a contrast agent. So we call Fig. 17.11 Film C or the angiographic radiograph.

Fig. 17.12 shows the result of Film B (the radiographic mask) and Film C (the angiographic radiograph) superimposed upon each other. The mask has a positive image and this image is also present in a negative version in the angiographic radiograph: in practical radiographic

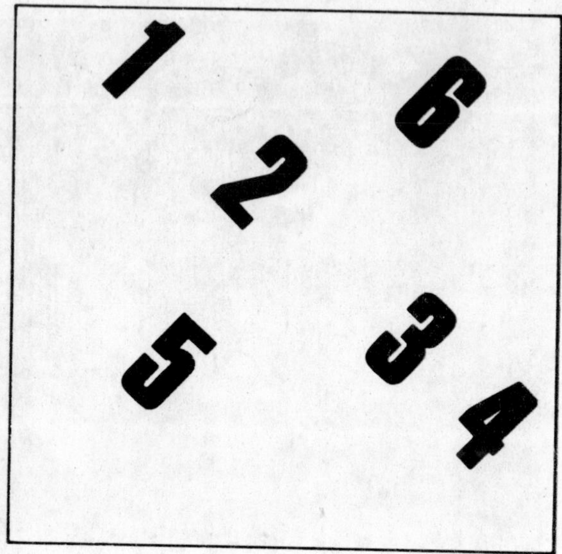

Fig. 17.9. Diagrams to illustrate subtraction.

Fig. 17.10. Diagrams to illustrate subtraction.

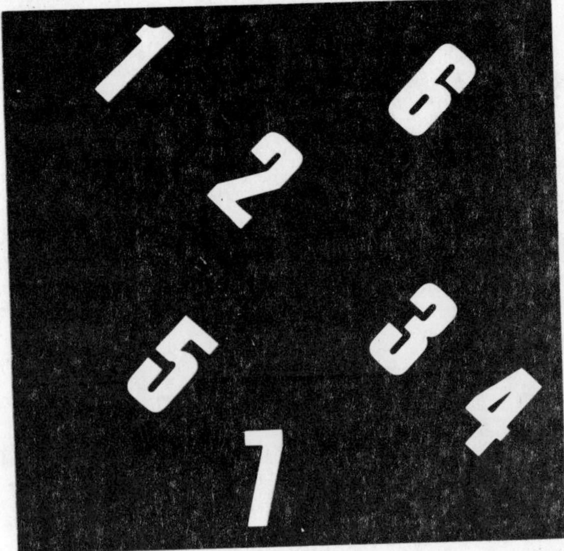

Fig. 17.11. Diagrams to illustrate subtraction.

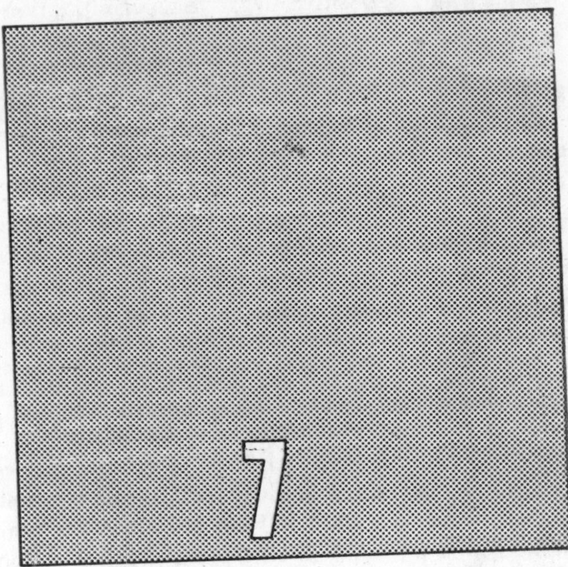

Fig. 17.12. Diagrams to illustrate subtraction.

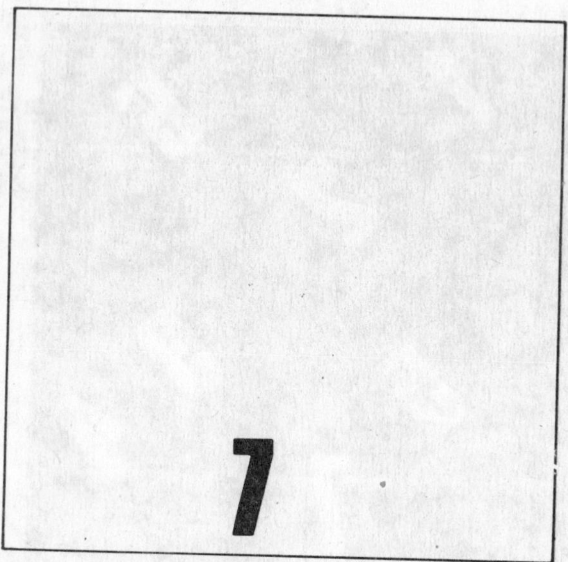

Fig. 17.13. Diagrams to illustrate subtraction.

examinations these shared images are the bones and soft tissues where no contrast agent is present. The positive-negative superimposition produces disappearance and all we can see in Fig. 17.12 is an image of what was present in Film C (the angiographic radiograph) but *not* present in Film B (the radiographic mask). So Fig. 17.12 shows the *difference* between the radiographic mask and the angiographic radiograph. Thus we see the contrast agent and nothing else

If the superimposed radiographic mask and the angiographic radiograph are used to make one more contact copy, the result is indicated in Fig. 17.13. This is Film D or the subtraction radiographic print which shows the contrast agent and nothing else. It is a positive image because the superimposition of the positive mask and the angiographic radiograph gave a negative image as shown in Fig. 17.17 and the contact copy is not made on reversal material.

To consider an example from cerebral angiography, an antero-posterior projection of the skull made before the injection of contrast agent (Film A, the basic radiograph) is used to produce a copy in the positive image (Film B, the radiochaptic mask). Film B is a positive and the tones in it are the reverse of those in Film A. Film A has 'white-grey' bones on a dark ground and Film B has 'black-grey' bones on a light ground. These are shown in Figs. 17.14 and 17.15.

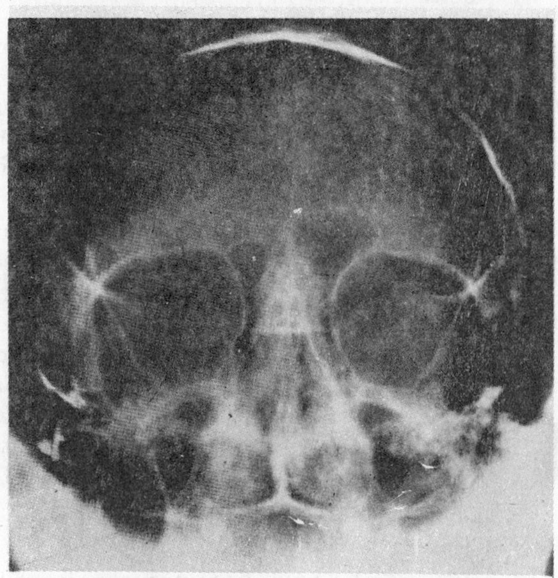

Fig. 17.14. Radiograph prior to the injection of contrast agent. This is the basic radiograph in the subtraction procedure.

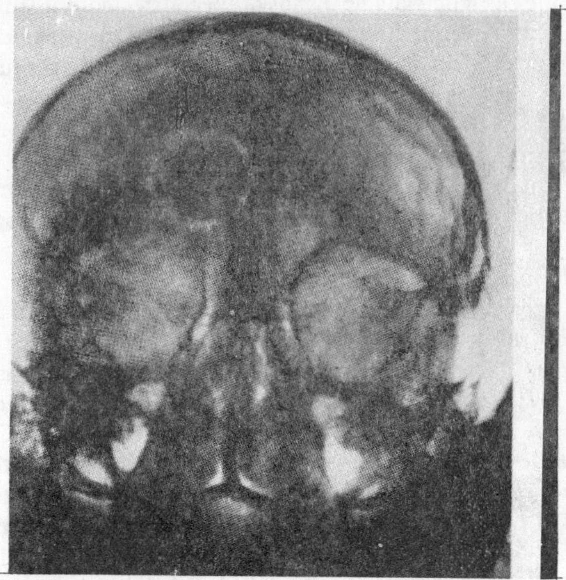

Fig. 17.15. Positive image copy of the basic radiograph. This is the radiographic mask in the subtraction procedure.

After the contrast agent has been injected, Film C (the angiographic radiograph) is taken. This is identical to Film A as regards (a) the projection; (b) the positions of the patient, the film and the X-ray tube; (c) the exposure factors. The only difference is that in Film C the blood vessels are outlined with contrast agent and in Film A they are not. Film C is shown in Fig. 17.16.

Film C (the angiographic radiograph) and Film B (the radiographic mask) are used together to make Film D which shows the subtracted image and is the final subtraction print. The positive image of Film B and the negative image of Film C cancel each other by superimposition of the two images. On printing through the positive-negative superimposition, Film D is made and this shows the parts of the radiographic image in Film C (the angiographic radiograph) which were not shared with Film B (the radiographic mask): these are the blood vessels outlined with contrast agent and shown clearly free of other structures. Film D is seen in Fig. 17.17.

MATERIALS AND EQUIPMENT FOR RADIOGRAPHIC SUBTRACTION

There is more than one way of obtaining a subtracted image. It can, for example, be done electronically by means of specialized equipment which is expensive to buy. The method we have indicated in the previous pages is a photographic one since it consists of contact printing through one film to another, using a light source for the exposure. This method is commonly practised in X-ray departments for it is easy to apply without specialized facilities. If subtraction is to be a valuable procedure, the final subtraction print with its subtracted image as in Fig. 17.17 must be available to the radiologist at the time that the report on the angiographic series is being made. So successful subtraction is of real use only when it can easily and quickly be undertaken.

There are two stages at which contact printing is done: (i) in making the radiographic mask from the basic radiograph; (ii) in making the final subtraction print from the superimposed radiographic mask and angiographic radiograph. Film materials suitable for making these two contact prints are available and have already been mentioned in Chapter 2. They are single-sided films with emulsion on one side only of the base and on the other side an anti-halation backing. They are usually described as subtraction films and in some cases may be differentiated as subtraction films for masks and subtraction films for subtraction prints. They are blue-sensitive films and they can be processed under the safelights and in the automatic processors found in X-ray darkrooms.

In addition to the special photographic materials to make the prints,

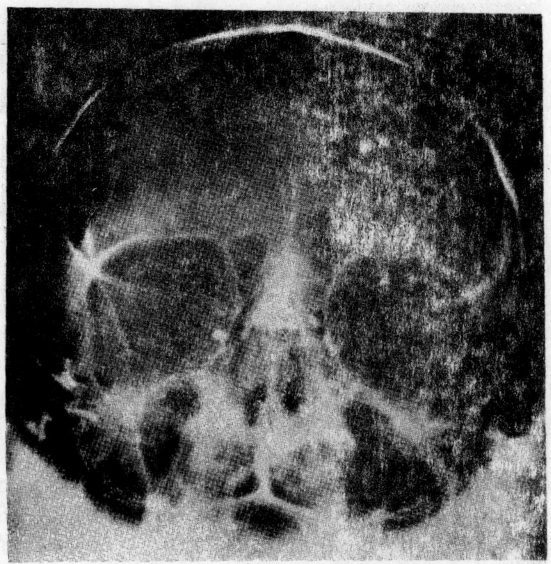

Fig. 17.16. Radiograph made after the injection of contrast agent in a cerebral angiogram. This is the angiographic radiograph in the subtraction procedure and is identical with the basic radiograph save for the presence of the contrast agent.

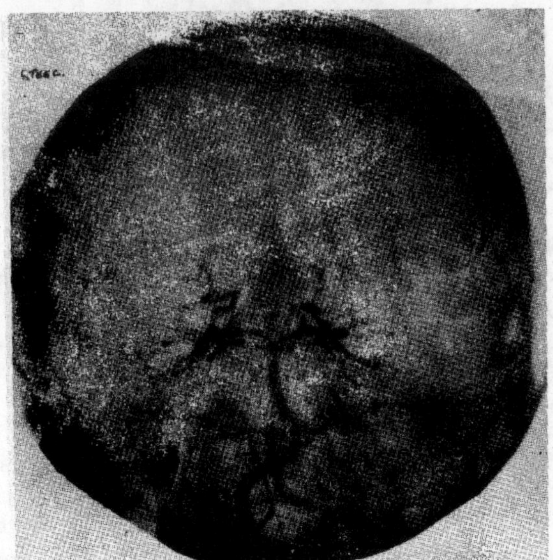

Fig. 17.17. The final subtraction print made by printing through the superimposed radiographic mask and angiographic radiograph.

equipment is required to hold the films for contact printing. This equipment is the same as we have already described (see page 505) for use in contact printing to make facsimile radiographs.

PROCEDURE FOR SUBTRACTION

(i) From the basic radiograph (that is, from the preliminary radiograph taken before the injection of any contrast agent) make a positive copy that is to be the mask. The selected basic radiograph should be of high quality, with optimum sharpness of outline and a long range of tones. A radiograph which lacks sharpness or has contrast which is very low or very high cannot make a satisfactory mask. Under safelights, a sheet of the subtraction film and the basic radiograph are placed in register in a contact printing device such as we have previously described. The emulsion side of the subtraction film must be in contact with the radiograph: the subtraction film has a code notch to make identification easy and when this is in the top right hand corner of the sheet of film it is usual to find that the emulsion aspect is then towards the holder. The radiograph must be placed against the glass of the printing device so that it is between the subtraction film and the light source to be used for the exposure. This light should be a low-wattage white light and not an ultra-violet source.

(ii) When the radiograph and the subtraction film are correctly set up and all is ready, the exposure is made. The exposure required varies with:

    (a) the densities of the basic radiograph;
    (b) the intensity of the light source used;
    (c) the distance between the light source and the subtraction film;
    (d) the characteristics of the subtraction film.

Dupont make the following suggestions about exposure when their Cronex Subtraction Film is being used: (i) in a printing frame at 6 feet distance from a 25 watt lamp, use an exposure which is approximately 8 seconds; (ii) in their Cronex Printer which has a 7·5 watt bulb as a light source for subtraction, use an exposure time of about 5 seconds. In the Cronex Printer the light source-to-film distance is fixed and is very much less than 6 feet.

(iii) Process the exposed subtraction film: this can be done in the same conditions that the department is using for its radiographic processing.

(iv) Assess the adequacy of the radiographic mask, resulting from this procedure. In making the assessment, you should realize that the greatest density in the basic radiograph and the greatest density in the radiographic mask should match. If the highest density within the image in the basic radiograph is greater than the highest density within the image in the radiographic mask, then the mask will be ineffective. So you should not accept a mask which is lacking in density because it has been underexposed. An overexposed mask with a density greater than the highest density within the image of the basic radiograph also loses masking capability. As in many other situations, practice helps recognition and it becomes not so difficult to appreciate a satisfactory mask as these words of advice may lead you at first to assume. If the mask is satisfactory, the next step in the total procedure can be made.

(v) The angiographic radiograph that is to be subtracted and the radiographic mask are taken and are carefully superimposed with the image of the one precisely covering the image of the other. The two films should be put in contact with the conventional viewing aspect of the angiographic radiograph facing *outwards* and the conventional viewing aspect of the radiographic mask at the back of the angiogram. For the required exact registration to be possible it is clearly essential that the preliminary basic radiograph (of which the mask is a positive contact copy) and the angiographic radiograph must have been taken in identical conditions with the sole difference that the second shows vessels filled with contrast agent. If the two images are not exactly superimposed the final result in the subtracted print will be a sculptured effect (bas relief) which looks striking but is not wanted in this case. If the tonal range of the radiographic mask does not match in reverse that of the angiographic radiograph, a ghost image of the bony parts may show in the final subtracted print: this may not be a disadvantage if it is not too obtrusive for it can help anatomical orientation in interpreting the image. If a contact printing frame is to be used to make the final subtraction print, an X-ray illuminator laid flat on a bench with its illuminated front plate horizontal is useful as an aid to superimposing the radiograph and the mask: if you try to achieve this superimposition against an illuminated surface which is vertical you add to your difficulties by engaging in a battle with the force of gravity! Once the precise superimposition has been achieved, the two films should be carefully taped together so that their relative placings do not shift. If a printer such as the Dupont Cronex Printer is to be used to make the final subtraction print, the required superimposition is easier. The Cronex Printer has its horizontal glass plate suitably illuminated from below by white light for the purposes of viewing and registration. Furthermore it has two sets of hold-down strips adjustable over the glass which make registration easy and save the tricky and time-consuming use of adhesive tape.

(vi) The last step is to use the superimposed mask and angiographic radiograph to make a contact print which is the final subtraction print as illustrated in Fig. 17.17. This print may be made on the same subtraction film that was used to make the radiographic mask: or it may be made on subtraction print film, which will give higher contrast in the result. When the superimposed mask-radiograph pair are put into the printing frame or printer and, under safelights, the subtraction film to be used is put in contact with the pair, the following points are important:

(a) the conventional viewing aspect of the angiographic radiograph, which is an outward face of the superimposed pair, must be against the glass plate of the printing assembly or printer;

(b) the emulsion aspect of the subraction (print) film must be in contact with the other side of the superimposed pair so that the pair is between the light source and the printing film.

(vii) When all is set up make the exposure to light. Dupont suggest that if their Cronex Subtraction Print Film is used, the exposure required to make the print is about the same as that used to make the mask on Cronex Subtraction Film. If Cronex Subtraction Film is to be used also to make the final print, then the required exposure is about twice that needed to make the mask.

(viii) Finally, process the subtraction print as the mask was processed.

Tabulated Factors in the Radiographic Image

Contrast here refers to *objective contrast*—that is difference between densities in different parts of the image.

Detail means *sharpness of outline* in the image. U_g means unsharpness arising from the geometry of image formation—i.e. geometric unsharpness. U_m means unsharpness arising from movement of the subject. U_s means the unsharpness arising from the use of intensifying screens.

Factor in image production	Any effect on image contrast?	Any effect on image detail?
Anode film distance (A.F.D.)	**No effect.**	**Yes.** (i) Alters U_g for given focal spot size and patient-film distance. (ii) Also an **indirect effect** since U_m may increase with A.F.D. because longer exposure times may be necessary.
Beam-limiting cone or diaphragm.	**Yes.** Reduces the volume of tissue irradiated and thus the amount of scattered radiation is less and contrast is improved.	**No direct effect.** An **indirect effect** because when very small fields are used it may be necessary to increase the exposure times and hence U_m may increase.
Compression of body part.	**Yes.** (i) The volume of tissue irradiated is less and thus the amount of scattered radiation is less. Contrast is improved. (ii) Lower kilovoltages can be used and hence there is increased differential absorption in different tissues. Contrast is improved.	**No direct effect.** An **indirect effect** as compression aids immobilization and thus lessens risk of U_m.

Factor in image production	Any effect on image contrast?	Any effect on image detail?
Developer Constitution Exhaustion Temperature Time.	**Yes.** These processing factors can increase or diminish contrast.	**No effect.** It is the **visibility** of detail which the developer alters and not the sharpness of shadow borders.
Exposure time.	**No direct effect.**	**No direct effect.** An **indirect effect** because longer times may increase U_m.
Film contrast.	**Yes.** Image contrast is enhanced if the contrast of the film material is high.	**No effect.**
Focal spot size.	**No effect.**	**Yes.** (i) U_g increases with focal spot size for a given A.F.D. and patient-film distance; (ii) Also an **indirect effect** as *small* focal spots may mean the use of low milliamperes and longer exposure times; hence U_m may increase. So in focal spot size what makes U_g small can make U_m very big. Larger U_g accepted to keep U_m small.
Intensifying screens.	**Yes.** (i) Increase contrast between low densities in the image. (ii) Absorb soft scattered radiation. (iii) Intensify the primary beam more than the long wavelength scattered radiation. (iv) Allow the use of lower kilovoltages. All these improve contrast.	**Yes.** (i) Very greatly reduce U_m by allowing the use of short exposure times; (ii) Add U_s but this is accepted in order to obtain the great reduction in U_m.
Kilovoltages used.	**Yes.** (i) Alters differential absorption in the tissues so that contrast increases as kilovoltage is lowered. (ii) Alters the amount of scattered radiation reaching the film; this increases as kilovoltage is raised and contrast is lowered.	**No direct effect.** An **indirect effect** because intensity increases with raised kilovoltage and hence shorter times may be used, resulting in less U_m.

Factor in image production	Any effect on image contrast?	Any effect on image detail?
Milliamperes.	**No direct effect.**	**No direct effect. An indirect effect** as high milliamperage (i) implies short exposure times which reduce U_m and (ii) implies larger focal spots which increase U_g for a given A.F.D. and patient-film distance. Increase in U_g accepted to lessen U_m.
Patient-film distance.	**No direct effect. An indirect effect.** When the patient is a long way from the film (air-gap technique) less scattered radiation falls on the film and contrast is improved.	**Yes.** U_g increases with patient-film distance for a given focal spot size and A.F.D.
Radiation contrast in the subject.	**Yes.** Image contrast increases with radiation contrast in the subject.	**No effect.** It is the *visibility* of detail which is altered by radiation contrasts in the subject and not the sharpness of shadow borders.
Secondary radiation grid.	**Yes.** Prevents scattered radiation from reaching the film and hence markedly improves contrast.	**No appreciable direct effect. An indirect effect.** (i) It may increase patient-film distance and hence also increase U_g; (ii) It may increase U_m as longer exposure times may be necessary.

Index